Robinson's Genetics for Cat Breeders and Veterinarians

Robinson's Genetics for Cat Breeders and Veterinarians

Fourth edition

Carolyn M. Vella
Licensed Judge, American Cat Fanciers' Association; Professional member of the Cat Writer's Association; Registered cat breeder

Lorraine M. Shelton
Research scientist, Southern California, USA; Registered cat breeder; Author and lecturer in the field of avian and feline genetics

John J. McGonagle
Licensed Judge, American Cat Fanciers' Association; Professional member of the Cat Writer's Association; Registered cat breeder

Terry W. Stanglein, VMD
Practising Veterinarian, Northampton, Pennsylvania, USA; Member, American Association of Feline Practitioners

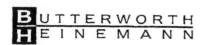

BUTTERWORTH HEINEMANN

EDINBURGH LONDON NEW YORK OXFORD PHILADELPHIA ST LOUIS SYDNEY TORONTO 1999

Butterworth-Heinemann
An imprint of Elsevier Limited

First published by Pergamon Press plc 1971
Reprinted 1973, 1975
Second edition 1977
Reprinted 1978, 1983, 1987
Reprinted with corrections 1988, 1989
Third edition 1991
Reprinted by REPP Ltd 1996, 1997, 1998
Fourth edition 1999
Reprinted 2000, 2002, 2003 (twice), 2005

ISBN 978 0 7506 4069 5

British Library Cataloguing in Publication Data
A catalogue record for this book is available from the British Library

Library of Congress Cataloguing in Publication Data
A catalog record for this book is available from the Library of Congress

Notice
Medical knowledge is constantly changing. Standard safety precautions must be followed but
as new research and clinical experience broaden our knowledge, changes in treatment and drug
therapy may become necessary or appropriate. Readers are advised to check the most current
product information provided by the manufacturer of each drug to be administered to verify the
recommended dose, the method and duration of administration, and contraindications. It is the
responsibility of the practitioner, relying on experience and knowledge of the patient, to determine
dosages and the best treatment for each individual patient. Neither the Publisher nor the editors/
contributor assumes any liability for any injury and/or damage to persons or property arising from
this publication.

The Publisher

Transferred to digital printing 2005

Contents

List of Tables

Preface

This book continues the pioneering work of the late Roy Robinson both in his three editions of *Genetics for Cat Breeders* (1971, 1977, 1991) and in his many articles. It seeks to expand the scope of these works in assisting the practicing veterinarian who is dealing with cats and cat breeders.

We concur with what Roy said in the Preface to his first edition:

> The writing of this book springs from the belief that the continued advancement of cat breeding relies upon an acknowledgment of modern trends in animal breeding. It should be recognized that the world of small animal breeding is discarding 'rule of thumb' methods for a more balanced program of scientific method and skilful breeding. The science of genetics has much to offer both to the theory and the practice of cat breeding. The thoughtful breeder should ponder on the fact that once his or her cats are provided with a good home, properly fed and receiving expert veterinary care, the sole hope of producing the superlative animal lies in the art of breeding.

As we worked on this book, we began to realize that the group known as 'cat breeders' is a very diverse one.

When we talk about breeding other animals, such as dogs, we can talk in terms of breeding for show purposes (both conformation and obedience), for work (herding, protection), or for enjoyment (as personal pets). However, cats are bred for a narrower range of purposes. While they compete in shows based on their conformation, that is how close to perfection they are when compared to a written standard, it would be absurd to conceive of obedience competitions. In addition, most cats are not bred for working; rather they seemed to have long been retired from their historical roles as mousers. That leaves two potential breeding goals: to produce specimens for competition or to propagate a breed for companionship, as 'pets'.

While that appears to be a narrow set of reasons, it is actually more complex than it seems. For example, breeders who breed their cats for exhibition/show competition also sell those cats which do not meet show standards as personal pets. There are also some breeders who do not show, but rather breed their cats solely to sell the kittens as pets. Others are seeking to create new breeds or varieties of cats, whether from combinations of existing recognized breeds, or by selectively breeding to preserve or develop unique characteristics that then breed true and healthy.

The Cat Fancy has not, until recently, had to deal with resuscitating a breed from extinction. Following World War II, however, cat breeders did do just that for numerous breeds, including the Birman, the Chartreux and the Norwegian Forest Cat. Now it appears that cat breeders will again have to do this with some minority breeds of pedigreed cats, most notably the Havana Brown.

Cat breeding, therefore, is an activity that encompasses a wide variety of different efforts. It is our belief that cat breeders and the veterinarians who work with these breeders are functionally geneticists. We believe that both groups must be well educated with respect to the genetics of the cats they all love. It is to assist those breeding and caring for all of these cats to do their job more scientifically, more rationally, and more compassionately, that we have undertaken this book.

To provide both breeders and veterinarians with the broadest range of information, we have reviewed not only the traditional sources for scientific literature and studies, but have conducted interviews with veterinarians, researchers and breeders. The results of these appear in our conclusions and assertions, in the references, and are the basis for some of the quotations which we have placed throughout the text. These will, we hope, serve to enlighten the discussions.

Knowledge about the field of genetics has grown exponentially from the time of Roy Robinson's first edition of this book. For decades, the discussion of genetics was limited to observations of populations. Now, geneticists are beginning to look at the actual molecular mechanisms behind the traits and diseases seen in the cat. Genetics has grown from being simply an exercise in statistics to being a study in chemical reactions.

One note for our readers: throughout the book, our examples use terms which are the same as or similar to recognized breeds or patterns. When we are discussing a breed itself, the context will be clear as to that. However, when we discuss color or pattern, e.g. Siamese or piebalding, we are using these in a genetic sense only. Breeds with the same or similar names *usually* manifest these traits. In addition, for those seeking to deal with problems which appear to be breed-linked, they should always remember that many of today's breeds have been created, revived or maintained through outcrossing to other breeds. Information on which breed(s) are 'in back of' which other breeds is both beyond the scope of this work, and is constantly in flux. If such information is needed, the readers can consult first with the technical appendix to Chapter 10 which details currently permitted outcrosses for breeds in the Federation Internationale Féline (FIFe) and the Cat Fanciers' Association (CFA), and then refer to some of the works cited in the bibliography or talk to the relevant breed club.

In updating this book, we have attempted to make it more user-friendly. For example, we have:

- Divided some topics, such as breeding practices, into several chapters.
- Removed text references to virtually all works which are already cited in the bibliography.
- Provided a glossary of relevant terms.
- Placed some important, but little used, materials in technical and historical appendices.

In order to deal with a work of this scope, each of us took primary responsibility for updating key areas: Carolyn for anomalies; John for breeding systems and inbreeding; Lorraine for color and breed genetics; and Terry for the veterinary perspective.

We hope you approve.

Carolyn M. Vella
Lorraine M. Shelton
John J. McGonagle
Terry W. Stanglein, VMD
December 1998

Copyright notice

We have adapted, with permission, portions of some of the following articles written by Roy Robinson:

Black-yellow mosaics, *Cat World™ International*, November/December 1990

Blood groups in cats, *Cats – The Official Journal of the GCCF*, 18 December 1992

Complex inbreeding, *Cat World™ International*, September/October 1996

Gene pools, *Cat World™ International*, July/August 1991

Genetics A to Z, *Cat World™ International*, May/June 1992

Genetics of the Ragdoll, *Cat World™ International*, May/June 1997

Glossary of breeding and genetic terms, *Cats – The Official Journal of the GCCF*, 24 January 1992, 7 February 1992, 21 February 1992, 6 March 1992, 20 March 1992, 10 April 1992, 12 May 1992, 22 May 1992, 17 July 1992, 21 August 1992 and 18 September 1992

Head conformation and bite, *Cat World™ International*, January/February 1996

How the queen optimises litter size, *Cats – The Official Journal of the GCCF*, 16 August 1991

Inbreeding, *Cat World™ International*, September/October 1991

Inbreeding and breeds, *Cat World™ International*, September/October 1994

Inbreeding in theory and practice, *Cats – The Official Journal of the GCCF*, 2 July 1993

Inbreeding within small groups, *Cat World™ International*, July/August 1994

Law of Descent, *Cats – The Official Journal of the GCCF*, 24 March 1995 and *Cat World International*, January/February 1996

More on inbreeding, *Cats – The Official Journal of the GCCF*, 14 October 1994

Numerically small breeds, *Cats – The Official Journal of the GCCF*, 10 June 1994

Pedigrees and inbreeding, *Cat World*™ *International*, November/December
  1995
Red Tabby, *Cat World*™ *International*, November/December 1994/January/
  February 1995
The cameo breeds – Part 1, *Cat World*™ *International*, May/June 1993
The cameo – Part 2 of 3, *Cat World*™ *International*, July/August 1993
White and white spotted cats, *Cat World*™ *International*, March/April 1995
These are copyright 1990 to 1997. All rights reserved.

Acknowledgements

Veterinarians

Dr Henry Baker
Dr John DePlanque

Dr Urs Giger
Dr M.D. Kittleson

Dr Susan Little
Dr Diana Scollard

Breeders/exhibitors

Carol Barbee
Barbara Belanger
Lynn Berge
Lisa Bressler
Ricky Burthay
Rosaline Dolak De
  Dan
Velta Dickson
Dorie Eckhart
Donna Einarsson
Eduardo Eizirik
Carl and Priscilla
  Eldredge
Prof Andrea Fischer
Kay Hanvey
LeAnn Harner
Terry Harris

Gwen Hornung
Joan Harvey
Dolores Kennedy
Rich and Nancy Koch
Marsha Lanier
Marianne Lawrence
Dr Heather Lorimer
Dr Leslie Lyons
Monique Malm
Candice Massey
Donatella
  Mastrangelo
Ebe McCabe
Kerrie Meek
James Mendenhall
Joan Miller
Ken Miller

Lynn Miller
Tony Morace
Jeanne Osborne
Lee Polk
Elizabeth Powell
Gene Rankin
Dolores Reiff
Sharon Riegner
Carine Risberg
J. Shartwell
Alisa Stark
Ron Summers
Kathy Thompson
J.W. Tromp
Kathie Von Aswege
Lori White
John Ypma

Others

The Staff and Instructors of the First International Feline Genetic Disease Conference at the School of Veterinary Medicine, University of Pennsylvania, and its sponsors, Ralston Purina and The Winn Foundation.

Thomas Dent and the staff of the Cat Fanciers' Association, Inc. (CFA) office, as well as the Cat Fanciers' Association Foundation, Inc. for research assistance and access to the CFA Foundation Library.

Lesley Pring and the staff of the Governing Council of the Cat Fancy (GCCF) as well as Debra Schofield of *Cats – The Official Journal of the GCCF*.

The staff of the Federation Internationale Féline (FIFe).

In dealing with methods of breed improvement, it is sometimes difficult to go beyond a general discussion, because only the breeder, working with a veterinarian, has all of the data from which to make correct judgments. In a sense, breed improvement is still at an elementary level, remaining more of an art rather than an exact science. It still entails gauging the worth of the individual cat by inspection, rather than by objective measurement and of then making decisions based on informed judgment rather than on a mechanical test such as a set number of matings or on the passage of a certain number of generations.

Many of the decisions that a breeder must make are based on personal observations. When all has been said and done, the occasion may arise when certain observations appear 'odd', that is they do not fit into the scheme of things. There are several potential reasons for this. One possibility which should always be considered is that a mistake has been made. A mistaken identification, an error in the breeding or registration records or an accidental mismating can often be the explanation for an otherwise 'impossible' situation. Remember, only saints are perfect – the rest of us all make errors. Only if mistakes **can absolutely** be ruled out, should the genetic explanation be considered to be not as accurate or as complete as it could be.

Alternatively, it can mean that something new has been discovered, such as the discovery of several genes for rex coats over the past three decades or the folded eared and curled ear mutants of more recent years. In this event, it is wise for the breeder to seek competent advice. Whenever unexpected results occur, it is **always** advisable to consult other people. The chances of discovering something novel are slim, but the possibility is always there.

Mendelism and genetics

The first accurate description of the principles of heredity was enunciated in 1866 by Gregor Mendel. As the scientific climate was not ripe for ready acceptance of his simple, almost blunt, account of these principles, Mendel's discovery languished until 1900. At this time, the prevailing ideas on heredity and evolution were being critically appraised by inquiring minds and biology was beginning to emerge as an experimental, as opposed to an observational, science. In about 1900, Mendel's work was acclaimed by three biologists, independently and more or less simultaneously.

It is common knowledge that Mendel carried out his experiments with a common flower, the sweet pea. Once the basic principles were grasped, there were many people who were eager to discover if his ideas applied to other plants and to animals. It was soon found that they did. The rules he developed applied, in most cases, with astonishing similarity. In others, these rules, with subtle variations, served to strengthen and to extend the principles he had formulated.

Mendel's Laws of Heredity, as his principles are known, have stood up to the test of repeatable experiment. Their generality for all species of plants and animals implied that they were fundamental. The study of heredity was known as 'Mendelism' until Bateson, in 1906, coined the word 'genetics' for the new biological discipline. Thus, heredity became a science, with principles which can be checked and with laws of real predictive value.

From the humble beginning of a man pottering around in a spare corner of his garden, genetics has grown to such an extent that research establishments are devoted to the subject. Today, no corner of biology or medicine can escape its impact. As this book is being written, new research in genetics, including that of cats, at the molecular level, and involving the mapping of DNA (deoxyribonucleic acid), continue to increase and refine our understanding.

It required decades for the foundations of genetics to be laid. Once the mechanism of heredity had been satisfactorily settled, it became obvious that former concepts such as those based on the 'percentage of blood' and the overestimated influence of remote ancestors had to be revised. Even the use of pedigrees in breeding became suspect unless one was very familiar with the ancestors listed and could recall their apparent worth. A tabulation of names, devoid of accurate description, is scarcely of any value at all except for intimating that the individual is derived from a well-known stock.

Nomenclature

The domestic cat is often referred to as *Felis domesticus*. The word *Felis* indicates that the animal belongs to the main genus of cats and the word *domesticus* indicates that it is a domesticated form. However, Carl Linne, the founder of scientific classification, has named the domestic cat as *Felis catus*. This designation is also often employed, more often than *F. domesticus*.

Everything would still be straightforward but for the fact that Linne singled out the blotched type of tabby (classic tabby) as *catus*, apparently neglecting the equally common mackerel type of tabby. In some people's eyes, the omission needed rectifying, so the mackerel tabby has come to receive the designation of *F. torquata*.

The name of *domesticus* appears the more appropriate even if, in strict scientific nomenclature terms, it is not precisely correct. As a designation, it certainly describes the present status of the cat.

It is unfortunate that the origin of the modern domestic cat is so obscure, for the animal must obviously be a domesticated form of a wild species. If the initial wild ancestor was definitely known, the use of its species in the name may seem preferable, even if *domesticus* is added. However, at present, the presumptive wild ancestor is not known with certainty, although there seem to be excellent grounds for arguing that it belongs to the *silverstri–lybica* species complex. The typical tabby pattern of these species is the mackerel type. For this reason it is customary to refer to the mackerel form as the 'wild type', from which the blotched (or classic) tabby pattern sprang as a mutant.

Origin and species hybridity

Early history

Few writers on the domestic cat can resist speculating on the origin of the cat. It is well known that the ancient Egyptians revered the cat and worshipped a cat-goddess. Egypt is commonly regarded as being a major center of origin, but whether it is the only center is perhaps open to question.

There was nothing to prevent anyone attempting to domesticate the cat anywhere and at different times. It is doubtful if the problem of its origin will ever be definitely solved. Like the dog, cats of wild origin, but of slightly less fearful disposition than the average, may have acted as food stealers or scavengers. Over time, they eventually may have been accepted or, at least, tolerated by humans. The cat's skill in keeping down rats and mice may have further ingratiated the cat in the human mind.

Mankind's acceptance of the cat (or the cat's acceptance of mankind) probably occurred at the hut or village level. There must have been sufficient genetic variation for docility or tameness within the species for the cat to become trusting of men and to breed either close to or within the village. Barter of animals probably occurred and cats may have become part of the paraphernalia of traders. In this manner, cats would have reached the towns and cities and probably would have acquired status as exotic pets. There would then have been selection against the wilder individuals and possibly in favor of color and pattern variations. Once accepted, the spread of the cat is more or less assured. Though not a prolific breeder, the cat is a persistent producer of litters and has a long span of reproductive life.

Egypt

Whatever the actual route, by 1600 BC, the cat was clearly domesticated and was regarded as a sacred animal in Egypt. Outside Egypt, for instance in Greece and Palestine, the cat was known, but was relatively uncommon, because the Egyptians did not allow them to be taken from the country. The Egyptians were also apparently not adverse to carrying off every cat they saw to Egypt. This could be a factor in the belief that Egypt is the center of origin of today's domestic cat.

Rome and beyond

In time, the cat lost its religious significance and its geographic exclusivity. The rise of Christianity caused the cat to lose its sacred position. The Romans carried the cat back to their homeland and throughout their empire. The cat was soon found in central Europe and even in Britain. The cat also traveled eastward, probably via Babylon, into India where it is known to have been domesticated for some 2000 years.

The assumption that Egypt was the unique birth center of the domestic cat is challenged somewhat by the parallel development of domesticated cats elsewhere in the world. In particular, there are indications that the Japanese have had (and possibly venerated) domestic cats, with a unique cork-screw tail, for more than 2000 years.

Originating wild species?

On the assumption that the Egyptians domesticated the cat, the problem becomes: from which wild species did the domestic cat descend? The Egyptians apparently kept a number of cats, among which were the jungle cat (*F. chaus*) and the African wild cat (*F. lybica*). One study of Egyptian mummified cats suggests that *chaus* may not have been domesticated in any true sense of the word, as these are poorly represented among the remains examined. The majority of skulls which the author examined belonged to a form smaller than *chaus*, yet larger than *lybica* or the present-day domestic cat. This form is named *F. lybica bubastis* and is thought to be derived from, or to be a race of, the widely distributed African wild cat *lybica*. Apart from size, the skulls of mummified cats and of *lybica* were closely similar. Curiously, there does not seem to be any existing known wild form which matches *bubastis* exactly. The above is the extent of the direct evidence for the origin of the cat.

However, another approach can be taken. This is to consider the number and distribution of wild species. The two most likely ancestral forms are *F. silvestris* and *F. lybica*, the European and African wild cats, respectively, on account of their size, characteristics and coloration. The former occurs in Britain, throughout Europe (except for Scandinavia), south-west Russia, Caucasia and Asia Minor. The latter occurs in most of the larger Mediterranean islands, much of Africa, Arabia, Turkestan and northern India. While some taxonomists are prepared to accept *silvestris* and *lybica* as two distinct species, each one is divided into a large number of geographical subspecies and races. These divisions are based mainly on differences of background color, intensity and distribution of striping, whether or not the striping is breaking up into spots and the clarity of the striping or spotting.

Thus, there is the diversity to be expected of a widely distributed species. In general, there is a north to south gradation of coat thickness, intensity of ground color and amount of tabby markings. Of the two, *lybica* displays the greater variation. If one examines these species complexes as a whole, it does not seem inappropriate to merge *silvestris* and *lybica* into one species, with geographical groups. A study has done this, giving *silvestris* as the embracive species name.

The results of interspecies hybridization affords another approach and, from a genetic viewpoint, the most interesting. Much of the literature on hybridization is very old and, unless a critical stance is taken, it is easy to believe that the domestic cat produces hybrids with practically any wild species. This could be so, but too many of the early claims are based on breeders' reminiscences and travellers' observations to be reliable. On the other hand, of course, if two species so different as the lion and tiger can be crossed reciprocally – tigron from the union of a male tiger and lioness and liger from a male lion and a tigress – then it is conceivable that a large number of the smaller cats might be capable of producing hybrids.

However, while the above cross is fairly easily obtained, the disparity between the two species is revealed by partial sterility. The male hybrids are thought to be completely infertile while the female hybrids are only partially fertile. These facts reveal the genetic remoteness of the lion and tiger.

Several sources of error have to be taken into account if claims of hybridity are to be taken seriously. Simple observation is not sufficient. Feral domestic cats abound in many parts of the world and many of them resemble wild species in color and temperament. The domestic cat is a variable creature and no variation of color or bodily proportions should be construed as positive evidence of alleged current or past hybridity. Only if a person has intimate knowledge of the animals concerned can a claim be entertained; yet even this is not conclusive. For a claim of hybridity to be conclusive, it is necessary for the parents to be confined and the matings controlled and visually confirmed.

Authentic hybrids between the domestic cat and various races (Scottish and European) of *silvestris* have been obtained on several occasions. In the majority of cases, the offspring are mackerel tabby in color and wild in temperament. In one instance, however, a male hybrid was observed to be 'as tame as a fire-side cat, so that after a while he was allowed out of his cage to wander about' (Gillespie, 1954). This is interesting because it denotes genetic variation for 'tameness', one of the prerequisites for domestication. The hybrids seem to be regularly fertile. This could be significant as it is usually indicative of a not too distant genetic relationship. Several of the domestic females carried mutant genes and these can be expressed by the hybrid genotype. Self black (the wild male was evidently a heterozygote), piebald with white spotting and Manx taillessness have been transmitted (the last two genes being dominant). Though the transmission and expression of mutant genes (the numbers were too few and the variation of expression was not closely studied), are not of great weight, again there is indication of some degree of genetic identity. Most of the hybrids possessed the bushy tail of *silvestris*, but this was not always the case, and, in one instance, the second generation showed variation in the amount of hair on the tail.

Alleged hybrids between the domestic cat and various races of *lybica* (both African and Indian) are claimed on several occasions in the older literature. More recently, fertile hybrids have been obtained between the domestic cat and the Steppe cat (*lybica caudata*) under controlled conditions. Furthermore, Pocock (1907) was able to produce hybrids between *silvestris* and an African race of *lybica*. These were typical mackerel tabby, similar to the parents. Two were eaten by the *lybica* mother shortly after birth while the surviving kitten at nine weeks was showing signs of having the well-covered hairy tail of *silvestris*. Thus, there is direct, as well as circumstantial, evidence that hybrids can be secured with *lybica*. If credence is given to these early accounts, there may be found stories of fertility and variable degrees of tameness for the hybrids.

Hybrids between the domestic cat and the Jungle cat (*F. chaus*) have been obtained. The hybrids are tabby in color and with somewhat more tabby striping than is apparent in *chaus*. Morphologically, the resemblance is closer to *chaus*, for the hybrid is larger, longer legged and shorter tailed than the domestic. The hybrid is apparently fertile, for daughter hybrids have been mated back to the *chaus* father and have reared litters. The hybrids appear to be well cared for and are said to be tame. Piebald white spotting, introduced by the domestic cat, showed the usual dominant expression on the hybrids (Jackson and Jackson, 1967).

Two further crosses may be noted because of the implication that they can be productive of hybrids. The crosses were between the domestic cat and the bobcat (*Lynx rufus*) and oncilla or little spotted cat (*F. tigerina*), two species from the Americas. In both instances, the hybrids tend to resemble the wild species, rather than the cat and were of wild disposition. Nothing is known of whether or not the hybrids were fertile. The intriguing aspect is that hybrids could be produced at all as the point of departure for the old and new world species must have been a vast number of years ago. Yet, despite this, the three forms can come together to produce viable offspring. The implication is that the production of offspring, per se, from the domestic cat and either *silvestris* or *lybica* loses some of its significance. Only the probability, if not certainty, that these offspring are fertile may turn out to be important for demonstrating genetic kinship.

No matter how much time is spent on detailed systematic examination of species appearance or how supposedly diagnostic features are compared, the crucial test of genetic relationship is that of crosses. The fact that the wild species and the hybrids are fearful and barely manageable is an unfortunate complication but one which can possibly be overcome. Already, certain European zoos are making determined attempts to breed and rear *silvestris* in captivity. The lack of kinship between the domestic cat and a wild species may show itself in one of two ways.

- The animals may copulate but no viable young are forthcoming.
- Young may be born but these are sterile either in one or both sexes.

These various possibilities are sometimes taken to represent different degrees of relationship. The former implying a more distant relationship than the latter.

However, the important item is that the putative wild ancestor of the domestic cat should be capable of producing fertile hybrids. Perhaps a clear cut answer may not emerge; for it is possible that the ancestral species may have become extinct or that the cat may be capable of producing fertile hybrids with more than one wild species.

There seems now little doubt that the present-day cat population of the world is probably a single genetic entity. By that, it is meant that cats brought together from the remotest localities will interbreed and produce fertile young. Even cats brought from Asiatic countries are fertile with European cats, in spite of the possibility that these have been separated since the early days of domestication.

One final point will be made: no matter how diverse the modern cat may be in coat color or body conformity, all of the variability can be

The only environmental factors which are known to affect the germ cells are X-rays, radiation and a wide variety of chemical mutagens. These agents do so by inducing chromosome aberrations and gene mutations. Furthermore, the mutation is entirely at random and occurs at a very low frequency. The possibility of increasing the mutation rate of certain kinds of mutants to bring about a desired change has been discussed among scientists, but the likelihood of this is remote and experimentation like this on pedigreed cats is never done by responsible breeders.

B: Timeline of cat breeds

Table 1.1 Timeline of cat breeds

Breed name	Area of origin	Accepted date(s) of origin
Abyssinian	Ethiopia	1860s
Alaskan Snow Cat – see Snow Cat		
American Bobtail	USA	1960s
American Curl	USA	1981
American Lynx	USA	1980s
American Shorthair	USA	1966. Previously Domestic Shorthair; first registered around 1900
American Wirehair	USA	1966
Australian	Australia	1946*
Australian Curl	Australia	1996. Discontinued 1997
Balinese	USA	1940s. Date of official recognition 1961
Bengal	USA	1963
Birman	Burma	Disputed, some say France in the 1930s
Bohemian Rex	Czech Republic	1994
Bombay	USA	1958. First official recognition 1976
British Angora	UK	1960s
British Shorthair	UK	1870s
Bristol		1970s
Burmese	Thailand	1350–1767. First official recognition 1936
Burmilla	UK	1981
California Rex	USA	1959*
California Spangle	USA	1971
Celonese	Sri Lanka	1984
Chartreux	France	Fourteenth century. First shown in 1931
Chantilly	USA	1967
Chausie	USA	1995?
Chinese Lop	China	1796*
Colourpoint British Shorthair	UK	1980s
Colourpoint European Shorthair	Italy	1982
Colourpoint Shorthair	UK	1947
Cornish Rex	UK	1950
Colourpoint Longhair (see Himalayan)		
Coupari – see Longhair Fold		
Cymric	Canada	1960s
Czech Curly Cat – see Bohemian Rex		
Devon Rex	UK	1960
Domestic Shorthair – see American Shorthair		

Table 1.1 Continued

Breed name	Area of origin	Accepted date(s) of origin
Don Sphynx – see Russian Hairless		
Dutch Rex	Netherlands	1969*
Egyptian Mau	Egypt	Early. First recognized in Europe in 1953
European Shorthair	Italy	1982
Exotic Shorthair	USA	1966
French Sphynx	France	1960s*
German Rex	East Germany	1946
Havana Brown (as 'Havana')	UK	1951
Himalayan	USA/UK	1950s/1920s
Italian Rex	Italy	1950*
Japanese Bobtail	Japan	Fifth to tenth century. Official recognition 1971
Javanese	USA/UK	1960s
Karakul	USA	1930s
Karel Bobtail	Russia	1990s?
Karellian Bobtail – see Karel Bobtail		
Kashmir	UK	1950s
Korat	Thailand	1350–1767
Kuril Bobtail	Russia	Recognition date 1990s? Existed prior to this
LaPerm	USA	1986
Longhair Exotic	USA	1990s
Longhair Fold	UK	1980s
Longhair Japanese Bobtail	Japan	1954
Maine Coon	USA	1860s
Maine Waves – see Rexed Maine Coon		
Manx	UK	Early. First shown in USA 1933
Marbled Mist	Australia	1997
Malay Cat	Malaya Peninsula	1881*
Malayan	USA	1980
Mei Toi	USA	1994
Mexican Hairless	USA	1902*
Missouri Rex	USA	1990s
Munchkin	USA	Recognition date 1991. Existed prior to this
Nebelung	USA	1990s
Norwegian Forest Cat	Norway	Early
Ocicat	USA	1964
Ohio Rex	USA	1944*
Ojos Azules	USA	1984
Oregon Rex	USA	1959*
Oriental Shorthair	UK	1950s
Peke-Faced Persian	USA	1930s
Persian	Iran	Early
Peterbald – see Petersburg Hairless		
Petersburg Hairless	Russia	1990s
Pixie-Bob	USA	1995
Poodle Cat	Germany	1994
Prussian Rex	East Prussia	1930s*
Ragamuffin	USA	1994
Ragdoll	USA	1960s
Renegade	USA	1997
Rexed Maine Coon	UK	1988
Russian Blue	Russia	Late 1800s
Russian Hairless	Russia	1987

Table 1.1 Continued

Breed name	Area of origin	Accepted date(s) of origin
Safari Cat	USA	1980s
Savannah	US	1997?
Savannah	UK	1997
Scottish Fold	UK	1961
Selkirk Rex	USA	1987
Serengeti	USA	1996?
Seychellois	UK	1984
Siamese	Thailand	1350–1767. May have first been shown in 1871
Siberian Cat	Russia	Early
Si-Rex	USA	1986
Singapura	Singapore/US	1971
Snow Cat	USA	1990s
Snowshoe	USA	1960s
Sokoke Forest Cat	Kenya	1977
Somali	USA/Canada	1967
Sphynx	Canada	1966
Spotted Mist	Australia	1976
Suqutranese	UK	1990
Thai-Bobtail	Russia	1990s?
Tiffanie	UK	1980s
Tiffany	USA	1967
Tonkinese	USA	1950s
Toy-Bobtail	Russia	1986
Turkish Angora	Turkey	Early
Turkish Van	Turkey	Early
Urals Rex	Russia	1991
Ussuri	Russia	1990s
Victoria Rex	UK	1972*
Wild Abyssinian	Singapore	1980s
York Chocolate	USA	1983

*Vanished breeds

Note: The breeds named here are not necessarily recognized by registries of pedigreed cats, but are listed here for information. The dates of origin are those which are generally accepted by breeders and fanciers as the dates (a) from which the breed can be dated as a distinct, natural breed, or (b) the dates from which the breed can be dated as descendants of cats selected to found the breed.

Source: J. Shartwell, Breeder/Exhibitor, Tony Morace, ACFA allbreed judge, updated by L. Shelton, co-author.

Chapter 2

Reproduction and development

Practical aspects of reproduction

Reproduction in the cat is a fascinating topic in its own right and one that we presume most breeders are familiar with. The majority of cats reproduce quite happily, if they are healthy. This section acts as a summary of the more practical aspects of the subject and forms a preamble to a more detailed discussion of what is actually transmitted from one generation to the next at the act of coitus. Additional resources can be found in the references at the end of this book.

Reproductive age

Under optimal conditions of husbandry and diet, sexual maturity or puberty in the female normally occurs between the ages of seven to 12 months, depending on a variety of factors, such as the month of birth and its growth rate. Exceptionally, a rapidly growing female may reach puberty as early as four months of age. Size is probably the governing factor, as one report says the female is capable of breeding when she weighs about 2.5 kg (5.5 lb). However, regardless of the actual onset of puberty, it is usually judged prudent not to breed from a queen until she is about 12 months of age.

The attainment of puberty is less obvious in the male, but is usually taken to be a month or two later than in the female. For medium and large cats, a weight level of about 3.5 kg (7.7 lb) is considered to be a convenient point. Queens will continue to produce litters until they are many years of age, although a figure of between eight and 10 years is the usual. The actual cessation of breeding is a gradual affair, usually accompanied by a rise of sterile copulations and decline in litter size. It is rare for a female to reproduce beyond the age of 14 years. Just as males attain puberty a month or so after females, they are also capable of breeding for a number of years beyond the latest age for the female.

Estrus and coitus

Estrus (heat) is the period in which the female is receptive of the attentions of the male. The duration is normally from five to eight days although persisting as long as 20 days. The period is marked by relatively distinctive behavior by the queen enabling an experienced breeder to judge the most advantageous time for the two animals to meet. For a day or two (the pre-estrus stage), the female becomes very affectionate, demands unusual attention, rubs herself against objects and indulges in playful rolling. There may also be howling and 'calling' although there are differences among various breeds in this respect.

The second stage is characterized by treading and the adoption of the coital crouch (flattening of the back and raising of the hindquarters). The coital crouch occurs in response to gentle stroking or a nudging of the genital region or the presence of a male. The queen is now fully receptive and coitus (mating) can occur. Successful intromission (penetration) is almost always accompanied by a loud cry or growl from the queen.

After the two cats have parted, the female usually engages in quite vigorous rolling, rubbing and licking, which then subsides into a short period of inactivity. They may resume mating within an interval of 15 or 30 minutes. Several matings per day for all but the last day of estrus may occur if allowed.

Litters may be born at any time of the year. The typical breeding period is from January to July (in the Northern hemisphere) or even somewhat longer. The natural winter pause, however, can be effectively reduced by the provision of artificial illumination to counteract the diminished hours of daylight. Two, or even three, litters can normally be produced per year, with the peak months being March to April and July to August (in the Northern hemisphere).

In the absence of coitus, the female usually shows recurrent estrus at intervals of 12 to 22 days although it is reported that some animals may have much more irregular cycles. An infertile mating is often followed by a pseudopregnancy which lasts about 30 to 40 days. After this the female comes into estrus again.

The cat is one of the few mammals in which the eggs are released by the ovary as a result of nervous stimuli provided by coitus. The gestation period is about 66 days, although the broad range of between 58 and 71 days has been recorded. Some latitude must be expected, however, to imprecise information on the actual day of the release of the eggs, especially for matings spread over several days.

The number of eggs released is probably in excess of the number of kittens born, due to intrauterine mortality of fetuses. Unfortunately, precise data on the extent of this mortality is lacking. A survey to determine weaned litter size revealed that the average litter consists of 3.9 kittens, with an extreme range of one to 10, based upon 5073 litters (19 813 cats). The size of the litter usually varies with the weight of mother, with heavier females tending to have larger litters than the lighter females. The sex ratio has been found to be 104 males to 100 females, based on 16 820 kittens.

The lactation period may vary from 50 to 60 days although partial weaning, particularly in catteries following an early weaning program, may begin before this. Complete weaning leads to a rapid end to the milk flow. While there is no estrus immediately following parturition (post-partum estrus), the estrus cycle usually recommences between two and four weeks after weaning, and can, on occasion, return even earlier.

Litter size

The ideal litter for a queen seems to be about four kittens. Statistics kept on pedigreed cats indicate that most breeds tend to produce litters of about this size. Few females seem capable of nursing more than this number unaided, particularly if rapid growth of the kittens is to be expected. Kittens from large litters can be transferred to queens with small litters or kittens may be supplemented with milk in a special cat feeding bottle. It must not be overlooked, of course, that the ability to suckle a complement of four young is inherited. Breeding stock should, therefore, only be chosen (as far as possible, after all other aspects, including overall health, are taken into account) from queens who have been 'good mothers' and who have reared kittens with a good record of growth.

Longevity

Stories abound of many cats living to a ripe old age, but people interested in feline geriatrics are reluctant to accept undocumented statements. A report on authenticated cases of cats living beyond 20 years shows a range of longevity from 19 to 27 years, with an average of 22 to 23 years. Unsubstantiated claims have gone even higher Unfortunately, the errors involved in recalling past events and establishing the age of an animal are notorious.

Genetic factors may influence most of the features discussed here. This means that line (strain) and breed differences exist. The Manx, for instance, usually has smaller litters than the average, because of the intrauterine mortality associated with the lethal gene found in the tailless condition.

Germ cell lineage

The cat as an entity commences life as the union of two germ cells. This occurs in the oviduct, a thin tube of tissue that conveys the egg (female germ cell) to the uterus on its release by the ovary. Though the act of coitus provides the stimulus, the eggs are not liberated until many hours have elapsed. The delay allows the sperms (male germ cells), which have been deposited in the vagina, to make their way to the site of fertilization. There, they either meet the eggs or are on hand for the arrival of the eggs.

Fertilization accomplished, the egg undergoes cleavage, passing through the morula and early blastodermic stages. Implantation is believed to occur about the 14th day. From this point on, growth and development are rapid and the tiny blob of protoplasm becomes transformed into a recognizable fetus. After about 66 days, the cat is expelled from the queen. It emerges as a young kitten, not fully able to fend for itself, but equipped with a sucking reflex to obtain nourishment from its mother.

As a new individual is created by the union of germ cells, it follows that their contents must form the material link between successive generations. The male and female germ cells differ greatly in size and structure, as befitting their different functions. The egg is relatively large and spherical, rich in nutrients to carry it over the developmental period from fertilization to implantation. On the other hand, the sperm is a fragile thing, microscopic in size and possessing a long tail, with just about enough energy for it to reach and enter the egg for fertilization. The function of the egg and sperm is to house a nucleus and to assure that two nuclei (one from the egg and one from the sperm) can come together and fuse.

Genetically, the important constituents of the two nuclei are the chromosomes. These are extremely small bodies, visible under the microscope. They are bearers of the hereditary material. Their joining up to form a common nucleus enables the egg to commence development as an independent entity.

In biological terms, the body of an individual is known as the 'soma'. It consists of myriad cells, all of which are concerned with either the structure or with the innumerable physiological functions necessary for sustaining life. The greater bulk of the somatic cells is not involved in reproduction, although some are indirectly. The reason for this is that, as the fertilized egg gradually changes into an embryo and then into a fetus, the various pathways of development become sorted out and then diverge at a progressive rate. A fundamental divergence is that between those cells that are destined to produce the soma and those cells that are destined to form the germ cells. Developmentally, once separation has occurred, growth can then be semiautonomous, subject only to the restriction that if growth is proceeding normally, the various processes must not become out of step with one another.

Heredity versus environment in the shaping of the individual

A careful distinction should be made between genetic endowment and subsequent development of an individual. Genetic endowment is completed at fertilization and is heredity in the strictest sense. That is, this represents the extent of the parental contributions. Development of the individual has yet to proceed. It is here where the genetically inspired growth processes and the effects of environment can interact.

In genetics, the environment has a wider, yet more technical, meaning than just that of the surroundings. All tangible non-genetic influences constitute the environment. At first, the developing individual has to contend with the maternal environment. Prenatally, that is provided by the uterus; postnatal'y, it is provided by the level of maternal care. Later, the developing individual has to contend with the impact of the physical world.

As an individual's development proceeds, it is buffeted on every side by environmental influences. The picture is complicated by the fact that the various characteristics that make up the individual are affected to different degrees by the innate genetic constitution. For instance, at one extreme, it could be argued that post-natal growth is largely governed by diet. If this is inadequate, a poorly developed and stunted animal will result. The animal may even languish, become susceptible to disease and die. On the other hand, somewhat similar results could follow if the individual is reared in cold, damp, surroundings.

These two examples are singled out because the two of the primary environmental factors on development are the diet and temperature. The former is obviously of great importance as growth is dependent on nourishing food. Yet, the dietary effect is almost entirely negative. Given adequate food, the growth is then largely governed by the genetic constitution.

At the other extreme, some characteristics are scarcely affected by the environment. To cat breeders, coat color and hair type are important attributes and these are almost completely controlled by heredity. True, the Siamese (pointed) pattern is modifiable to some extent, as the temperature of the cat's environment influences the amount of pigment deposited in the hairs. That is, the intensity of the color is impacted, but the presence or absence of pointing is not. This is the exception that tends to prove the rule, for only one particular series of genes (of which Siamese is a member) is affected in this way. In general, it is almost impossible to modify the color by environmental factors.

A third point is worth mentioning to complete this discussion. This deals with developmental error. Developmental error arises from accidental quirks and irregularities of development peculiar to the individual that cannot be easily attributed either to genetic or to environmental causes. This source of variation is of little concern for practical responsible cat breeding, though it is advisable for breeders to be aware of its existence. Any variation of this nature is relatively small. The variation of piebald white spotting provides a good example of this. Though the variation can be described in broad terms, such as bicolor or van pattern, no two white marked cats are exactly alike. In part, this is due to the erratic development of the white areas during embryonic growth, so the particular pattern is a feature of the particular individual.

The chromosomes

As the chromosomes within the germ cells are the hereditary material that is passed on from generation to generation, the mechanism by which this is achieved will be discussed in more detail. Two sorts of cell division are involved:

- Mitosis – ordinary cell division.
- Meiosis – two special divisions that lead up to the formation of the germ cells.

The treatment here is admittedly oversimplified to bring out the essential similarity and to show that meiosis is a subtly modified form of mitosis.

Mitosis

In ordinary mitotic cell division, which takes place during growth or to replace worn out or damaged tissue, the membrane containing the nucleus dissolves away. At that time, the chromosomes (38 in the cat) orient themselves so as to form an ordered line-up in a plane across the center of the cell. This is a period of intense activity within the cell. Soon, each chromosome has given rise to a partner, alike to it in all respects, by a process of self-copying, cloning.

The chromosomes lie in close proximity for a while and then begin to move apart. Each of the 38 chromosomes behaves in the same manner. The two groups tend to move in unison and eventually huddle together at each end of the cell. A nuclear membrane forms around each group, to bring into being two nuclei. The cell may constrict between the nuclei, or simply construct a cell wall. The nuclei are now contained in separate cells and these increase in size, until they are identical to the previous single cell.

The mitotic divisions are responsible for the growth of the soma, cell by cell, until the tissues, bones and various organs are built up. They are also responsible for the formation of the gonads, which are formed at the appropriate stage of embryonic development. The fact that the gonads are formed so early in life does not mean that they are immediately functional. Rather, functionality does not occur until many months later, when somatic growth is almost completed and the animal attains puberty. It does mean, however, that the gonads are semi-independent of the soma, remaining inactive until, under the influence of hormones, they become active and begin to produce germ cells. It is at this stage that the mitotic divisions are transformed into the slightly more complicated meiotic divisions.

Meiosis

As in mitosis, meiosis begins by dissolution of the nuclear membrane and the orderly line-up of the chromosomes. However, instead of the chromosomes behaving as separate bodies, they now come together in pairs. The pairs of chromosomes then exchange genetic material at cross-over points. Examination reveals that the pairing is not at random, but only involves those chromosomes of similar size and shape. It is clear that the 38 chromosomes are, in reality, 19 pairs of chromosomes (that is, two of each kind). This explains why pairing can occur, as different chromosomes as a rule behave independently of each other.

Whatever is the attraction that brings the similar chromosomes together, it soon wanes, and the repellent starts. The chromosomes move apart towards opposite ends of the cell and the 19 chromosomes remain bunched together while a nucleus forms around them. A cellular wall divides the cell and the two new cells are formed. This is the first meiotic division. A second division follows which is essentially a mitosis. There, the chromosomes line up, but do not pair. Instead, a partner chromosome is formed by self-copying, and the chromosomes fall apart to form separate nuclei. The appearance of a cellular wall results in two new cells. Note that this division only involves 19 chromosomes.

The important meiotic division is the first. During this stage the mixing of genetic material occurs so that no two germ cells then contain the same genetic material. But, for purposes of this book, the most important aspect is the reduction in number of chromosomes that takes place during meiosis. There are 19 different chromosomes in the somatic cells of the cat but, as each one is present twice, this gives a total of 38. This number, 38, is the diploid number (the reduced number of 19 is denoted as the 'basic' or 'haploid' number).

The products of meiosis are transformed into germ cells, each containing 19 chromosomes. The transformation is more or less direct for the male, with the meiotic divisions leading to the production of sperms. The transformation is less direct for the female, although the end result is the same, the production of a fertilizable egg nucleus containing 19 chromosomes. The union of two germ cells, male and female, each with 19 chromosomes, restores the diploid number of 38 and gives an individual the full complement of genetically determined characteristics, half from the mother, half from the father.

The necessity of reducing the somatic chromosome number by half should now be apparent. If this did not occur, the number of chromosomes would double in each generation, which would be absurd. However, the substitution of meiotic divisions just before the production of the germ cells is an elegant mechanism to maintain a constant number of chromosomes.

The arrangement of the chromosomes in pairs is also part of the genetic mechanism. It is not sufficient that the germ cells should receive any random collection of 19 chromosomes, but rather they receive the same basic 19 in every cell. The line-up ensures that this occurs by sending one of each pair to opposite ends of the cell. However, the chromosomes may be jumbled up in the cell before a division, the meiotic line-up effectively sorts out the pairs.

The diploid–haploid alternation is confined to the germ cells, the soma invariably containing 38 chromosomes (except for accidents of division). These accidents tend to be rare but, when they do, they can lead to abnormalities. The production of the tortoiseshell male cat, to be discussed in a later chapter, is one such instance.

The latest information on the haploid number of chromosomes for both the small and large cats is given in the technical appendix to this chapter. It shows that the haploid number of 19 for the domestic cat is by no means exceptional. Indeed, detailed studies by karyologists (people who study chromosomes) have shown that the majority of felids possess a similar number. They have also shown that the sizes and shapes of the individual chromosomes do not appear to differ a great deal between species. This probably explains why it is possible to obtain hybrids between many of the species, even if the hybrid may be sterile.

Sex chromosomes and sex determination

Each of the normal complement of 19 pairs of chromosomes in the cat differs from the others. Some pairs are larger than others and some a different shape. In general, the chromosomes that make up each pair match; they are identical in size and shape. The reason for this, of course, is that each chromosome is represented twice in the somatic cells, hence their selfsameness is no cause for surprise. According to the latest examinations, there are nine pairs of large chromosomes and nine pairs of medium to small chromosomes.

What is interesting, however, is that in addition to the above, one pair of chromosomes is not identical. Their most obvious difference is in size. One is a medium-sized chromosome while the other is quite small. Why should this be? A clue may be found in the fact that the inequality is confined to the male. Observations have shown that the female has 10 pairs of medium to small chromosomes while the male has nine pairs plus the unequal sized pair. It may be deduced that the latter are associated with sex. In fact, they are sex chromosomes. This makes the pair rather novel.

So, to distinguish the other chromosomes from these, all of the ordinary chromosomes are called 'autosomes'. The sex chromosomes themselves are further distinguished by calling the medium-sized chromosome the X and the smaller chromosome the Y. As the Y chromosome is carried only by the male, it is commonly referred to as the 'male' chromosome. Therefore, using the symbols indicating the sex chromosome makeup of the two sexes, the male is XY and the female is XX.

A confirmation that the unequally sized sex chromosomes are a true pair is provided by a study of meiosis in the male. In the line-up of chromosomes, the sex chromosomes can be seen to pair up and migrate to opposite ends of the cell. This means that the two cells formed by the division are not fully identical. Each cell contains a set of identical autosomes, but one cell contains an X chromosome while the other has the Y. These cells are transformed into sperms. It follows that there are two sorts of sperm, those carrying an X and those carrying a Y. Furthermore, as the cell divisions are proceeding continuously, the two sorts of sperm are produced in equal numbers.

In the female, on the other hand, this differentiation of the germ cells cannot occur as the sex chromosomes in this sex are an identical pair. At meiosis, the XX sex chromosomes come together at the line-up, and separate in the usual manner. But it does not matter which member of the pair ends up in the fertilizable egg nucleus. The result is always the same: the egg will contain one X chromosome. When the egg and sperm unite at fertilization, the sex chromosome constitute of the individual will depend upon the sperm. The egg contributes one X, but the sperm contributes either an X or a Y. The two sorts of sperm occur in equal numbers, so two sorts of individual are formed at fertilization: those with XX chromosome and those with XY chromosome. The former will develop into females and the latter into males. The cycle of sex chromosome reduction and reconstitution is mediated in the male.

To put it another way, sex is determined by the X and Y chromosomes. The male is of constitution XY and the female is XX. The male produces both X and Y chromosomes, while the female produces only one (X). These unite at random to give an expected 1:1 sex ratio among the offspring.

This in turn means that the sex of the individual offspring is determined by the male. It is also determined at the moment of fertilization. The XY

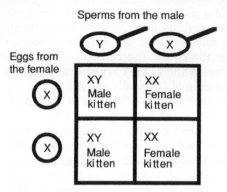

Figure 2.1 Sex development

and XX chromosome constitution of the embryo will see to it that the developing sex organs will be appropriately male or female (Fig. 2.1).

Sex development

Sex is initially determined by the XY or XX constitution of the individual and in the vast majority of cases, subsequent development of the embryo is perfectly normal. However, in some cases the normal development is upset and one of a variety of anomalies may arise. Anomalies tend to be rare and this is an indication that the cause is an exceptional event.

In some instances, the abnormality will be independent of the sex chromosome constitution. These will either be due to accidents of development or be caused by genes on the autosomes. For example, a not infrequent anomaly is unilateral or bilateral cryptorchidism, that is a disruption of the descent of testes into the scrotum. As a male with one testis fully descended (unilateral cryptorchidism) is usually fertile and will sire both male and female kittens, this indicated that his XY constitution is unimpaired. The defect is clearly one of development. The cause of this anomaly is discussed in Chapter 4.

On the other hand, some sex anomalies are known to be caused by unusual sex chromosome constitutions. These cases are of particular genetic interest. Whereas the Y chromosome may carry very few genes, the X may carry a fair number. It is not possible to say how many because their discovery is dependent upon the rare event of mutation. Yet, one X-borne mutant has been known in the cat for a very long time. This is sex-linked orange, the gene responsible for the tortoiseshell pattern. The reason why this pattern ordinarily occurs only in the female is due to sex-linkage. The genetic situation is fully discussed later in Chapter 4, but one aspect of it is relevant at this point. Tortoiseshell males do occur on rare occasions and one of the explanations for their appearance postulates an abnormal XY constitution. This suggestion can be checked by examination of the chromosomes and this has been done for a number of cases.

The simplest case of a male tortoiseshell is the presence of an extra X to produce XXY. This curious and anomalous constitution could occur from mistakes during meiosis or in the mitotic divisions that occur after fertilization. Whatever the cause, the cells of the individual have gained an extra X chromosome. While a XXY constitution can produce an externally normal male, the animal is usually sterile.

Other unusual constitutions have been found in cats. These include mixtures of XX and XY cells, of XY and XXY cells, and of XY and XXY cells, together with yet more complex combinations involving a Y with several X chromosomes. Individuals with mixtures of different cell types are known as mosaics. Overall, the Y chromosome is so strongly male-inducing that the individual possessing it develops as a male, despite the number of X chromosomes that also may be present. However, the price paid is that these males are sterile.

In contrast to the above are individuals with only one X chromosome, a constitution that is written as XO. These individuals are able to live, are females, but are sterile. They typically fail to come into estrus, a feature that is the most obvious external sign of the anomaly.

Almost all of the anomalous constitutions involving the Y chromosome were discovered because they produced the rare tortoiseshell male. The reason is the chance occurrence of the orange gene *O* on one of the X chromosomes. Without the presence of an *O* gene, these cats would be simply infertile males.

However, some tortoiseshell males are actually fertile. There are two mechanisms by which these can be produced.

- A frequently recurring mosaic is a mixture of XX and XY cells, a type that is represented as XY/XX. This constitution is easily understood because the cat is a mixture of male and female chromosome constitutions. However, it is possible to have a mosaic of the type XY/XY, a mixture of two male chromosome constitutions. Such a cat can be a tortoiseshell should one of the X chromosomes carry the *O* gene. Whereas the XX/XY mosaic is sterile, the XY/XY mosaic is fertile.
- The second mechanism draws upon the concept of somatic mutation. A body cell can mutate in a similar manner to a germ cell. A mutation on the X chromosome of a male cat to produce an orange gene *O* will result in a tortoiseshell. The form most commonly encountered is a red tabby, with variably sized patches of black pigmentation. These have been produced by a mutation from *O* to *o* in the body cells of the red tabby. These males are fertile and they usually breed as a red tabby. An account of the sex-linked inheritance of the orange gene *O* is given in Chapter 4.

Technical appendices

A: Basic data on reproduction and the life cycle of the domestic cat

Table 2.1 Basic data on reproduction and the life cycle of the domestic cat

Item	Average	Typical variation
Puberty, males	12 months	6–14 months
Puberty, females	9 months	4–21 months
Estrus cycle	12–22 days	7–40 days
Estrus	5–8 days	3–20 days
Gestation period	66 days	58–71 days
Weaned litter size	3–9	1–10+
Secondary sex ratio	104:100	75:100–130:100
Breeding period	Mid-winter–summer	Year-round
Cessation of breeding	8–10 years	To 14 years

Note: These ranges are approximations only. Both research and observation indicate that there can be wide differences among breeds as to averages and typical variations for all of these measurements. Within breeds, the averages tend to be more consistent and the range of variation tends to be narrower

B: Haploid number of chromosomes for selected cat species

Table 2.2 Haploid number of chromosomes for selected cat species

Common name	Zoological name	Haploid number
African golden cat	Felis aurata	19
African wild cat	Felis lybica	19
Blackfooted cat	Felis nigripes	19
Bobcat	Felis rufs	19
Caffer cat	Felis ornata	19
Caracal lynx	Felis caracal	19
Cheetah	Acinonyx jubatus	19
Clouded leopard	Neofelis nebulosa	19
Domestic cat	Felis catus	19
European wild cat	Felis silvestris	19
Fishing cat	Felis viverrina	19
Flat-headed cat	Felis planiceps	19
Geoffroy's cat	Felis geoffroyi	18
Jaguar	Panthera onca	19
Jaguarundi	Felis jaguarondi	19
Jungle cat	Felis chaus	19
Leopard	Panthera pardus	19
Leopard cat	Felis bengalensis	19
Lion	Panthera leo	19
Margay cat	Felis wiedi	18
Northern lynx	Felis lynx	19
Ocelot	Felis pardalis	18
Pallas's cat	Felis manul	19
Pampas cat	Felis colocolo	18
Puma	Felis concolor	19
Rusty spotted cat	Felis rubinginosa	19
Sand cat	Felis margarita	19
Serval	Felis serval	19
Snow leopard	Panthera uncia	19
Temminch's golden cat	Felis temmincki	19
Tiger	Panthera tigris	19
Tiger cat	Felis tigrina	18

Note: Those species inhabiting Central and South America have 18 instead of 19 chromosomes possessed by the Old World species. The cause of this is a fusion between two of the smaller chromosomes to form a larger chromosome during the course of evolution. This has effectively reduced the chromosome number by one

Chapter 3

Principles of heredity

Introduction

The basic laws of heredity are relatively simple. They can be reduced to two concepts:

1. The law of separation of the genes in the germ cells.
2. The law of independent assortment of the genes in various crosses.

Add to these the phenomenon of linkage (which is actually an extension of the second law), then most of elementary genetics is easily covered.

The very simplicity of the bare bones of heredity may be a factor operating in their disfavor. Some people may feel that this model of genes and their heredity cannot explain everything in the development of a complex mammal such as the cat. This aversion is understandable but mistaken. The cat is indeed a complex organism and it must be admitted that a detailed study of feline genetics can certainly lead into deeper waters. But, no matter how complex an organism may be, it can always be broken down into simple attributes for expository purposes. In genetics, these are conveniently referred to as inherited 'characters' or 'traits'. Some oversimplification is inevitable, but this does give an insight into the mechanisms behind the heritable characteristics that define the differences between individual cats.

As the principles of heredity can be explained to a large extent without reference to the chromosomes, such approaches have been taken in the past. It should never be forgotten that the DNA and the chromosomes that they comprise constitute the material basis of heredity. In the early days of genetics the hereditary determinants present in the cells were known as 'factors'. In modern terms, the factor is now the 'gene'. In essence, genetics is concerned with tracing the path of these genes as these are transmitted from parent to offspring. The effects of genes on the growth, function and appearance of the individual will also be discussed. Genes control just about every aspect of the life of a cat.

Genes and alleles

The gene may be visualized as a minute section of a chromosome, made up of deoxyribonucleic acid (DNA) in a double helix structure. Genes are responsible for producing the protein molecules that make up a cat's body and allow it to function. Each chromosome consists of some thousands of genes, along with sections of DNA that control the expression of the genes and some sections that have functions as yet unknown to us. As complex as the function of DNA is, it is comprised of only four building blocks:

- A – adenine.
- T – thymine.
- C – cytosine.
- G – guanine.

These building blocks are molecules called nucleic acids. A chromosome can be visualized as a string of beads, with each bead representing one of these nucleic acids. If you picture DNA as four colors of beads on a string, it would take a strand 3000 miles long to represent the entire genome (genetic makeup) of the cat.

The DNA strands of the chromosomes reproduce an exact copy of themselves during cell division. The duplication is so good that many hundreds of thousands of daughter genes are produced before a mistake occurs and an inexact copy is then made. The creation of an inexact copy is known as a mutation; the altered gene is referred to as a mutant. The original gene and its mutant form are both referred to as 'alleles'. The two genes, the original and the mutant, are said to be 'allelic'. That is because one has originated from the other and, therefore, must occupy the same position in the chromosome. This position is the 'locus' of the gene on the chromosome. The concept of the locus is important in genetics because each chromosome contains some thousands of loci; each capable of producing a characteristic mutation or series of mutations. When a mutation occurs, the gene may no longer produce the protein that it is responsible for, or it may produce a defective form of that protein. A single change in 'color', or deletion of just one of those beads on the 3000 mile long strand, may represent a mutation. That mutation may produce anything from a benign change in a cat's color to a deadly disease.

The occurrence of mutations is so uncommon that, for most practical purposes, the event can be ignored. Nevertheless, all of the existing colors and coat types of the cat, as well as all of the inherited diseases, have come into existence as a result of mutation. An indication of the rarity of mutations is that the number of mutant varieties is so few in spite of the millions of cats bred all over the world. Only two dozen or so mutant genes are definitely known. One reason for this is that a cat with a unique mutation may not be viable and may die before or shortly after birth. With more benign mutations, a cat displaying a new variety may not be particularly attractive at first sight. Instead of being carefully nurtured and developed, it may be destroyed out of hand as a 'freak' or permitted to expire without support. This sort of behavior certainly results in a loss to science and possibly to the Fancy.

The inherited colors of the cat provide excellent illustrations of the principles of heredity. It should be remembered that genetics is not concerned merely with color or coat types. To a greater or lesser extent, the genetic constitution controls the following:

- The development of the animal.
- The cat's behavior.
- A cat's proneness to certain afflictions and disease.
- A cat's reproductive ability.

However, the simpler aspects of genetics may be explained more easily using coat colors as examples, than by using less sharply defined traits.

Simple inheritance

The original, wild type coloration of the cat is the ubiquitous tabby pattern and it has been established that the pattern consists of two components. These are:

1. Areas in which the hair fibers are banded or ticked with alternating black and yellow pigment.
2. Areas in which all-black hairs predominate and the yellow band is reduced to the very base of the hairs, if it exists at all.

The first component is identical to the drab yellowish-brown agouti coat that is found in numerous animal species. The second represents the melanistic overlay (bars, spots, rosettes or reticulation) which is a characteristic feature of the cat family. Tabby pattern, therefore, consists of two co-existing systems of pigmentation or, more likely, a background of agouti, with a superimposed system of stronger black pigmentation.

One of the first mutants to be found in the cat was probably that of self black. This occurred so long ago that it is now futile to speculate just when the event occurred. It is of greater practical importance to know how this mutant color is inherited. This knowledge, determined circa 1918, may be used to demonstrate the transmission of any single gene. The self black color comes into existence by a change in one of the genes controlling the agouti background. In the black individual, none of the hairs display yellow pigment. The hair fibers are primarily black, the color fading to a smoky gray at the lower regions of the hair shaft.

A pure breeding strain of tabby cats will, by definition, produce only tabby kittens. Similarly, a pure strain of black cats will produce only black kittens. If, however, animals of the two strains are crossed, all the offspring will be tabbies. Despite their tabby appearance, these offspring are carriers of the black trait (as indicated by their parentage). That means the black color will reappear in subsequent generations. Should these resultant tabbies be bred together, the next generation will consist of tabby and black offspring in the ratio 3:1. However, if the tabby offspring are mated back to the black parent, the ratio of tabby to black kittens will be 1:1. A mating could also be made back to the pure tabby strain, but little would be gained (as far as appearance goes) as all of the kittens would be tabby.

For purposes of discussion, the following symbols are used:

- The initial generation, before crossing, is symbolized as P (for parental).
- The first cross generation is designated as F_1 (the first filial generation), and the subsequent generation as F_2 (the second filial generation).

Subsequent matings are known as backcrosses (BC) and it is usual to indicate to which parent or strain the backcross is made. Of these crosses, the F_1 and F_2 are the most informative from a genetic viewpoint, although the backcross also has its uses.

In a preceding chapter, it is stated that the chromosomes are presented in pairs in the somatic or body cells, but only once in the germ cells. As the chromosomes are composed of genes, it follows that the genes must be present twice in the individual's body cells (one copy of each gene in each chromosome), but only once in the germ cells (the sperm or the egg). This explains the ratios of tabby and black kittens in the above example. The ratios are generated by the random fusion of germ cells carrying different alleles. At this stage, it is convenient to introduce the symbols for the various genes, as these greatly facilitate the discussion. It is customary to choose as symbols the upper and lower case letters of the Latin alphabet.

The symbol adopted for the agouti gene is A and its mutant form (non-agouti) is a. Normal genes and their mutant alleles share the same letter. As each individual contains two copies of each gene, the pure breeding tabby is symbolized by AA and the pure breeding black will be symbolized by aa. The germ cells contain only one copy of each gene, either A or a, depending on the strain. The F_1 tabby offspring must have the genetic constitution Aa because it is the result of the fusion between the A germ cell of the tabby parent and the a germ cell of the black parent.

The F_1 animals of constitution Aa produce two kinds of germ cells: those carrying A and those carrying a. The cell divisions that lead up to the formation of germ cells are essentially impartial and any particular germ-cell is just as likely to receive allele A as it is to receive allele a. The result is that the F_1 animal will form both A and a bearing germ cells in equal numbers. When two F_1 individuals are mated together, the germ cells will unite at random, one egg with one sperm. The chances of fusion of an A sperm with an A egg (to produce an offspring AA) is as likely as that of fusion with an a egg (to produce an offspring of genotype Aa). Similarly, the chances of fusion of an a sperm with an A egg (to produce an Aa offspring) are as likely as that of fusion with an a egg (to produce an aa offspring). These four possibilities are illustrated in the simple diagram in Fig. 3.1.

Figure 3.1 shows that the following offspring are produced: one AA, two Aa and one aa.

The first genotype (AA) represents a pure breeding tabby, the second (Aa) is a tabby capable of producing black offspring, and the last (aa) is

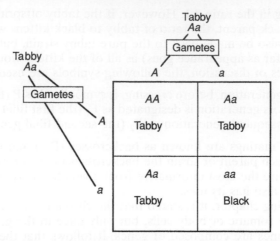

Figure 3.1 The possible outcomes from mating two F_1 heterozygous tabbies; to illustrate the 3:1 ratio of tabby to black for the F_2. Note that among the tabby offspring, one third will be homozygous AA and two thirds will be heterozygous Aa

a black. The AA and Aa tabbies, although different in genetic constitution, are of identical appearance. Hence they should be grouped together. When this is done, a ratio of three tabbies to one black is obtained. This ratio has been confirmed by experimental breeding and may be verified by any breeder who is willing to make the necessary effort. The 3:1 ratio has been described as the fundamental ratio of heredity.

At this point we must introduce several important concepts. The recovery of black individuals in the F_2 generation, resulting from the fusion of an a containing germ cell from one parent and an a containing germ cell from the other parent, is said to be due to the 'random assortment' of the alleles A and a. To use another term, it is due to the 'segregation' of gene a in the F_2. In genetics, the germ cells are called 'gametes'. The individual that results from the fusion of two gametes is termed a 'zygote'. Two types of zygotes exist. There is the true breeding or 'homozygote' of constitution AA or aa and the impure or 'heterozygote' of constitution Aa. This designation is used in describing any pair of alleles.

The fact that homozygous (AA) and heterozygous (Aa) tabby cats cannot be distinguished visually indicates that the influence of allele A predominates over the actions of allele a. When this occurs, allele A is said to be 'dominant' to allele a and, conversely, allele a is 'recessive' to allele A. The dominant versus recessive nature of an allele is indicated by the choice of symbols. **By convention, when one of two alternate alleles is dominant to the other, the dominant allele is given the upper case letter**. In this example, the agouti allele is symbolized by A while the recessive non-agouti allele takes the symbol a. By adhering to this guideline, it is easy to determine which is the dominant or recessive allele.

The phenomenon of dominance means that although the two tabbies AA and Aa are of identical appearance, they have a different genetic constitution. The outward appearance is referred to as the 'phenotype' and the genetic constitution as the 'genotype'. Even for the simple case of homozygous versus heterozygous tabby, it is important to make this distinction. Although the two tabbies have a similar phenotype, their genotypes infer quite different breeding capabilities. The first will produce only tabby offspring, while the second is capable of not only producing tabby, but black kittens as well.

The backcross of the F_1 to the black parent is an interesting mating. The black parent can only produce one type of gamete (a) whereas the F_1 individual produces two, namely A and a. The offspring, therefore, will consist of tabbies (Aa) and blacks (aa) in a 1:1 ratio. Figure 3.2 shows how the expected outcomes from the backcross can be determined. All of the tabbies that are produced will be carriers of black by virtue of their parentage. In this respect, they are identical heterozygotes to the F_1 individual.

Gametes from tabby *Aa*

	A	a
Gamete from black *aa* a	Aa Tabby	aa Black

Figure 3.2 The expectation from mating an F_1 heterozygous tabby to a black; to illustrate the 1:1 ratio of tabby to black

The existence of both homozygous and heterozygous tabbies in F_2 generation means that it is impossible to determine genotype by mere inspection of the phenotype. The most that can be inferred is that at least one A gene must be present, resulting in the cat being a tabby. It is customary to indicate ambiguities of this nature by inserting a dash sign (-) in the genotype. Therefore, A- denotes that the individual may be either AA or Aa. Parentage is a helpful guide in determining the genotype. When one parent exhibits the recessive phenotype, its offspring that exhibit the dominant form are called 'obligate carriers', as they must have received one copy of the recessive allele from this parent.

The situation is different for a recessive trait. A recessive phenotype cannot be expressed unless the responsible allele is in homozygous form. The fact has two general implications:

1. When an individual exhibits a recessive trait, the genotype relating to it is easily symbolized.
2. When two homozygous individuals are bred together, they will breed true for that trait.

In the present example, the black individuals produced either by the F_2 or the backcross, can only have the genotype aa. Therefore, should they be mated together, they will only produce black offspring.

The inheritance of non-agouti is quite straightforward and raises no special challenges. The trait of interest 'disappeared', as it might be put, in the F_1 but 'reappeared' in the F_2 and BC in its original form. Neither the agouti, nor the non-agouti, gene 'contaminated' each other as a consequence of being in close juxtaposition in the F_1. On the contrary, the various tabby or black offspring remained clearly tabby or black in appearance, displaying no evidence of any blending of the characteristics. This aspect may be generalized to include all cases of simple gene inheritance, not only non-agouti, but all those subsequently described in this book.

Checkerboard diagrams

The previous section described the inheritance of two alleles at the same locus (the agouti gene). The symbol A, used to represent the dominant agouti allele, may also be used to denote the agouti locus. The cat has 19 pairs of chromosomes, each one of which is composed of some thousands of gene loci. Consequently, it is important to know what happens when animals are bred together which are heterozygous for two or more mutant genes carried by different chromosomes.

A second gene is that for dilution of color, a common mutation in the cat. The gene causes a modification of the arrangement of pigment granules in the hair fibers, with the result that the coat appears slate-gray or bluish. Dilution is inherited as a simple recessive (symbolized d) to the gene producing dense pigmentation (symbolized D). A true breeding black cat is a densely colored animal of genotype DD, while a blue is a diluted variety of genotype dd. The F_1 of a cross between these is black, with the genotype Dd. In the F_2 generation, the blue color will recur in the ratio of three black to one blue. In other words, the mode of inheritance is similar to that of agouti versus non-agouti. This may be verified by substituting the symbols D and d for A and a, respectively, in Figs 3.1 and 3.2, and calculating the incidence of black versus blue kittens.

As the a and d alleles do not exist at the same gene locus, it is possible for a cat to be homozygous for the recessive form of both genes, resulting in the genotype $aadd$. When this occurs, the result is the non-agouti blue (self or solid blue). So what will happen when this blue is crossed with a tabby having the genotype $AADD$? As the a and d genes are independent, both will be present singly in each gamete as ad. Similarly, the gametes produced by the tabby will be AD. The F_1 from crossing the above will have the genotype $ad + AD = AaDd$. It will be a normal tabby in appearance since the A and D genes are dominant to a and d, respectively. In the F_2, the genes will sort independently and recombine at random to produce ratios of nine tabby, three blue tabby, three black and one blue.

The easiest method of deriving the potential results from a cross involving two or more mutant genes is with the aid of checkerboard diagrams. The diagrams of Figs 3.1 and 3.2 are checkerboards of a sort, but these fail to demonstrate the full power of this technique. Checkerboards are simple to construct and faithfully represent the random assortment of genes of interest and the complete range of expected genotypes.

There are a few basic rules for the construction of a checkerboard diagram. All the possible types of gametes are written along two sides of a square; those from one parent along the top and those from the other down the left side. Vertical and horizontal lines divide the square into as many columns and rows as there are different gametes. Within each cell are now transcribed the gene symbols at the head of the column and those at the side of the row in which the cell resides. To complete the diagram, it is merely necessary to examine the genotype of each cell and to write in the corresponding phenotype. Counting the incidence of the various phenotypes will give the expected ratios. The checkerboard is a useful tool and provides a valuable exercise in the manipulation of genes and for grasping the essence of the basic mechanism of heredity.

You must take care to ensure that the allele content of the gametes is correct. Each gamete can carry only one of each pair of alleles; and each allele of each pair must included when the combinations are made up. For example, the cross of a homozygous tabby ($AADD$) with a blue ($aadd$) gives the F_1 of $AaDd$, an animal doubly heterozygous for a and d. Four different gametes will be produced by this genotype: $AD + Ad + aD + ad$. Each gamete contains one allele of each of the two genes. The essential principle is that all possible combinations of A versus a in respect to D versus d must be formed. Once the number and composition of the gametes are determined, the procedure is straightforward, as shown by Fig. 3.3. The next step is to establish the phenotypes that correspond to

Gametes from tabby $AaDd$

		AD	Ad	aD	ad
	AD	AADD Tabby	AADd Tabby	AaDD Tabby	AaDd Tabby
	Ad	AADd Tabby	AAdd Blue tabby	AaDd Tabby	Aadd Blue tabby
Gametes from tabby AaDd	aD	AaDD Tabby	AaDd Tabby	aaDD Black	aaDd Black
	ad	AaDd Tabby	Aadd Blue tabby	aaDd Black	aadd Blue

Figure 3.3 A checkerboard diagram for two pairs of assorting mutant alleles. The expected ratio is 9:3:3:1 for the four phenotypes. Note the various homozygous and heterozygous genotypes within each phenotype

each genotype. This is achieved by considering the dominance relationships between the pairs of alleles. Alleles A and D are dominant to a and d, respectively, and produce their effects independently. This means that:

- The genotypes $AADD$, $AaDD$, $AADd$ and $AaDd$ are tabby.
- The genotypes $AAdd$ and $Aadd$ are blue tabby.
- The genotypes $aaDD$ and $aaDd$ are black.
- The single genotype of $aadd$ is blue.

The 9:3:3:1 ratio arises from the fact that some genotypes occur more than once. If the frequencies of the various genotypes are examined, it will be seen that these, too, have consistent ratios to one another. For instance, the number of heterozygotes and homozygotes, with respect to any dominant gene, will be in the ratio of 2:1 for an F_2 generation precisely as noted earlier for the segregation of one gene.

Any individual that displays one or more recessive characters will be homozygous at that locus. Therefore, all of the non-agoutis must be aa and all of the dilutes must be dd. This is true whether the individual is blue-agouti (A-dd) or a self blue ($aadd$). The latter phenotype is a combination of two recessive characters and, therefore, this cat must be homozygous for both a and d. It is not possible to be equally confident in the genotype of individuals displaying one or more dominant characters. In the present case, for example, a blue-agouti kitten that appears in the litter may have either of the two genotypes $AAdd$ or $Aadd$. These ambiguities are represented by dashes in the genotype. Thus, the genotypes corresponding to the phenotypes observed in the above F_2 offspring would be written as follows:

- Nine A-D-.
- Three A-dd.
- Three aaD-.
- One $aadd$.

Another example of the checkerboard is one representing the expected results from backcrossing the F_1 $AaDd$ to the self blue ($aadd$). The same four colors will be produced, but in the ratios of 1:1:1:1 as shown by Fig. 3.4. The perceptive reader will no doubt observe that this result is a direct extension of the 1:1 ratio seen in the backcross with one gene. The ratio

Gametes from tabby *AaDd*

		AD	Ad	aD	ad
Gametes from blue *aadd*	*ad*	*AaDd* Tabby	*Aadd* Blue tabby	*aaDd* Black	*aadd* Blue

Figure 3.4 Expectations for backcrossing a double heterozygote to the double recessive to illustrate the 1:1:1:1 ratio

Gametes from tabby *AaDd*

		AD	Ad	aD	ad
		AADd	*AAdd*	*AaDd*	*Aadd*
	Ad				
Gametes		Tabby	Blue tabby	Tabby	Blue tabby
from					
blue					
tabby		*AaDd*	*Aadd*	*aaDd*	*aadd*
Aadd	*ad*				
		Tabby	Blue tabby	Black	Blue

Figure 3.5 Expectations for a cross in which one gene is assorting at a 3:1 ratio and another at a 1:1 ratio; to illustrate the 3:1:3:1 ratio

of the four colors of offspring accurately reflects the random combination of genes that form the gametes produced by the F_1. The self blue is homozygous for two recessive genes and therefore can only produce gametes with the genotype *ad*. Any F_1 gamete carrying one or more dominant alleles will produce that dominant trait in the resultant offspring.

It is possible to have another type of backcross when two genes are involved. This occurs when one gene is heterozygous in one parent but homozygous in the other. Such a cross will be of the type *AaDd* (tabby) X *Aadd* (blue-tabby). The offspring will be expected to occur in the ratio of three tabby, three blue-tabby, one black and one blue, as shown by Fig. 3.5. In effect, the 3:3:1:1 is a combination of the 3:1 and 1:1 ratios.

A more extensive checkerboard is shown in Fig. 3.6. This depicts the expectations for an F_2 generation involving the simultaneous assortment of three recessive genes. The third gene is *l*, a mutant allele that produces long hair and is inherited independently of *a* and *d*. The F_1 shown here could be the result of a cross between a tabby of genotype *AADDLL* and a blue long hair of genotype *aaddll*.

The F_1 parents are triply heterozygous (*AaDdLl*) and the F_2 offspring will be represented by the body of the checkerboard. The eight phenotypes can be expected to occur in the ratios of 27:9:9:9:3:3:3:1. The interesting aspect is that, while the diagram may appear formidable at first sight, closer inspection reveals that this is simply a duplication of the steps described for the previous checkerboards.

The ratios discussed in this and other sections represent only the theoretical expectations for the various matings. This does not mean that in a litter of four kittens, for example, three will be of the dominant type and one will be of the recessive. Or that after a total of 16 kittens have been bred, exact 9:3:3:1 ratios will be obtained. Unfortunately, random chance intervenes in the same way that prevents an exact 50:50 ratio of

Gametes from tabby *AaDdLl*

Gametes from tabby *AaDdLl* (side)

	ADL	ADl	AdL	Adl	aDL	aDl	adL	adl
ADL	AADDLL Tabby	AADDLl Tabby	AADdLL Tabby	AADdLl Tabby	AaDDLL Tabby	AaDDLl Tabby	AaDdLL Tabby	AaDdLl Tabby
ADl	AADDLl Tabby	AADDll Tabby LH	AADdLl Tabby	AADdll Tabby LH	AaDDLl Tabby	AaDDll Tabby LH	AaDdLl Tabby	AaDdll Tabby LH
AdL	AADdLL Tabby	AADdLl Tabby	AAddLL Blue tabby	AAddLl Blue tabby	AaDdLL Tabby	AaDdLl Tabby	AaddLL Blue tabby	AaddLl Blue tabby
Adl	AADdLl Tabby	AADdll Tabby LH	AAddLl Blue tabby	AAddll Blue tabby LH	AaDdLl Tabby	AaDdll Tabby LH	AaddLl Blue tabby	Aaddll Blue tabby LH
aDL	AaDDLL Tabby	AaDDLl Tabby	AaDdLL Tabby	AaDdLl Tabby	aaDDLL Black	aaDDLl Black	aaDdLL Black	aaDdLl Black
aDl	AaDDLl Tabby	AaDDll Tabby LH	AaDdLl Tabby	AaDdll Tabby LH	aaDDLl Black	aaDDll Black LH	aaDdLl Black	aaDdll Black LH
adL	AaDdLL Tabby	AaDdLl Tabby	AaddLL Blue tabby	AaddLl Blue tabby	aaDdLL Black	aaDdLl Black	aaddLL Blue	aaddLl Blue
adl	AaDdLl Tabby	AaDdll Tabby LH	AaddLl Blue tabby	Aaddll Blue tabby LH	aaDdLl Black	aaDdll Black LH	aaddLl Blue	aaddll Blue LH

Figure 3.6 A complex checkerboard to illustrate the assortment of three genes. Despite the size of the diagram, it is constructed in the same manner as simpler checkerboards

head to tails in a small number of tosses of a perfectly balanced coin. The ratios are more closely approximated if a large number of young are bred. This is admittedly difficult for the cat. But, in very prolific animals (for example, mice or hamsters), the theoretical ratios can be attained more closely. The fact that exact ratios cannot always be obtained with small numbers of offspring does not invalidate the usefulness of this technique. Most events occur in this world as a matter of relative probabilities and animal breeding is no exception. The usefulness of the theoretical probabilities resides in their value for planning experimental crosses and, in a wider sense, as a guide to breeding programs.

To check the accuracy of a checkerboard, it is helpful to know the maximum number of different gametes that can be produced by an individual heterozygous for a given number of genes. An individual heterozygous for only one gene will produce two different gametes. For an individual heterozygous for two genes, the number will be four; for three genes, the number is eight; for four genes, the number is 16; for five genes, the number is 32. The number of different gametes doubles with each additional gene. The number of progeny that comprise the expected ratio for an F_2 generation is the number found above multiplied by itself. Heterozygosity in both parents at one gene requires calculation of four offspring, two genes require 16, three genes require 64, four genes requires 256 and five genes requires 1024. This series of figures should be sufficient to indicate how the sizes of the successive checkerboards would have to escalate in order to represent all of the expected animals. For more than a handful of genes, the task rapidly becomes impractical. This aspect constitutes a challenge in animal breeding. This is because it frequently means that it is not possible to determine quickly all of the results to be anticipated from particular crosses.

Dominant and recessive mutations

The majority of mutations of the cat are inherited as recessive alleles to the wild type gene. The wild type gene is the gene normally present at the locus in the wild animal from which the domesticated cat evolved. However, exceptions do occur and no account would be complete without a mention of the possibility of dominant mutant alleles.

The most obvious example of dominant inheritance is provided by a gene that is responsible for the yellow-eyed white (additionally, often causing blue or odd eye color, as will be discussed later). Typically, the coat is fully white or white but for a few small patches of color confined to the head. The symbol for the allele is W; the wild type gene being represented by w. The white cat may have either the WW or Ww genotype. If two of the latter animals are mated together, a ratio of three white to one colored is obtained, regardless of any other coat color genes that may be assorting simultaneously (see Fig. 3.9 page 41).

Detection of the homozygous dominant

A practical problem that can face the breeder is that of deciding whether or not a particular cat may be heterozygous for a particular recessive gene. In principle, the solution is clear. Suppose you want to discover if a black animal is heterozygous for blue dilution (carries blue). Test breeding would consist of mating this cat to a blue. If only black kittens are produced, the breeder may assume that the animal is a homozygote (DD). However, if even a single blue kitten is produced (regardless of how many black siblings), the animal is a heterozygote (Dd).

In practice, test breeding can be misleading. A heterozygous animal may produce a number of black kittens by chance, even if it is not heterozygous. The situation is analogous to tossing a coin and obtaining only heads. Statistics tell us that equal numbers of heads and tails can expected to occur over a large number of tosses. But this does not prevent a string of either heads or tails from occurring occasionally. The difficulty can be overcome, however, by stipulating that more than a certain minimum number of black kittens must be produced before it is concluded that the animal is homozygous. In this manner, the risk of being wrong can reduced as much as possible. Should five offspring be bred, with none of the kittens being blue, the risk of error is 3 per cent (also stated as a 97 per cent confidence level). This is a reasonable level of certainty, but not as stringent as might be desired if the establishment of homozygosity is an important goal. The production of seven black offspring in a row is a better indicator, as the risk error is reduced to about 1 per cent. This is equivalent to mating 100 known heterozygous black cats, producing seven kittens from each, and finding that one individual has produced only black offspring. Column A of Table 10.5 gives the probabilities of being wrong for various numbers of black kittens per tested individual.

The black/blue example is purely illustrative. The same problem would arise if it is deemed necessary to test for a wide variety of other outcomes. For example, to test a tabby for heterozygosity for non-agouti, or a normal coated animal for either long hair or one of the recessive rex coats. In each case, it is convenient to test mate the cat with one that is homozygous for the allele that it is suspected of carrying. A test could also be carried out by mating the animal with a cat known to be heterozygous for the recessive gene in question. This procedure is not as efficient, as it requires the production of far more offspring, and is thus not recommended for those cases where the direct test can be performed.

Incomplete dominance

All of the mutant alleles described thus far share a common property. All of them are inherited as complete recessives or as complete dominants. This is certainly the usual situation but a small number of mutant genes exhibit incomplete dominance. In these cases, the usual 3:1 ratio is modified to a 1:2:1 because the heterozygous cat has a unique phenotype instead of being indistinguishable from the homozygous dominant.

The most frequently quoted case of incomplete dominance in the cat involves the piebald form of white spotting, as found in the tortoiseshell and white (calico) cat or a large proportion of mongrel cats. The piebald allele is symbolized by S, and the corresponding allele is s for non-spotted. The heterozygote, Ss, is usually mildly or moderately spotted (of grades 1 to 4 in Fig. 9.1) with white appearing on the stomach and fore parts of the body. The homozygote is much more extensively marked with white (grades 4 to 7). When two cats of genotype Ss are mated together, the offspring will segregate as follows:

- One extensively spotted.
- Two moderately spotted.
- One non-spotted.

These correspond with the production of offspring having the genotypes SS, Ss and ss, respectively. Unfortunately, the inheritance of white spotting is not the best example of incomplete dominance because the two phenotypes, Ss and SS, are not always readily distinguished. The expression of white is very irregular and the genotypes Ss and SS can have overlapping degrees of white spotting. Nevertheless, the principle should be clear. A somewhat better example is given in the following section on multiple allelism. There the 1:2:1 breeding behavior of the dark phase Burmese, light phase Burmese (Tonkinese) and the Siamese is discussed (see Fig. 3.8, page 39).

Multiple allelism

A gene locus may mutate to produce a new allele on more than one occasion. Each separate event could give rise to the same mutant but this is not usually the case. Although new mutations occur only rarely, each one is capable of producing a distinctive phenotype. Therefore, it would be possible for a succession of different alleles at one locus to develop over a period of time. While the number of alleles that may occur for any given locus is almost unlimited, geneticists are wary of recognizing new mutants as distinctive alleles until sound evidence is generated.

Each series of alleles is given an appropriate name. For example, one important series in mammalian genetics is known as the albino locus. The reason for this name is that the most commonly known allele is the pink-eyed albino. It is not unusual for one or more alleles of a series to be incompletely dominant to each other, especially those at the bottom of the scale of dominance. Yet another property is that the series often affects one particular feature in a progressively severe manner.

The number of alleles that has been reasonably established for the albino series in the cat is five. These may be listed as follows:

- Full color C
- Burmese c^b
- Siamese c^s
- Blue-eyed albino c^a
- Albino c

The symbols used to represent members of an allelic series consist of the same base letter (to denote that all of the alleles belong to the same locus) with suitable superscripts for each allele. In this case, the base symbol is c. The names of the alleles are taken from those breeds in which the allele is considered a characteristic feature. The normal (unmutated) gene is C and the four other alleles represent mutant forms. No matter how many alleles may be known for a locus, only two may be carried by any particular individual. For example, a black heterozygous for Burmese or for Siamese will have the genotypes Cc^b or Cc^s respectively. It cannot be heterozygous for Burmese and Siamese simultaneously, as this would imply a genotype of Cc^bc^s requiring three chromosomes in the cell instead of two. However, a light phase Burmese (Tonkinese) may be heterozygous for Siamese, with the genotype c^bc^s. If this cat is crossed with a tabby heterozygous for c^s, the following offspring are to be expected: two tabby, one light phase Burmese (Tonkinese) and one Siamese. Full details are shown in Fig. 3.7. The explanation for the three colors resides in the random assortment of the alleles c^b and c^s versus C and c^s, and the

Gametes from Tabby Cc^s

		C	c^s
Gametes from Tonkinese $c^b c^s$	c^b	Cc^b Tabby	c^sc^b Tonkinese
	c^s	Cc^s Tabby	c^sc^s Siamese

Figure 3.7 Expectations for a cross involving three alleles assorting independently. Note that only two alleles can be present in one individual. The result is the breeding of three colors in the ratio 2:1:1

dominance relationships between the alleles. This example illustrates the care that has to be exercised in the interpretation of breeding results.

The dominance relationships between the various alleles are summarized in Table 3.1. The allele C, for full color, is dominant to all of the mutant alleles but these, in general, are not fully dominant to each other. The allele showing this most clearly is c^b, where c^bc^b is often noticeably darker than c^bc^s. Thus, the two phases of Burmese (Tonkinese) can differentiated by most Burmese breeders. It is sometimes stated that there is a small amount of overlapping of phenotypes, such that a c^bc^s may be very similar to a dark c^sc^s or a light c^bc^b. This may be true but this does not overturn the principle. It must be admitted that the effects of the c^a and c alleles have not been investigated in all combinations. But c^s, c^a and c are so close that it is doubtful if a radical phenotypical difference is produced by the substitution of c^s by c^a or c. If there is a difference, it will be in the direction of a slightly paler phenotype than the corresponding c^s combination. Preliminary observations indicate that c^sc^a is somewhat lighter than c^sc^s, but that the difference between them is subtle. It did not seem worthwhile to stress this point in the table by separating c^sc^a from c^sc^s.

Another cross between members of the series is worthy of attention. This is between two Burmese of the light phase (Tonkinese). The genotype of this color is aac^bc^s. When bred together, these will produce

Table 3.1 Phenotypes produced by combinations of the albinistic series of alleles

	Appearance	
Genotype	With agouti	With non-agouti
CC, Cc^b, Cc^s, Cc^a, Cc	Tabby	Black
c^bc^b	Sepia tabby (dark)	Burmese (dark)
c^bc^s, c^bc^a, c^bc	Sepia tabby (light)	Burmese (light/Tonkinese)
c^sc^s, c^sc^a, c^sc	Tabby Siamese	Siamese
c^ac, c^ac^a	Blue-eyed albino	Blue-eyed albino
cc	Pink-eyed albino	Pink-eyed albino

Gametes from light Burmese $c^b c^s$

	c^b	c^s
Gametes from light Burmese $c^b c^s$ — c^b	$c^b c^b$ Dark Burmese	$c^b c^s$ Light Burmese
c^s	$c^b c^s$ Light Burmese	$c^s c^s$ Siamese

Figure 3.8 The expectations from mating two light phase Burmese; to illustrate the 1:2:1 ratio of an incompletely dominant gene

dark phase Burmese, light phase Burmese (Tonkinese) and Siamese in the ratio of 1:2:1. Fuller details are illustrated in the checkerboard of Fig. 3.8.

A second series of alleles is a more recent discovery. These are the determinants of the black and brown pigments and are represented as follows:

- Black B.
- Brown b.
- Cinnamon b^l.

The allele present in the ordinary tabby or non-agouti cat is B for black pigmentation. This gene has mutated to brown (b) and light brown (b^l) alleles. The b allele is responsible for the ordinary brown or chocolate color as found in the Havana Brown or chocolate Siamese. The color is a rich deep chocolate. The second allele produces a lighter cinnamon brown. The order of dominance is that B is dominant to both b and b^l, and that b is dominant to b^l.

It had been theorized in the past that the tabby patterns exist as a single allelic series:

- T^u (ticked).
- T (mackerel).
- t^b (blotched or classic).

However, recent breeding studies (Lorimer, 1997) have revealed that at least three gene loci are responsible for tabby pattern in the cat:

- The first determining if the cat is ticked tabby or not (T^u versus t^a).
- The second determining mackerel versus blotched/classic tabby pattern (provisionally Mc versus mc).
- A third determining spotted pattern versus non-spotted (provisionally S_p versus s_p).

Masking of genes

An important phenomenon of gene behavior is epistasis, also known as masking. The term dominance has a special meaning in genetics. Its use is restricted to those cases where one of two alleles at the same locus predominates over the other in the heterozygote. However, the effects of some genes are so overriding that they are able to conceal the presence of genes at other loci. **This 'masking' effect is not the same as dominance**. The distinction should be carefully noted as it is easy to confuse the two.

An example of the effects of one gene masking those of another is that of non-agouti over the various tabby alleles. The masking is virtually complete, so that while a black cat must carry tabby alleles in its genotype, one would scarcely think so to judge from its uniformly black coat. However, a 'ghost' pattern of tabby striping can often be seen in the coat of the young kitten and sometimes in the young adult under certain lighting conditions. Sometimes, the type of tabby can even be distinguished. This implies that the masking effect need not necessarily be complete at all stages of growth or at all times to be considered an example of epistasis. It also confirms that the black cat does indeed carry a tabby pattern, although its presence may not be obvious.

Another classic example of masking is the effect of the dominant white allele, W. Because this gene is responsible for lack of pigment-producing cells in the skin, none of the coat colors present in the genotype are expressed. If a blue ($aaddww$) is paired with a white of genotype $AADDWw$, (masking tabby) the F_1 will be expected to consist of half tabby ($AaDdww$) and half white ($AaDdWw$). It is not obvious where the tabbies came from, as the blue does not carry the agouti allele nor the allele for dense coloration. The answer, of course, is that both genes were introduced by the white parent. The white coat color might give the impression that the animal lacks the ability to carry any color genes at all, but this belief is erroneous. The animal is white because it carries a gene that prevents the expression of pigment of any color in the coat, even though the genes themselves are present.

This phenomenon can be further illustrated by calculating the possibilities from crossing $aaDdww \times AaDdWw$. The expectations are: nine tabby, three blue-tabby, three black, one blue and 16 whites. As an exercise, the reader could work out the checkerboard of possible genotypes for himself or herself, particularly to verify that for every one of the 16 colored individuals there is a corresponding white individual of the same genotype masked by the epistatic W allele. This should emphasize that white cats may have almost any underlying genotype.

Should two heterozygous white cats, which are also heterozygous for another gene, be mated together, the 12:3:1 ratio of Fig. 3.9 will be obtained. In this example, the two cats are heterozygous for non-agouti. Because of the epistatic nature of W, the assortment of the A and a genes can only be seen in the 25 per cent of offspring with colored coats. The other 75 per cent will be white animals except possibly for an occasional spot or two of colored fur on the head. As a matter of practical interest it is often possible to determine the underlying genotype from these spots. Those with tabby spots will be of genotype AA or Aa and those with black

Gametes from white *AaWw*

	AW	aW	Aw	aw
AW	*AAWW* White	*AaWW* White	*AAWw* White	*AaWw* White
aW	*AaWW* White	*aaWW* White	*AaWw* White	*aaWw* White
Aw	*AAWw* White	*AaWw* White	*AAww* Tabby	*Aaww* Tabby
aw	*AaWw* White	*aaWw* White	*Aaww* Tabby	*aaww* Black

Gametes from white *AaWw* (left vertical label)

Figure 3.9 The 12:3:1 ratio which comes into being from the masking effect of the dominant *W* gene

spots will be *aa*. This minor point is mentioned because it is wise to be continuously on the look-out for clues that can establish the genotype.

The masking of the effects of one pair of alleles by another produces a characteristic ratio in the F_2. This ratio may be seen in the interaction of non-agouti and the tabby alleles. Suppose that a blotched tabby (*AAmcmc*) is mated to a black of genotype *aaMcMc*. The F_1 will be tabby (because of the dominance of *A* to *a*) and will express the mackerel tabby pattern (because of the dominance of *Mc* to *mc*). The genotype is *AaMcmc* and four types of gametes will be produced: *AMc + Amc + aMc + amc*. It is necessary to construct a checkerboard of 16 squares to show all possibilities in the F_2 as shown in Fig. 3.3. The expected offspring are nine mackerel tabby, three blotched tabby and four black. This ratio is due to the necessity for the dominant agouti allele to be present for the pattern of tabby striping to be discerned. Unless extensive ghost striping makes it is possible to determine the nature of the tabby pattern carried by the black kittens, these will have to be lumped together into a single group.

Unless one is aware of the existence of epistatic genes, certain results may seem mystifying. For example, in the cross of a blotched/classic tabby

Gametes from mackerel tabby   *AaMcmc*

	AMc	*Amc*	*aMc*	*amc*
AMc	*AAMcMc* Mackerel tabby	*AAMcmc* Mackerel tabby	*AaMcMc* Mackerel tabby	*AaMcmc* Mackerel tabby
Amc	*AAMcmc* Mackerel tabby	*AAmcmc* Blotched tabby	*AaMcmc* Mackerel tabby	*Aamcmc* Blotched tabby
aMc	*AaMcMc* Mackerel tabby	*AaMcmc* Mackerel tabby	*aaMcMc* Black	*aaMcmc* Black
amc	*AaMcmc* Mackerel tabby	*Aamcmc* Blotched tabby	*aaMcmc* Black	*aamcmc* Black

Gametes from mackerel tabby *AaMcmc*

Figure 3.10 The 9:3:4 ratio that results from the simultaneous assortment of two mutant genes, one of which masks the expression of the other

cat of the genotype *AAmcmc* to a black cat of the genotype *aaMcMc*, the F$_1$ are mackerel striped tabbies, *AaMcmc*. This could catch a breeder by surprise, since the only apparent tabby animal is blotched and this pattern is recessive to mackerel. The confusion is cleared up once it is understood that the black color could be masking the mackerel allele. Adding to the confusion is a common erroneous belief that tabby is dominant to black. This is not strictly true and this belief could be misleading. Although the *A* allele of the tabby is dominant to the *aa* alleles of the self black, this agouti gene acts independently from the pattern genes.

The study of epistasis, or masking, reinforces a point made earlier in respect to dominance, namely, the importance of making a distinction between the genotype and phenotype. The animal's appearance is not always an indication of its breeding potential. The genetic caliber of the individual lies not so much on appearance but on the quality of the offspring. For this reason, it is advisable to supplement a judgement based on a cat's appearance with consideration of its parentage.

Mimic genes

Two or more independent mutant genes may have identical or closely resembling phenotypes. This sort of parallel behavior is not due to

Gametes from normal *RrRere*

	RRe	Rre	rRe	rre
RRe	RRReRe Normal	RRRere Normal	RrReRe Normal	RrRere Normal
Rre	RRRere Normal	RRrere Devon rex	RrRere Normal	Rrrere Devon rex
rRe	RrReRe Normal	RrRere Normal	rrReRe Cornish rex	rrRere Cornish rex
rre	RrRere Normal	Rrrere Devon rex	rrRere Cornish rex	rrrere Devon-Cornish rex

(Gametes from normal *RrRere* — left axis)

Figure 3.11 The expectation for the F$_2$ generation from animals heterozygous for the two rex genes; to illustrate the 9:7 ratio of normal:rex

coincidence, but is an indication that many traits are governed by numerous genes. Any one of these may mutate into an allele that brings about a similar change in phenotype. Such alleles are rather loosely referred to as 'mimics'.

An example of this in the cat is the occurrence of multiple rex mutations. The most well-known are the Cornish and Devon rexes, each of which are inherited as recessives. Recessive genes that produce the same phenotype may be tested by crossing the two forms. If they are genetically identical, the offspring will resemble the parents, but if they are independent, the offspring will be normal. Experience showed that crosses between the two rexes produced normal coated kittens; therefore, the two genes are genetically distinct. The symbols for the Cornish and Devon Rex mutant alleles are *r* and *re*, respectively.

The cross between the two rex mutants deserves to be discussed in more detail. The genotypes for this cross are *rrReRe* (Cornish rex) × *RRrere* (Devon rex) to give an F$_1$ with the genotype *RrRere*. Each parent has contributed a wild type gene (i.e. *R* or *Re*) and this explains the abrupt disappearance of the rex coat. Should the F$_1$ offspring be interbred to produce an F$_2$, the ratio of normal coated to rex coated cats will be 9:7. This curious ratio occurs because the two rexes are of similar appearance making it difficult at times to distinguish one form from the other. The double rex combination (*rrrere*) will be a rex and probably will be identical to one of the other rexes. The reader may like to work through the appropriate checkerboard (Fig. 3.11) to assure himself that the expected ratio is indeed that of 9:7 of normal and rex kittens.

Mimic genes are of interest to geneticists because meticulous examination often reveals subtle differences that are valuable in understanding how characters develop. In practical breeding, however, they can be a nuisance. For instance, unless careful breeding records are kept, it is possible for the mutant forms to become confused. It could be a serious mistake to cross two similar forms with the expectation of recovering each type at a later date. If the descendants of such crosses are recklessly distributed, the occasion may arise when two animals are mistakenly identified as having the same recessive form. When they are bred together, however, they produce offspring of the dominant phenotype. This is likely to cause dismay and even to cast doubt on the validity of the rule that recessive traits always breed true.

The rule is not violated, of course; it only seemed to be so because of the similar phenotype produced by each gene. As the genes actually belong to different loci, the reversion to the normal phenotype is to be expected. Other cases of mimicking genes may be discovered in the future – an obvious candidate is blue dilution. In the mouse, several distinct diluting genes have been identified which, when interbred, produce wild type offspring. Some of these mimic blue dilution closely and could be easily confused. Suppose such a situation existed in the cat. The occasion would eventually arise when two apparently blue individuals are mated, only to produce black kittens. This could mean that one parent was homozygous blue dilution, but the other was carrying a different diluting gene. **It must be emphasized very strongly, however, that few people may be willing to accept the existence of two independent diluting genes unless it can be convincingly shown that a mismating (or double mating) has not occurred**. This is not always as easy to rule out as one might think.

The multiple recessive

Is there a limit to the number of mutant genes that can be combined together? Simply answered, not as a rule. There are perhaps two qualifications to be made with regard to this statement. Both involve practical considerations of what is possible and what is not. Some mutant genes confer a slight reduction in the viability of the individual that, while not being particularly noticeable in isolation, may reveal itself more obviously when combined with another mutation. Sooner or later, these health consequences of this reinforcement effect could bring the practice of combining the two traits to a halt. However, no effects of this kind have yet been observed for the cat.

The second qualification has to do with the problem of lack of differentiation between certain genotypes because of epistasis. This is especially true for color mutations. With some combinations, each additional gene will result in a reduction in color until a nearly or completely white animal is produced. The cat with the greatest number of recessive genes is the lilac Siamese of genotype *aabbcscsdd*. If the gene for long hair is added, the lilac Colorpoint will result, of genotype *aabbc^{s}c^{s}ddll*. A Cornish rex version could be produced, of genotype *aabbc^{s}c^{s}ddrr*. From crosses between these, the lilac Siamese long haired Cornish rex of *aabbc^{s}c^{s}ddllrr* could be derived. Phenotypically, this animal would have lilac Siamese coloration, with the fine hair and curved whiskers of the long hair rex.

Expressivity and impenetrance

One of the delights or nuisances of animal breeding, depending upon one's point of view, is that no two individuals are exactly alike. This variation is seen in both wild type and mutant traits, but appears to be more common in the latter. The existence of this variability has led to the concept of 'expressivity' as a means of describing the range of expression of certain traits. Some mutant phenotypes are relatively stable while others vary considerably. A character that shows wide variability is that of piebald white spotting as illustrated by Fig. 9.1.

The *S* gene is semi-dominant; that means that the heterozygotes and homozygotes often have different phenotypes. Expression of the spotting, however, is extremely variable, particularly for the heterozygote *Ss*. This variation can be assessed by plotting the number of individual successive grades of spotting as a curve on a graph. This could be termed the 'expressivity profile'. A curve for one strain of cats could be different from another and, thus, indicate that the expression of the trait may vary not only between individual cats but also between strains.

If a character is extremely variable, then it is conceivable that some individuals could fail to express the character at all and appear as normal, despite having the mutant genotype. This curious phenomenon can even potentially occur for a character that is not known to be exceptionally variable. The terms 'incomplete penetrance' or 'partial manifestation' are used to represent this situation: the character has failed to be manifested even though the genotype indicates that it should. Fortunately, impenetrance is not a common characteristic of the color genes known at present. All of these manifest regularly and to expectation. An example of impenetrance, however, is the probable existence of a minor spoiling gene that produces a small white spot or clump of hairs on the breast or lower belly. The size of the spot is variable and it is possible that some animals, which ought to exhibit the spot, do not. These are solid in color. Such animals are called 'normal overlaps' because, though of normal coloration, they have a mutant genotype and thus will indeed breed as a mutant.

Though coat color genes, as a rule, exhibit regular penetrance, this is not true for other genetic anomalies. It is not unusual for these to display impenetrance. The inheritance of tail kinks or nodulation could be an example and even such breed defining traits as wirehair or folded ears exhibit this phenomenon. A possible reason for this is that the body of an animal has the surprising ability to repair itself. This is particularly true when a defect makes an appearance early in development, before the tissues are so well formed that timely and self-regulating growth cannot swing into action to rectify the defect. In many individuals a genetic disruption persists and eventually produces a defective individual. In another individual, however, the disruption may be overcome with the result that an outwardly normal appearing individual is produced. The variability in the severity of many abnormalities is due to the same process; only in these cases, the self-rectification has only been partial. In both cases, the gene causing the disruption is present and, particularly in the case of the apparently normal individual, this should not be overlooked.

Genetic fingerprinting

An event of some interest to breeders is the discovery that minute but variable sections of the chromosomes can be portrayed as a series of dark bars on a photographic film. The most significant finding of this discovery is that the bars are unique to each individual, and have therefore been called 'genetic fingerprints'. The pattern of bars resembles the computer 'zebra' codes found on many retail items and for this reason they have also come to be known as 'genetic bar codes'.

The individual bars are inherited from parent to offspring in a consistent manner. The uniqueness of the bar codes for each individual and the heritability of the patterns have immediate practical applications. For instance, they may be used to determine decisively cases of uncertain or disputed paternity. In the past, they could have been used to indicate that a certain stud could not have sired a specific kitten. Now, it is possible to state that only a certain stud could be the sire. Genetic fingerprinting is available as a service from a commercial laboratory by arrangement with a vet. The usual procedure is for the veterinarian to take small samples of blood from the dam and each potential sire for submission to the laboratory.

Other recent advances in molecular biology, the study of genes at the molecular level, include the development of the feline genome map at the National Cancer Institute of the United States. Mapping is the process of determining where each gene is located on the various chromosomes. Each species of animal has a unique set of genes, arranged in a unique manner. Cats are quite similar to humans in their genetic makeup, much closer than either mice or dogs. The comparison of the genetic makeup of different species is called comparative genetics.

It is important to prepare a map of the feline genome so that it can be compared to the known genetic makeup of other species. As there is more known about the genome of mice and humans, researchers can use what is known about those species to provide 'candidate genes' for similar diseases in cats. Genes in the cat are often in approximately the same order as genes in the human, with a bit of rearranging, different spacing, etc. For instance, the gene that causes the dominant form of polycystic kidney disease has been mapped in both mice and humans. This can give researchers clues about where to possibly look for such a gene in the feline genome.

Right now the map of the feline genome is considered 'low resolution', but the goal is to map 300 different genes as well as 300 other segments of DNA known as 'microsatellites'. Microsatellites do not code for a particular protein, as genes do. Genes are known as the 'type I marker' for a particular disease. Finding the specific gene for a disease requires a great deal of time as well as a large financial investment. It is easier to find a microsatellite associated with a gene of interest, a type II marker. A good type II marker will have a 90 to 95 per cent probability of being associated with a particular disease causing gene.

Microsatellites consist of tandem two to six pairs of nucleic acids in a repeat motif. Genes do not vary widely in their composition, as they have an important function: to create a specific protein correctly. Any mutation may result in that protein not being constructed correctly, resulting in an animal that may not be able to survive. Microsatellites, on the other hand, are highly polymorphic (having many forms), a result of their high mutation rate. They have no known function, so when mutations occur, they do not have any adverse effect on the individual. This results in mutations being passed on to the future generations, creating a great degree of variety at these loci among a population. There are approximately 100 000 microsatellites, randomly distributed, in each genome.

At this time, the feline genome project has isolated 30 cat specific microsatellites. These are enough to perform some genetic procedures already: DNA fingerprinting, paternity testing, determining the level of inbreeding in a group of cats and conducting various population studies. The analysis of the DNA from a particular cat can indicate what 'breed group' a cat might be a member of (Persian versus Oriental, for example). Examination of DNA through the analysis of microsatellites can also be a tool for historians to track the migration of humans throughout the world. People have always loved cats and have taken them with them wherever they go. The result is that a cat from one part of the world shares similar DNA with a cat that has been taken to another part of the globe. Examination of mummified Egyptian cats could also give us insight into the origins of the domestic cat.

Future research will result in tests for gene mutations that will have almost 100 per cent accuracy. This will be most valuable in attempts to eliminate deleterious, disease causing mutations. It will also help to ascertain the genotype for more positive traits of interest in an individual, thus assisting the breeder in making better decisions regarding their breeding program. Advances in molecular biology have resulted in a gradual shift in the focus of study. It has moved the study of genetics from the examination of population statistics to an examination of the trait producing genes themselves. These advances will eventually permit breeders, researchers and veterinarians to resolve ongoing debates dealing with hereditability in areas ranging from anomalies to susceptibility to certain cancers and from the reasons for particular birth defects to the likelihood of reaction to certain vaccines.

Technical appendix

A note on Mendel's distribution and statistics

In discussing the likely outcome of breeding situations, geneticists use a variety of tables, such as the checkerboard tables used throughout this work, to illustrate expected outcomes. The key term here is expected.

In statistical terms, every combination of a sperm and an egg is a random event. That means that the expected outcomes demonstrated by the checkerboard tables apply to each such combination. But it can be expected, in the long run, that the distribution of results would be as predicted. However, these tables cannot apply to every kitten or even to every litter, as the odds are applicable to each kitten in the litter.

Let us give a very simple example. If we have four coins, each with heads and tails, and flip all four at once, statistics tells us that the expected outcome, over time, would be that 50 per cent of them would be heads and 50 per cent tails. However, each set of tosses is independent of all other tosses. Thus, we could get four heads, three heads and one tail, etc. But, if we do this, say 1000 times and record the results, the average would be expected to be two heads and two tails. When this is applied to breeding cats, while an expected distribution of a litter of four might be 1:2:1 for a particular combination of characteristics, in any given litter, all four kittens may instead have the same characteristic. The ratios apply over time, and not to each kitten or even to each breeding.

Chapter 4

Impacts of heredity

- Manifold effects of genes
- Linkage
- Sex-linked heredity
- Sex-limited expression
- Continuous variation
- Threshold characters
- Abnormalities

Manifold effects of genes

Some genes seem to modify only one discreet trait while others appear to influence the expression of several characters simultaneously. In the latter case, it is said that the gene has 'pleiotropic' action. The concept of pleiotropism is intimately bound up with the depth of analysis of gene action. Superficially, many genes will exhibit pleiotropic effects to a lesser or greater degree. For example, if eye color and coat color are treated as separate characters, then the Siamese gene could be regarded as pleiotropic because of its effect on both eye color and coat color. Yet, if the pigmentation of the animal is considered as a whole, there is no pleiotropism. This is because the blue eye and whitish sepia coat are both due to the same cause, the severe impairment of pigment formation brought about by the c^s allele.

A more accurate example of pleiotropism is demonstrated by the dominant white gene. The most obvious effect of this gene is to produce white coat color. It does so in 100 per cent of cases, i.e. all cats with the gene have white fur. However, the gene also is capable of producing blue eyes and deafness, but does not do so in every cat. Thus, it may be said that the gene is 'pleiotropic' in that it affects three diverse characters: Coat color, eye color and soundness of hearing. The gene is completely 'penetrant' for coat color but 'impenetrant' for eye color and deafness.

It is probable that at the biochemical level no gene is truly pleiotropic. A gene may appear pleiotropic because analysis of the effects have not been taken far enough to reveal the fundamental action of the gene. In the example of the dominant white gene, all three effects could stem from a common cause, as yet unknown.

Linkage

The cat has 19 pairs of chromosomes and each one contains some thousands of genes. While the number of known mutations are small, the chances are that these will be borne in different chromosomes. The inference for practical breeding is that the various mutants will be inherited independently of each other.

However, this situation changes if two mutations happen to occur in the same chromosome. The model of independent assortment will no longer hold completely. So, in crosses, the two genes tend to stay together as these are transmitted from one generation to the next. This 'staying together' is termed 'linkage' and the two genes are said to be 'linked'. The probability of linkage is an attribute that is based on the physical distance between two genes on a particular chromosome.

None of the known mutations of the cat are believed to be linked. Regrettably, this is not due to experimental tests for linkage but rather to a complete absence of such tests. It is traditional to assume that genes are inherited independently until it is definitively proven that two genes are linked. As more mutations are discovered and progress is made in the mapping of the feline genome, the chances of finding linkages increase and more cases will undoubtedly become evident. For this reason, it is wise to be aware of the possibility of linkage and to be on the look-out for possible instances.

Two types of linkage have been described:

- In the first type, two genes are located in the same chromosome, and therefore will frequently be inherited together.
- In the second type, the two genes are in different members of the pair of chromosomes. When the genes are present in the same parent, they will be transmitted separately far more often than they will be inherited together. In this case, the genes are not recombining as freely as they would if they are inherited independently. The two genes are then said to be in 'repulsion'.

In the first form of linkage, the two genes are behaving as if they are coupled; in the second form, they behave as if they are repelling one another.

The special cell divisions that lead to the formation of gametes require that the pairs of homologous chromosomes come in close proximity and form intimate contact at certain points along their length. During this process, internal stresses are induced which are relieved by spontaneous breakage and rejoining of the DNA strands. In a proportion of cases, the rejoining is between constituents of partner chromosomes, with the result that the two homologous chromosomes have exchanged segments of DNA with each other. The exchange of material between homologous chromosomes means that blocks of genes have been conveyed from one chromosome to the other or, to use the appropriate term, they have 'crossed over'. This exchange process is known as 'crossing over'. The frequency of the separation of genes on the same chromosome arm will depend upon the relative distance between the two genes. The greater the distances, the greater the chance that the genes will be separated when one crosses over to the homologous chromosome. Therefore, it is possible for two genes to be 'loosely' or 'closely' linked. When two genes are closely linked, the absence of random assortment may become noticeable.

The whole topic of linkage is important in the study of genetics and most genetics textbooks discuss the subject in depth. However, in applied genetics (such as cat breeding), the phenomenon of linkage may introduce a frustrating challenge. For example, consider the case where a breeder is working to create a new color variety of an existing, well-established breed by attempting to isolate a color mutation from the rest of the contributing breed's phenotype. In this case, the intrusion of linkage can be annoying. The breeder may find that this proves to be more difficult than anticipated because unwanted traits of the contributing breed are being carried along with the desired color mutation.

Sex-linked heredity

The cat is one of the few mammals that exhibit the presence of a sex-linked trait that dates from the dawn of genetics. The unusual tortoiseshell pattern of some female cats and the great scarcity of similarly colored tortoiseshell males has been cited in most books on animal genetics.

It was stated in Chapter 2 that the sex of the individual is determined by a pair of special chromosomes: the X and the Y. These chromosomes carry gene loci that can mutate, in the same manner as those borne by the ordinary chromosomes. There is a vital difference, however. A mutant allele carried by a sex chromosome will be associated with gender and will display the inheritance pattern of 'sex-linkage'. This describes the mutant that produces 'ginger' or red pigmentation and which is indirectly responsible for the mosaic pattern of the tortoiseshell.

The gene responsible for the ginger cat is known as orange and is symbolized by O. The color is produced by an alteration in the animal's pigment physiology so that only yellow pigment is produced instead of a mixture of yellow and black in the tabby and black for the non-agouti. The word yellow is used in a general sense to include all cream, yellow and red pigmentation. Yellow is the technical term for the pigment granule that produces all of these colors. In this mutation, the black tabby striping is replaced by red striping of the same pattern, while the intervening agouti areas become yellow or rich beige.

The sex linkage of O becomes apparent when the segregation of the gene is determined for the various matings. The male has only one X chromosome; consequently, he can only be either O (yellow) or o (non-yellow). On the other hand, the female has two X chromosomes; consequently, she may be one of three genotypes: OO (yellow), Oo (tortoiseshell) or oo (non-yellow). The tortoiseshell cat, therefore, is a heterozygote at this locus. It is unique in that its coat reflects the influence of both the O and o genes in different parts of the animal at the same time. The yellow areas correspond to O and the non-yellow areas to o.

To predict the results of matings with sex-linked genes, it is necessary to know the gender of the particular cat that is contributing the O allele. For convenience, all of the possible matings with the orange mutation are illustrated in Table 4.1. The possible genotypes for the offspring can be determined with the aid of checkerboard diagrams, as shown by the examples of Figs 4.1 and 4.2. The reader may find it a valuable exercise to sketch checkerboards for all of the crosses mentioned in Table 4.1. Remember, with sex-linked genes the male can only transmit one allele

Table 4.1 Expectations for the possible matings of yellow and tortoiseshell cats

		Expected offspring	
Dam	Sire	Males	Females
Yellow	Yellow	Yellow	Yellow
Black	Yellow	Black	Tortoiseshell
Tortoiseshell	Yellow	Yellow	Yellow
		Black	Tortoiseshell
Tortoiseshell	Black	Yellow	Tortoiseshell
		Black	Black
Yellow	Black	Yellow	Tortoiseshell
Black	Black	Black	Black

Note: In the above table, black is used as a euphemism for all non-yellow colors (e.g. black, tabby, blue, etc.)

Gametes from tortoiseshell
female *Oo*

		O	*o*
Gametes from yellow male	*O*	*OO* Yellow female	*Oo* Tortoiseshell female
	Y	*OY* Yellow male	*oY* Black male

Figure 4.1 The assortment of the sex-linked *O* gene. Note that *O* can only be transmitted in half of the sire's gametes, the ones responsible for producing female gender in a particular kitten

(*O* or *o*) in 50 per cent of gametes; the other 50 per cent carry a Y chromosome that does not possess a *O* locus.

In these examples, the word black has been used to denote all non-yellow colors. Keep in mind that 'black' can mean tabby, blue, seal point, chinchilla, chocolate and other colors; the common denominator of these is that they are 'non-yellow'. The mutant alleles producing these colors will be inherited independently of *O*; the assortment of these may have to be taken into account to determine the full potential for any cross or series of crosses. The procedures to follow are those for ordinary inheritance, as shown by the checkerboards described earlier, in combination with those for sex-linkage.

The non-agouti mutation has no effect on the production of yellow pigment. This means that the red or cream cat of genotype *aaO* (male) or

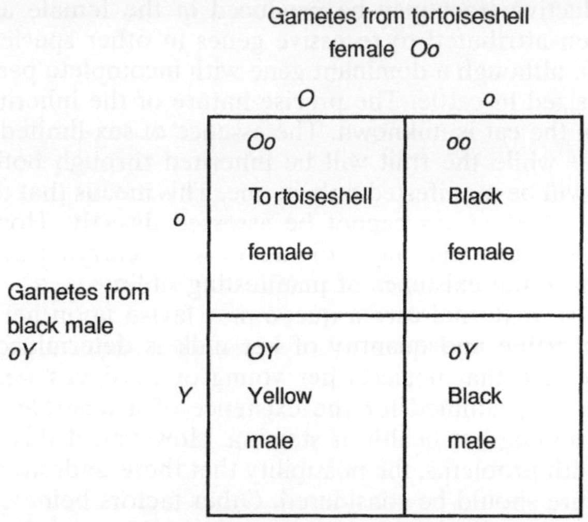

Gametes from tortoiseshell
female *Oo*

	O	*o*
o	*Oo* Tortoiseshell female	*oo* Black female
Y	*OY* Yellow male	*oY* Black male

Gametes from
black male
oY

Figure 4.2 A second example of assortment of the sex-linked *O* gene. Note that the wild type allele *o* can only be transmitted in half of the sire's gametes, with the other kittens receiving the male gender determining chromosome Y

aaOO (female) is identical in appearance to that of *A-O* or *A-OO*. Therefore, it may be stated that the *O* allele masks the expression of the genotype at the *A/a* locus. This fact can be verified by crossing a yellow male of genotype *AAO* to a black female of genotype *aaoo*. The offspring will consist of tabby males and tabby tortoiseshell females. As the black female cannot carry agouti, the offspring must have gained the gene from the yellow parent.

The patchwork coloring of the tortoiseshell provides direct visual evidence that the yellow gene can mask the expression of non-agouti. It is possible to breed both tabby and black tortoiseshells of genotypes *A-Oo* and *aaOo*, respectively, where the yellow areas in the two cats have the same exact appearance, despite the contrast between the black/tabby areas. One could not ask for a better demonstration of the epistatic nature of *O*.

Sex-limited expression

There is another form of sex associated heredity that, unfortunately, is sometimes mistaken for sex-linkage. This is where the expression of a gene is confined to one sex although the gene itself is carried by one of the ordinary chromosomes. No clear-cut instance of sex-limited expression of a gene affecting coat color has been reported for the cat, although examples are afforded by other characteristics.

Cryptorchidism is the failure of one or both testes to descend into the scrotum. It appears to be due to one or more genes. It is believed to be a heritable defect that is sex-limited to the male, although abnormalities of the reproductive tract may be produced in the female as well. This defect has been attributed to recessive genes in other species (e.g. goat, pigs and dogs), although a dominant gene with incomplete penetrance has been hypothesized in cattle. The precise nature of the inheritance of this abnormality in the cat is unknown. The essence of sex-limited inheritance is the fact that while the trait will be inherited through both sexes, the characteristic will be manifested only in one. This means that the genotype of the non-manifesting sex cannot be assessed directly. However, some idea of the probability that any individual can be carrying the defect can be obtained from the existence of manifesting siblings.

The quality of maternal care a queen may lavish upon her kittens and the nutritional value and quantity of her milk is determined in part by heredity. A female that neglects her young or produces weak offspring should always be examined for the existence of a possible ailment that may be undermining her health or stamina. However, if this examination reveals no health problems, the possibility that these undesirable traits are genetic in nature should be considered. Other factors being equal, such a queen should not be used for breeding, and possibly her offspring as well should be excluded from the breeding program. It should not be imagined, however, that these traits are inherited solely from the mother. A son of a poor mother may be equally likely to pass on these undesirable qualities to his female offspring. A male cannot express any real forms of maternal instinct but, nevertheless, he may carry the genes responsible for determining this.

Continuous variation

The type of heredity described in previous sections is known as discrete or discontinuous inheritance because the characteristics involved are sharply defined. For instance, no one could confuse a tabby cat with a black nor, after a modicum of experience, a mackerel with a blotched striped tabby. Yet, no traits are inherited in this nature. Many characteristics are known which vary continuously from one extreme form of expression to another. A good example is the variation in intensity of yellow pigmentation, which can range from light 'ginger' to rich, mahogany red. Although, a major genetic mutation is required to create the yellow cat, there is a wide variation in intensity of expression that is inherited independent of this.

A sizable part of the variation seen in the traits seen in cats is inherited, although the proportion may vary from character to character. In this respect, continuous variation differs from the discontinuous. With discrete heredity, the overwhelming effect of one mutation can conceal the incidental background variation, whether inherited or not. With continuous characters, on the other hand, the incidental background variation can be observed and it is not always wise to assume that all of the observed variation is inherited. However, it is also unwise to go to the other extreme and assume that none of the variation is inherited. The true situation lies in between: some of the variation is genetic and the remainder is not.

The heredity of variable expression can be due to the presence of multiple genes with similar effects. The effect of any one gene is small relative to the total spectrum of variation. Though the action of each individual gene is small, the total effect is cumulative. So an individual that carries a number of these genes is phenotypically different from an individual that carries only a few. Because numerous genes with minor effects are involved, the inheritance of continuously varying traits has the appearance of being a blending of characteristics. The genes themselves do not blend, of course, but assort in the same manner as genes with major effects. It is only the phenotype that shows blending in the form of offspring that are generally intermediate to that of either parent, with the production of the odd individual that strongly deviates from the average. Characters controlled by many genes are termed 'polygenic', and the genes concerned are known collectively as 'polygenes'. The important point to remember is that many, not just a few, polygenes are intimately involved in producing a polygenic trait. In addition, the effect of each one is small compared with the cumulative effect of the group. Those genes with large individual effects (i.e. ordinary alleles) are 'major genes' in this terminology.

It is convenient to speak of polygenes as possessing 'plus' and 'minus' effects with respect to the expression of a character. To continue with the example of the variation of intensity of yellow, the ginger mongrel cat may be visualized as possessing minus polygenes. This is in contrast to the rich coloring of the exhibition (show quality) red tabby that is produced by plus polygenes. These extreme forms often breed relatively true; ginger cats rarely produce other than ginger young and vibrant red tabbies often produce vibrant red tabby offspring. The color may vary but, in general, this is the case. The reason is that they are at opposite extremes of the spectrum of yellow color expression, due to a large number of the polygenes sharing a common direction of influence, either plus or minus. Should the two forms be crossed, the offspring would be expected to be somewhat intermediate between the two parents, richer in color than the ginger but less vivid than the show quality animal. Interbreeding these crosses would be expected to produce a generation of widely variable expression of intensity of yellow color. Most would be intermediate in color but a number will approach either the ginger or the red coloration of the grandparents. Should the intensity of yellow be divided into grades and the parentage of animals of each grade be tabulated for a large number of offspring, the result could be similar to Fig. 4.3.

The checkerboard of Fig. 3.6 illustrates the behavior of polygenes. In this example, three polygenes are hypothesized in the production of a particular trait. The plus alleles are represented by capital letters and the various minus alleles by small letters. In this oversimplified model, the ginger grade of yellow can be symbolized by the genotype $aabbcc$ and the vibrant red grade by $AABBCC$. To keep the picture simple, assume there is no dominance of any of these alleles. Also assume that the variation of intensity of yellow can be divided into seven grades (from 0 for ginger to 6 for the most intense red). The F_1 will be of an intermediate color (grade 3) and have the genotype $AaBbCc$. When these are interbred, the polygenes will assort and combine at random to produce 64 potential genotypes as shown by Fig. 3.6 (by substituting the symbols A, B, C, etc.

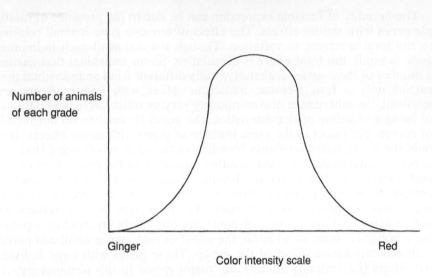

Figure 4.3 Idealized curve illustrating how the frequencies of animals, graded for intensity of yellow, might be distributed in the F_2 generation of a cross between a ginger and a show quality red

for the genes A, D, L, etc. of the checkerboard). Suppose that each plus polygene increases the intensity by one grade. Thus, the genotype *aabbcc* will be of grade 0 and the genotypes *Aabbcc*, *aaBbcc* and *aabbCc* will be of grade 1, and so forth. Proceeding in this manner over the whole range of genotypes, the 0 to 6 grades will be found to occur in the frequencies of 1, 6, 15, 20, 15, 6 and 1, respectively. Figure 4.3 shows this expectation in an idealized form. The curve on the figure is of the general type that occurs when numerous factors are operating to determine the expression of a character. This is commonly known as the bell-shaped curve. Even with a hypothetical, oversimplified example of 64 individual genotypes, the shape of the curve can be seen in a plot of the expected frequencies.

If the F_1 generation is backcrossed to the red parent, the expectation is a range of grades from 3 to 7, with the majority of offspring being of the intermediate grades 4 and 5. Similarly, if the F_1 are backcrossed to the ginger, the range of variation will be from grades 0 to 3, with the majority of offspring being of the intermediate grades 1 and 2. The average expression of the trait in each case will be a grade of yellow that is halfway between that of the parents. This is a typical result of continuous or polygenic heredity. Although the majority of offspring will in be in-between the coloration of two parents, there will also be some individuals that will be either paler or darker than either parent. Any breeder who has had occasion to breed together yellow cats of various intensities will probably have noticed this phenomenon.

The above example is a deliberate simplification of the mechanism of polygenic heredity. Apart from the obvious probability that many, rather than a few, polygenes are usually involved, any of the attributes of genes with major effects could be influenced by polygenes. The complexities of polygenic inheritance have been competently tackled and anyone wishing for further information should review works cited in the bibliography.

Polygenic variation may be conveniently divided into two types:

- The 'pure' state, where no major genes are involved.
- A state where variation is seen in combination with the presence of a major mutant gene.

The heredity of body size, head shape, ear size and other components of general conformation falls into the first category. No major genes are known to effect any of these features. Assuming that diet is adequate and the cat receives sufficient exercise for full development, the size and shape of the body is due to polygenic influences. 'Size and shape' is an abstraction, of course, encompassing many individual features. A cat may have a cobby or long, tubular body, it may heavy or lightly boned, have short or long legs and so forth. These are the components of 'type' as it is referred to by the Cat Fancy.

Polygenic modifiers

A common form of variation can occur when a major gene is also involved. In the prior example, for instance, of variation in intensity of yellow coloration, the presence of the O gene is required. This has led to the practice of referring to polygenes as 'modifying' genes. Although the yellow color is due to O, the form of expression of O is due to modifying polygenes or 'modifiers' for short. Another trait that shows variation is long hair. This character is primarily due to the mutant l allele, but the longhaired mongrel differs greatly from the show quality animal. Polygenes are at work, modifying the length and texture of the coat of the longhaired cat. A third example, which has captured the attention of breeders, is the variation in the depth of color of blue cats. The basic genotype for these cats is $aadd$, but the blue color can vary appreciably between breeds and between individuals of those breeds. This type of variation is also due to polygenes. Black cats also vary in depth of color but to a lesser extent than do blues. Therefore it may be said that the polygenes involved are modifiers of the expression of the blue gene.

Some people have proposed that in cases where the expression of a gene (in particular, a mutant trait) is dependent upon the presence of modifiers, these polygenes will have no effect on the alternate allele (particularly, the wild type). The variation in the shade of blue is an obvious example. Superficially, all blacks are the same color. Upon closer inspection, however, it can be observed that black cats do vary in intensity, although certainly not to the same extent as blues. The polygenetic modifiers of the dilute gene probably modify the black phenotype as well, but not to the same extent as it influences the coloration of the blue. The action of these modifying polygenes is subtle in the black phenotype but accentuated in the blue. This aspect makes it rather difficult to determine the presence of any desired dilution polygenes in the black. On the other hand, it is fairly obvious that a light blue carries those polygenes that lighten color (minus alleles), while a dark blue will carry those of opposite tendency (darkening or plus alleles).

In a similar manner, the coat length polygenes may have a greater effect when combined with *l* than with the wild type allele *L*. The polygenetic modifications of hair fiber length and structure are accentuated when the fiber has already been lengthened by the *l* gene. It is as if the normal, stabilized development has been upset by the introduction of the mutant allele, allowing for the possibility of further influence by other genes. This would explain the relative minor effects of the polygenes on the wild type phenotype while greater effects are produced in the mutant phenotype.

A definable group of polygenes can be treated as a genetic entity in its own right. For instance, if the group is combining or interacting with more than one gene, identifying this group as modifiers of one specific gene or phenotype will no longer be appropriate. The polygenes responsible for the intensity of yellow pigmentation apparently behave in this manner. In addition to their effects on the yellow phenotype, the quality of the yellow pigment seen in the agouti band of the show quality brown tabby and the Abyssinian, when compared with the mongrel tabby, can be attributed to the actions of this group of polygenes. Variation in the presence of yellowish or tawny suffusion (tarnishing) in some silvers could also be part of this series of variation. The intensity of yellow pigmentation is controlled by polygenes, whether or not this occurs in a cat that is fully yellow, or in one that is only partially yellow, like the tabbies. The show quality silver displays no tarnishing. This implies that selective breeding has operated against yellow pigmentation, decreasing its presence to the point of total elimination.

The polygenes that decrease the production of yellow pigment may reveal themselves in an interesting manner. When a show quality silver is crossed with a normal tabby, the tabby offspring are often unusually pale in color, because of the weak color of the agouti band. It is as if the yellow coloration has been diluted (the black pigmentation is normal). It is likely that the polygenes carried by the silver are inherited in a typical blending manner. This means that although *I* is completely dominant to *i*, the intensity of yellow pigmentation may be diluted by the action of the polygenes contributed by the silver parent. This sort of polygenic behavior is not unusual whenever the phenotype of one of the parents has been selected for extreme expression of any particular feature.

Identified polygenes

A few groups of polygenes have been identified in the cat.

- The first are the group affecting the intensity of yellow, known as the 'rufus polygenes'.
- The second are those modifying the depth of blue pigmentation (dilution group).
- A third group could be those modifying the depth and warmth of chocolate pigmentation, as found in the chestnut brown.

The variation here is akin to that of the blue as it is possible to have light and dark chocolate colored animals, when the corresponding blacks scarcely differ. If the dilution and chocolate groups of polygenes are identical, the dark blue and rich chocolate animals would carry identical polygenes that darken the color. It is by no means certain that the rufus polygenes are independent of the dilution group. Those polygenes that deepen the yellow to red could be the same as those which darken the other colors. For most purposes, the rufus and dilution groups can be treated as independent, but it is wise to be aware that this may not be so.

Another group of polygenes is that responsible for influencing eye color. This trait exists on a spectrum from deep, violet blue to dark, almost brown, copper. There are undoubtedly polygenetic modifiers of eye color. Another group to be mentioned is that controlling the amount of agouti ticking in the tabby areas of the coat. This is variable and controlled to some extent by polygenes. As far as is known, the ticking polygenes produce no effect upon a non-agouti background.

Almost any feature of the cat that can be sensibly analyzed will be found to vary, although not all of the variation will be genetic. The range of phenotypes vary from feature to feature and from strain to strain for the same feature. This explains in part why successful results can be obtained with some individuals and strains but not with others. Most phenotype variation, in general, will be controlled by polygenes. All breeding animals in a population or breed may be homozygous for one or more particular traits, where a major gene (or genes) becomes the basic genotype for all individuals. Subsequent modification of the phenotype will depend solely upon manipulation of the various groups of polygenes.

Threshold characters

Polygenic inheritance is usually associated with characters that vary smoothly from one extreme of expression to the other. However, it is possible for polygenic variation to be involved in a type of discontinuous variation that, at first sight, may be thought to be under the control of a major gene. The simplest way to explain this is to visualize a build-up of polygenes. When this build-up reaches a certain level, it causes a process to be carried past a 'developmental threshold' so that a new phenotype appears. This sort of character is called a 'threshold character'.

Alternatively, it is possible that a developmental process may fail to be carried through to completion because there are insufficient plus ('upregulating') polygenes. Figure 3.6 may be used to demonstrate the underlying principle. Suppose that a vital physiological reaction requires the presence of a certain number of plus polygenes to proceed and that a population of cats may be represented by Fig. 3.6. In this figure any individual may contain from one to six plus polygenes, together with a small number of deficient individuals (the 0 class). If the presence of at least one plus polygene is sufficient for full completion of the reaction, then only the zero class individuals will not function normally; in other words, the failure rate will be about 2 per cent. However, suppose at least two plus polygenes are required, then both the 0 and 1 classes will be involved and the incidence will rise to about 11 per cent. Therefore, if many polygenic loci are involved and the essential polygenic complement varies from strain to strain, it becomes apparent that the incidence of a threshold character could vary within wide limits.

a breed operates concurrently through selection and mating systems to create and maintain certain genetic characteristics. However, these rationalizing activities are then superimposed upon two types of processes: gene mutation and recombination, and chromosome assortment and crossing-over. These processes have the effect of injecting more variety and complexity of combinations while the efforts of the breeder seek to control and reduce them. In essence, all the breeder can do is to improve the odds of obtaining a desired outcome. The underlying natural processes prevent the breeder from ever asserting total control and predictability.

Random mating

As a prelude, it is wise to consider what random mating, which is the antithesis of inbreeding, means. Most mongrel cats are representatives of random mating only in the sense that there is an absence of affirmative control. With pedigreed cats, the situation is radically different. The breeders control their matings and the breeders should carefully regulate the choice of cats used. If the various breeders are working together in informal groups or networks, then the overall randomness quickly vanishes.

Remember that true random mating, in a strict statistical sense, implies that there will be the odd mating of brother to sister and other, less close, breedings of related cats over time. In the case of pedigreed cats, some, but certainly not all, breeders may assiduously avoid the closer breedings. Therefore, the assumption of random mating at the breed level is not unreasonable.

Random breeding versus random bred

Random breeding literally means that the probability of any male cat being bred with any female cat is a directly related function of the number of females in the population. Which cat breeds with which cat is a matter of chance. So if there are 1000 females, the chance of breeding any one of them is 1:1000. Sib mating happens at random too. If there are two sibs among the 1000 females, the chances of a sib breeding are 2 in 1000 or 1:500. That is, it is not likely, but it is not impossible.

Random bred, on the other hand, is a way in which breeders of pedigreed cats often refer to cats that are not pedigreed. But, just because a cat is not pedigreed does not automatically mean it is not inbred. In fact, the so-called random bred cat may not be randomly bred. Take, for example, a small colony of barn cats. The cats in such a colony will, within a very short time, tend to become a highly inbred colony because the number of potential mates is limited by geography to those in barn. Say, one male has access to two females and produces four kittens per breeding, two females and two males. There are two breeding, the first year and no kittens die. By the next year, there are now nine adult males: the original stud, four males by female 1 and four by female 2. The eight younger males are either half-brothers or full brothers. There are now also 10 whole females: the two (unrelated) queens and four females by each queen and the original stud. Generally in such an environment, a dominant male, usually the oldest and strongest, would tend to force the younger males away from any female that goes into heat. So unless all of the females went into heat at once, only one male, the dominant male, would be breeding this group of females. If the remaining male is, for example, the original stud, then 80 per cent of the next breedings that occur in that colony would between the original stud and his own daughters. That is because they now make up eight of the 10 whole females. As can be seen, as this pattern continues, this population will rapidly become very highly inbred. So those cat breeders who seek to inject so-called random-bred cats into a breeding program in the hopes of improving genetic vigor may well be doing just the opposite.

Breeding systems

In the case of Singapuras, I very definitely think they should breed true. I have never had anything else come from mine, and would not wish it to happen. This is due to severe culling when the breed was established.
                                     James Mendenhall, Singapura breeder

Selection

The phenotype of the individual cat is made up of a large number of genetic characteristics of varying expression. The ideal cat is one in which the expression of each of these characteristics is just right, in the eyes of the breeder. This means that an intermediate expression will be required for some characteristics, but an extreme expression required for others. The expression of these characteristics is controlled by selective breeding, of which there are several kinds of systems.

The simplest is based on the choice of the individual cat itself. But selection programs can take in whole families and even extend into progeny testing.

Side by side with selection, and reinforcing the process, there is the system of mating used. The systems of mating can include inbreeding of strong or moderate intensity, the matings of like to like, and the grading up of poor quality animals.

These are some of the tools that are at the disposal of the breeder. How these tools may be used, and, more importantly, which are most suitable for particular situations, is the subject of the balance of this chapter.

Selective breeding is by far the most potent factor in trying to control genetic characteristics, whether the type chosen is straightforward selection, with no frills, or one of several more sophisticated variations. The evidence for this power is demonstrated by the very existence of many breeds of cats, particularly as they differ in body conformation. Body conformation, which cannot be so easily manipulated, is one of the real bases of breed differentiation.

Selection by itself is not very efficient in eliminating heterozygous genotypes, the producers of deviating forms. Inbreeding is consistently

Obviously, some of the above items can only be seen after the cat has been bred. This means that a breeder will have to delay certain parts of this selection process until the cats are mature enough to breed.

Reproductive performance is so important that it may be thought super-fluous to have to mention the topic. Unfortunately, in the sorting out of the many traits that have to be selected, some breeders do not always give reproduction the priority it deserves. It is poor practice to breed a superla-tive strain only to find that it is properly held in low esteem because of either poor health or poor reproduction.

The most spectacular results from this practice occur when it is possi-ble to select for a single, well-defined characteristic, while ignoring all others. These are situations that produce the nice arcing curves of the results of selection found in some genetic textbooks. In most cases, the practical cat breeder may have to settle for less. There are several reasons for this, of which three in particular are key:

- The first is lack of facilities, space, or time. If a breeder intends to breed cats, he or she should tackle the job properly, and make full use of the available facilities.
- The second reason is to have a clearly defined objective in mind from the start. For most people, this will mean seeking to produce cats excelling in all of the fine qualities of the breed they choose. This, in turn, means a close study of the written standard of excellence for the breed as well as a visual and physical study of those cats judged to be the best available. The breeder should now critically evaluate his or her own breeding stock against the standard and compare them with these animals. This is the moment of truth. The more objective the compar-ison, the more quickly can something be done to correct any failings that are evident.
- Thirdly, the breeder is almost never in a position where he or she can concentrate entirely on one characteristic. The breeder must consider all sorts of characteristics simultaneously to achieve all-round excel-lence. There are three methods of dealing with this problem: the tandem method, the independent culling levels method and the total score method.

The tandem method

Under the tandem method, it might seem feasible to work on one feature at a time. The breeder would then proceed to deal with the next only when the first has been raised to a sufficiently high standard. The main objec-tions to the tandem method are two. The first is the time required to produce worthwhile results for several characteristics. The second is the real danger that the progress achieved with the early characteristics will be lost while the breeder is dealing with the later ones.

Independent culling levels

A second procedure is to decide that any cat that falls below a given standard in any one characteristic will be removed from (or kept out of) the breeding program. This method is easy to apply and can be surprisingly effective, provided the breeder does not weaken in his or her resolve. As the culling levels rise with the improvement of the strain, so the selection becomes more stringent. Note, however that the culling level need not be the same for each characteristic. Some characteristics are not so important while others may need more drastic selection to realize the same results. The responsible breeder should consider all of these aspects. The more well thought out the plan of action, the greater the overall improvement is likely to be.

An advantage of this method is that it necessitates a careful appraisal of the number of characteristics that can be dealt with and of their variation. The number of characteristics that can be effectively managed is limited. This means that the breeder has to establish priorities and then adhere to them. It requires analysis of the manner in which the chosen characteristics vary individually to be able to grade the cats as being either above or below the culling level. The most serious objection to this method is that, on occasion, it may be too ruthless. It may be unwise to totally reject a cat possessing several admirable qualities just because it falls below a certain culling level in only one characteristic. To counter this argument, a third more flexible method has been devised.

It should be kept firmly in mind that when breeders of pedigreed cats refer to culling, they mean the practice of spaying or neutering a kitten (or cat) that does not measure up to the standard being applied to that kitten (or cat). It in no way signifies that healthy kittens or cats which fail to meet the standard are killed.

Total score

This is probably the most efficient of the three options. In company with the preceding method, it requires that the contribution of each characteristic to the ideal cat be carefully assessed. The breeder should grade the variation of each characteristic by a convenient scale of points. The composition of the scale should be as accurate as possible without becoming unduly complex. Even a simple grading of very poor (1), poor (2), average (3), good (4) and very good (5) gives a five-point numerical scale. It is better, however, to score each cat against a 10-point judging scale. The scale ranges from 1 for the lowest to 10 for the highest grade of expression of the characteristic. The value of the scale depends largely on the competence of the breeder in grading his charges. It is best to base the grading against on the written competition standards. These provide numeric scales, with the relative weights that the judges must give to various physical features of that breed.

Now, with the total score method, the need to impose a limit on the number of characteristics is not quite as important as in other methods. It is probably best to include as many as possible, because it is difficult to foretell if a minor feature may turn out to be of major importance. It could become useful to be able to check on how a particular minor feature has been varying in past generations.

In practice, a working limit is set by the amount of time that a breeder can devote to calculating the index. The reason why a large number of characters can be considered is because the next step is to rank these by a system of 'weights'. These are numerical coefficients that reflect the relative importance of the various traits, in the breeder's estimation. These are used because the mere point scoring of expression of each characteristic cannot take this factor into account.

The scale of points assigned should be relatively unchanging, provided it is objectively drawn-up in the first instance. That is another reason to use the scoring system used by cat registries, as the breeder can change his grading if the scoring of the breed changes. On the other hand, it may be necessary to change the coefficients from time to time to give greater emphasis to certain characteristics. For example, if a certain feature is showing no signs of continuing improvement, the coefficient for it could be increased so that individual cats with exceptionally good expressions of that characteristic would score slightly higher. However, breeders should not change the values of the coefficients except for very good cause. A good cause is not the inability of a breeder to achieve a satisfactory expression of a possible characteristic with existing breeding stock.

The working of this method in application can probably be best explained by an illustration. There is no special basis for the choice of the coefficient for health, as this must be chosen for all breeds. However, the characteristics and the points assigned to them are taken from the official standard for the Somali by the Cat Fanciers Association (US).

Suppose the following characters are graded:

- Health (condition) (H).
- Head shape – including eye shape and ears (HS).
- Body build – including tail (BB).
- Coat texture and length (CT).
- Color – including ticking and eye color (CL).

Now, the relative importance of these seven features might be assessed as follows, with all but health based on the points assigned by the breed standard:

Total score = 25 HS +25 BB + 20 CT + 30CL

That is, head shape is considered to be just as important as the body and so forth. **Health is ranked as the most important and is a separately handled item**. If a cat fails to achieve a certain level of health, it is removed from further consideration in the breeding program. So, for purposes of this example, any cat with a health rating of less than eight is automatically excluded from further consideration.

To calculate the total score, the breeder evaluates each cat and grades it on a 10-point scale for each set of characteristics. In this case, the maximum total would be 1000. However, no cat would be expected to attain this level of absolute perfection.

Table 5.1 shows how eight cats might be evaluated according to the above formula. Cat A scores highly because it happens to be exceptionally good in the important characteristics HS and BB although it is mediocre in other respects. Compare the score with that for cat C that graded highly for several but slightly lower on others, thus producing a slightly above average score. This shows how the coefficients adjust the point rating in this respect. The best all-round cat is A, followed closely

Table 5.1 An example of calculating total score as an aid to selective breeding (see text for meaning of abbreviations and source of weighting)

Cat	Point grading for each set of characteristics					Total score
	Health	HS	BB	CT	CL	
A	10	10	10	6	5	780
B	9	8	7	7	7	725
C	10	6	7	7	8	695
D	10	6	6	7	8	670
E	9	6	6	7	7	650
F	6	7	7	8	7	730
G	10	5	6	6	5	555
H	9	5	4	4	5	445

by B. Individuals C, D and E tend to be similar, that is, somewhat above average cats. Without the total score, it might be very difficult to rank these in order of preference. This aspect reveals the discrimination possessed by the method.

It should be noted that cat F is a fine animal except that it had suffered an attack of an undefined sickness that makes its health suspect. This fact has removed the cat from further consideration. Had the cat been healthy, its score would have been 730, or second to cat A.

The table thus indicates the ranking of the eight cats for potential value to the breeding program based on the total score. If three animals are required for the next generation, these would be A, B and C.

Compare this ranking with that generated by the use of independent culling levels. As only three individuals are required, the culling level will have to be rather high. If all animals that score grade 5 or less for any set of characteristics are eliminated, then cats B, C, D and E remain. If all animals that grade 6 or less are eliminated, then only cat B remains. Thus, the culling method does not possess the fine discrimination shown by the total score technique.

It is important to note that, under this method, cat A is totally rejected. This is because cat A grades poorly in several sets of characteristics, in spite of its exceptional rating in the important traits HS and BB. A refinement would be to vary the culling levels, being more stringent against the important sets of traits and less so against the less important. To do this, however, the breeder is shifting the practical application of the culling method closer to that of the total score, but without quite gaining the flexibility of the latter. It might be worthwhile to employ the total score without such additional adjustments.

The total score technique is only an aid to selection. Its value is limited by three factors:

- The ability of the breeder to define the characteristics that are important for the task in hand.
- The breeder's skill in grading.
- The correct balance among the weighting coefficients. While it is possible to learn the calculations necessary to use this method for the first time, a 'feeling' for a soundly constructed score only comes with experience.

The example given above may be simplistic in that it may be useful to consider more characteristics, such as eye color or temperament. Also, using the standards of excellence as a source for scoring, it should be feasible to subdivide those being considered. Color (CL), for instance, could be further analyzed and subdivided in terms of depth of color, quality of the ticking and clarity of markings.

Family selection and progeny testing

Selection is normally practiced on an individual basis. However, selection may also be applied with a litter or a series of litters from the same parents. If 'familial' selection can be carried out, it enhances the effectiveness of the process. It can be applied whether the method used is culling levels or the total score option. The total score option, however, lends itself more easily to familial selection, as it provides a numerical value from which to generate an average.

Ordinary selection usually ignores familial relationships, as the superior animals are chosen from all litters being considered. However, a critical appraisal should take note of the capability of certain pairings to produce offspring consistently above the average of other pairings. This appraisal can take one or two forms: either noting which pairings have the highest number of young above a certain level of excellence, or deriving an average.

Should the total score be in use, you can calculate an average by adding the individual scores and then dividing by the number of young. The parents with the highest average are clearly those producing the better offspring. Future kittens should be obtained from these parents and preference should also be given to their offspring.

Indeed, to carry familial selection through to its logical conclusion, those parents that have produced inferior litters should be altered, as should their offspring, thus removing them from the breeding program. The effectiveness of familial selection stems from the fact that the selection is acting somewhat more efficiently on the genetic constitution than is possible by selection that is based on individual phenotype.

This can also be applied to situations when there are a limited number of cats breeding in differing combinations. Some of these combinations may consistently produce kittens that have a higher average than others. Those breeding combinations that have produced the inferior offspring need not be repeated.

These differences can be deliberately exploited to reveal differences in breeding capability. Normally, queens cannot be analyzed in this manner. That is because individually it is impossible to obtain enough kittens in a reasonable time to provide a fair sample. However, in theory at least, two or more stud males can be evaluated this way. The procedure is to obtain a round of litters with several females from one male and another round of litters with the same females from a second male.

A comparison of the quality of each round of litters could indirectly reveal the breeding ability of the different males. This is 'progeny testing' in one of its more direct forms, whereby the breeding worth of a male is determined by the average quality of his offspring.

Two or more separate lines composed of a few breeding cats could be dealt with in a similar way through 'group selection'. Begin with more than one separate line of a few individuals. Then, at an appropriate stage, make a comparison to ascertain if one line or group has made greater improvement than the other. The inferior line can be abandoned by altering the cats and developing two separate lines from the remaining line.

The stud male and grading-up

The stud male cat is the most important whole member of the cattery. This is neither because of his sex nor because some characters are inherited more strongly via the male. Rather, the reason is statistical. A stud male can sire many more kittens than a queen can ever hope to produce. It follows, therefore, that a breeder should be particularly choosy in the choice of stud males.

Fortunately, it is possible to be more selective of males. This is because fewer males are required, while the breeds tend to produce males and females in approximately equal proportions. This means a breeder can and should insist on at least as high a standard for the male as for the best of the queens. Actually, the breeder should insist on even a higher standard whenever possible.

For a number of practical reasons, not every breeder can keep a whole male cat as a part of the cattery. To compensate for this, breeders may make their whole males available for stud service. In the past, stud service was relatively open. However, now there are relatively fewer whole males at open stud; rather, stud service is more often negotiated among a relatively small group of breeders. The most common exception to this is the placing at open stud of whole males that have achieved particular prominence in competition.

The use of outside stud service benefits the owner financially, and the Cat Fancy as a whole by helping to raise the overall quality of the breed. When financial, geographical, genetic and health circumstances warrant it, there should be no hesitation in taking advantage of the services of these males.

The only problem is which male to use? The fact that the male is a well-known grand champion does not necessarily mean that he is the most suitable animal. He may have the same faults (despite his grand championship status) as the owner of the queen is seeking to correct in his or her own stock. It is good policy to visit shows and examine the various males competing to assess the good and bad features of each one. One or more should emerge as the appropriate mate for certain queens and then arrangements can be made for stud service.

Queens may be taken to males at open stud for various reasons. Probably the most common is a desire for general improvement in the breeder's lines, particularly if the queen is not outstanding in any way. Improvement in this manner is known as 'grading-up'. Grading-up is a term that can be used to denote most policies of mating average queens to superior studs or, less frequently, to taking superior queens to average studs. These matings are sometimes repeated for more than one generation (backcrosses) in an attempt to firmly impress the superior qualities carried by the male onto the breeder's lines.

This may not always be successful, or even desirable, as this aspect is highly dependent upon the degree of pure breeding of the superior animal. This problem is discussed in more detail later in the next chapter as 'pureness' of breeding is closely related to the amount of inbreeding which the superior stock has already undergone. The breeder should immediately stop any backcrossing if either of the following situations occurs:

• A general improvement is no longer occurring.
• The undesirable traits are beginning to emerge.

However, leaving this aspect in abeyance, grading-up is the quickest method for the improvement of mediocre lines and one that can be easily recommended to the novice breeder. Superb competition (show quality) cats are usually scarce and expensive, so the beginner often has to be content with lesser cats. This does not mean that they are of poor quality and not appropriate as the basis for a new breeding program. If correctly mated through grading-up, cats derived from a reputable line should produce very good quality kittens.

Another important reason for sending queens to outside males is to improve specific traits. If the breeder's animals have many good qualities already, extreme care must be taken not to upset these while the new or improved features are being incorporated. The whole situation has to be handled very carefully, both in the proper choice of mates and in the subsequent breeding. Unlike general grading-up, these outcrosses are not necessarily immediately repeated, as it is not a general improvement that is being sought. Much will depend upon whether the specific trait shows a desirable change and if this can be incorporated into the lines without either deteriorating or losing the good points it now has. To do this, it may be better to interbreed the offspring, rather than to outcross again.

The next moves do not lend themselves to any worthwhile generalization. Only the breeder, with full knowledge of his cats, their pedigrees, and his own breed can decide what to do in each case. So much depends on the problem in the line being addressed and the line's response to the outcross. If the offspring show deterioration in desired qualities, this may be a sign that the outcross has not been successful and an outcross to another male, unrelated to the first, might be the best policy.

Selection for intermediate versus extreme expression

Selection of characters falls into one of two categories:

• Selecting for an intermediate degree of expression.
• Selecting for extreme expression.

As many different characteristics make up the ideal cat, both sorts of selection may be operating at the same time. This is unfortunate, as the two forms of selection require different handling if each is to achieve the maximum possible success.

Intermediate expression

In the case of intermediate expression, the selection entails removing cats that deviate most from the optimum from the breeding program. More than anything else, it is a matter of fixing the character so that as many cats as possible possess it. The quickest means of achieving this is by close inbreeding, keeping in mind that many breeds are already closely inbred.

Extreme expression

Selection for extreme expression, on the other hand, implies striving for something not yet obtained or found in only a few individuals. Extreme expression is displayed only by genotypes containing a large number of genes having either plus or minus effects with regard to the character (depending on which end of the scale is being considered). These genotypes are only formed by gathering together the appropriate plus or minus genes that are scattered throughout the general breed population. Logic tells us that this must be the situation, otherwise the extreme expression would be common. This, in turn, means searching for and then breeding with any cat with a phenotype tending in the right direction. Breeders do this in the hope that different polygenes are brought in and combined to produce kittens of more extreme expression than that of both of the parents. To achieve this, it is desirable to have individuals heterozygous for as many genes as possible, despite the fact that the selection tends to pick out homozygotes. In other words, too early a decrease in the proportion of heterozygotes hinders the free recombination of genes that is essential for the formation of the extreme phenotypes.

Here lies the conflict between these. Put in another way, to fix intermediate expression, the heterozygotes should be eliminated; however, to realize ever more extreme expressions, the maximum number of heterozygous loci is required. Given the fact that breeders do not have an unlimited number of cats that can be accessed, nor an unlimited number of generations to achieve desired ends, a compromise must be found.

The most common compromise usually takes the form of a moderate amount of inbreeding, combined with intense selection. The hope is that there will be a steady fixation of intermediate characters, but that this fixation will not occur too quickly. The hope is that there can also be some progress towards extreme expression in other characters at the same time. The interface is the breeding program that can be so managed that the amount of inbreeding can be high, moderate or weak. How the breeder can manage this is the main topic of succeeding sections.

Inbreeding

Ordinarily speaking, inbreeding means the pairing together of any closely related cats. In practice the actual mating should be specified, as this determines the relative intensity of inbreeding. Some forms of inbreeding can be regarded as very close, others as less so and still others as quite mild. A rate of inbreeding can be roughly calculated for most systems of mating and can thus be used as a measure of its strength. This is an advantage, as in some limited circumstances it might be desirable to inbreed closely and, in others, significantly less closely.

Inbreeding is more correctly seen as the act of mating individuals of various degrees of kinship. But what does the process of inbreeding actually achieve? If continued for generations, it produces ever increasing homogeneity in the offspring. Genetically the offspring become more and more alike in appearance and general behavior. This is because the common ancestry causes many of the same genes to be received by different individuals. The limitation in the number of different ancestors and the absence of outcrossing are the key factors in this process. Through inbreeding, there is a tendency for the offspring to receive the same genes from each parent and to become progressively more homozygous.

The proportion of homozygotes in any interbreeding group of animals is known as 'homozygosis'. Conversely, the proportion of heterozygotes is known as the 'heterozygosis'. These two terms are the opposite sides of the same coin, but both are used because some people like to speak of an increase in homozygosis, while others speak of a decrease in heterozygosis. In reality, they are essentially the same thing. Crudely put, the proportion of homozygosis represents the 'purity' of the group while the heterozygosis represents the 'impurity' of that group. In this context, a group can mean either a line or an entire breed.

Sib mating

One of the closest forms of inbreeding is that of full brothers and sisters; the mating of siblings, or sib mating for short. As the inbreeding in sib mating is intense, easily appreciated and can be quickly put into practice, the consequences of repeated sib mating have been carefully investigated.

The breeding system is simple enough. It requires that the best individuals from the same parents are mated. The cats do not have to be from the same litter to be considered a sib mating. The result of that breeding is an immediate decrease in the amount of heterozygosis as shown by Table 5.2.

The interpretation of Table 5.2 is as follows: after one generation of inbreeding, the proportion of heterozygosis is 75 per cent of what it was before inbreeding began. After two generations, the amount is 63 per cent and so on. After 10 generations, the reduction has reached 11 per cent.

The figures in the table are those expected, calculated for each generation starting from scratch. The successive values show that the decrease

Table 5.2 The steady decrease of heterozygosis for successive generations of sibs mating

Generation	Percentage of heterozygosis
1	75
2	63
3	50
4	41
5	33
6	27
7	22
8	17
9	14
10	11
11	9
12	7

is a little uneven for the first few generations, but that the ratio of decrease becomes relatively constant later on.

For convenience, the initial unsteadiness is usually ignored and a constant ratio of decrease considered characteristic of this type of inbreeding, sib mating. So, the ratio could be regarded as an average over the generations and, for sib mating, the ratio is 81 per cent.

This ratio somewhat overstates the decrease for the early generations. As will be seen later, the ability to describe the intensity of inbreeding by a simple ratio (an index) has some advantages. This is true particularly when the relative usefulness of close versus mild inbreeding and other problems must be discussed.

There is one other system of pairing that has a very similar effect on heterozygosis to sib mating. This is where certain offspring are chosen to pair with the younger of its two parents. A given individual is mated twice, once to its younger parent and once to its own offspring. For example, suppose the queen was the younger parent, then a suitable son would be selected as her next stud. From the offspring of this breeding, a daughter would be chosen to continue the line and so on. The ratio of decrease of heterozygosis is also about 81 per cent per generation, approximately the same as for sib mating.

Although the two systems of mating have about the same ratios, they should not be intermixed if the object of the inbreeding is to bring about the maximum amount of homozygosis in the shortest time. This is because when the two systems are intermixed, the ratio is 84 per cent whenever a changeover is made from one system to the other.

Another system of mating is where a male may be mated to two of his own half-sisters, who are also full sisters of each other. Three individuals are involved in each generation and two series of litters.

The procedure is as follows. A male is paired with two females. The goal is to produce at least two litters, or series of litters, if a wider range of offspring are desired, provided the same male and female are being paired. From these litters the breeder chooses the next generation. From one litter, a male is selected while the other litter contributes the two females.

The system is self-perpetuating. This is because it should not be difficult to find two females per generation, while the rearing of two litters (or sires) allows a wider choice of offspring per generation than is possible with either sib mating or mating back to the younger parent (one litter or single series). The ratio of decline of heterozygosis is less than that for the latter systems but still significant, about 87 per cent.

Closed catteries

The above methods of inbreeding are often referred to as regular, because the cats are paired according to a set of predetermined rules. However, if inbreeding is desired, a more flexible system may be desirable. Many breeders have at least one stud and a number of queens. Inbreeding may be practiced with these, provided the cattery is closed to outsiders. That means no new stock is brought in and no queens are sent out for stud service. The queens and studs for the next generation must be chosen only from litters born within the stud. From here, no specific rules require that certain animals be mated to others. This allows the maximum freedom of pairing.

This 'closed cattery' method of breeding is similar to that used by many breeders. It differs from other types of inbreeding and random breeding not only in the exclusion of outside influences, but also in that there is no overlapping of generations. In this system, each male and his circle of queens are chosen fresh each generation. That means that any backcrossing of daughter to the father, for example, will result in a retardation of the trend towards homozygosis. In general, the matings are between half brother and sister if the numbers of males are small.

The closed cattery method will naturally lead to a decline in heterozygosis simply because of the limited number of parents within each generation. In fact, the intensity of the inbreeding directly varies according to the number of parents, as shown in Fig. 5.1. This figure gives values for the ratio of the decline of heterozygosis for different combinations of studs and queens. When studying this figure, a clear tendency is apparent. The decline in heterozygosis is appreciable only if the number of males and females are kept quite small. From a practical viewpoint, the

Percentage of heterozygosis in closed cattery system

# of Queens	1	2	3	4	5	# of Studs
1	81%	2				
2	85%	89%	3			
3	86%	91%	92%	4		
4	87%	92%	93%	94%	5	
5	87%	92%	94%	95%	96%	6
6	87%	92%	94%	95%	96%	96%
7	88%	93%	94%	95%	96%	96%
8	88%	93%	95%	96%	96%	96%
9	88%	93%	95%	96%	96%	97%
10	88%	93%	95%	96%	96%	97%
15	88%	95%	95%	96%	97%	97%
16+	89%	94%	96%	97%	98%	98%

Figure 5.1 The ratio of decrease of heterozygosis for various numbers of males and females for the closed cattery breeding system. To use, trace across from the number of queens to the column which has the appropriate number of studs at its head

number of males is the important item. With one stud and one queen, the only possibility is sib mating; the figure shows this has the quickest decline of heterozygosis. With one stud and successive additions of unrelated queens, the decline can still be relatively rapid up to about six queens. It is possibly not all that fast for larger numbers of queens. The situation changes rather abruptly even for the addition of one extra stud male. The value of the ratio rises until the decline is so small that very many generations are required to reduce the heterozygosis. In effect, the degree of inbreeding is then so minuscule that it need scarcely be considered as such.

The decline of heterozygosis over the generations can be estimated by successive multiplication of the appropriate ratio for any size of closed cattery. The use of the ratio slightly over estimates the decline for the first few generations, but is accurate enough to provide a legitimate comparison between catteries of different sizes. For example, the decline for a typical cattery of one male and five females will go approximately as follows: after one generation, the amount of heterozygosis is reduced to 87 per cent of what it was formerly; after two generations, the proportion remaining is 76 per cent (87 per cent times 87 per cent); and after five generations, it falls to 50 per cent.

Table 5.3 shows the number of generations it takes before a cattery composed of different numbers of males and females will lose 50 per cent of the initial level of heterozygosis. The fewer generations required to do this, the more effective is the system in achieving inbreeding. Sib mating is obviously the most efficient. However, the effectiveness of the other systems is inversely related to the number of animals involved. The more cats involved, the longer it takes to produce significant inbreeding.

The fact that inbreeding can be accomplished quickly does not mean that it is necessarily desirable. The question whether or not to inbreed can be a difficult one to answer. However, one thing is certain: if a breeder wishes to found his own lines with its own particular characteristics and with uniformity of offspring, some measure of inbreeding is essential. A high level of homozygosis cannot be attained in any other manner. Selection alone cannot do this.

Table 5.3 The number of generations required to halve the proportion of heterozygosis with various breeding systems

System	Number of generations
Sib mating	3
1 male and 2 sisters	5
1 male and 3 females	5
1 male and 5 females	5
1 male and 8 females	6
1 male and many females	6
2 males and 6 females	9
2 males and many females	12
Group of 4 cousins	9
Group of cousins	19

Selection may appear to do this because the parents may be alike in appearance as the breeder has started by selecting a certain type. But the kittens' appearances will vary, with only the occasional individual tending to resemble both of the parents. Inbreeding is necessary to 'fix' the specific characteristics that are being selected. The appropriate genetic term for this is 'fixation' of genes.

There is little doubt that inbreeding is valuable in stabilizing the results of selection. **Inbreeding, if any, should be deferred until after the selective breeding program**. As Roy Robinson noted,

'There is something to be said for deferring inbreeding for a few generations, largely because the most significant results of selection are usually achieved during the early stages. Later, it is often a case of consolidating gains and seeking to make improvements which are less easily realized. This is where the inbreeding could commence.'

Differences between alternatives

However, this is not the whole story. It is useful to examine more closely what inbreeding can do. In practice, there are two systems to consider seriously. These are sib mating and the closed cattery method, usually centering on one or two specially chosen stud males in each generation.

Sib mating is the most intense form of inbreeding and thus produces the most rapid increase of homozygosis. From the viewpoint of fixing a characteristic, it produces the quickest results. However, this fixing of characteristics is double-edged. While it may be desirable to have fixed particular characteristics, the breeder must remember that once these are fixed, further progress is impossible. The characteristics of the line are frozen in one mold, and further selective breeding will have little or no effect.

Should the cats of the resulting line be healthy and of a high order of excellence, the fixation may be considered to be an advantage. Yet the cost of doing this must be carefully considered. **No matter how excellent the strain may be, some faults are likely to be present. These faults, visible or not, are then fixed as well**. What happens is that the rapid increase in homozygosis fixes both good and bad points with fine impartiality. On balance, the good points may predominate, if the prior selective breeding has already picked out the better individuals and these have left their impact.

Now, suppose the increase in homozygosis has occurred less rapidly? In other words, if a less intense form of inbreeding had been adopted, it would have been possible to do two things:

- Emphasize the good features of the strain line further.
- Eliminate a greater number of the bad points before too much fixation had occurred.

A balance has to be struck between a rate of increase of homozygosis that will bring about the fixation of identifiable desirable traits and yet allows time for the elimination of the undesirable. This is where the closed cattery system has the advantage, because the intensity of inbreeding there is invariably less rapid and intense than that of sib mating.

In most cases, the closed cattery system of breeding centers around one or perhaps two males. More than two males may be used, but then the rate of loss of heterozygosity is very slow; possibly too slow except for very long term breeding programs. Should one male and a number of females constitute the cattery, the inbreeding will then be moderately high, with the actual level being determined by the number of whole females (Fig. 5.1).

Within each generation, the actual individuals retained for breeding will be determined both by the method of selection employed (see previous section) and by the number of females required. A fair number of kittens should be obtained from each possible pairing of male and female so that the intensity of selection can be reasonably high. In this way, the two main factors in cat breeding will be operating at the same time:

- One shaping the general appearance and quality of the line (selection).
- The other tending to fix these characteristics (controlled inbreeding).

With the closed cattery stud system, the temptation may be to backcross the daughters to the father, rather than to choose a stud male for the next generation. The breeders should always resist this temptation, unless the existing stud male is especially outstanding in a critical respect. If backcrossing is undertaken, then the movement towards homozygosis is held up, particularly if the backcross occurs during the earlier stages. This, in turn, could mean a delay in the establishment of the strain by a generation or two. It is difficult to generalize further in matters like this as the key to responsible breeding is the ability to be flexible and to knowledgeably balance the results of one process against those of another.

Often it may prove to be impossible to maintain a constant number of breeding cats in each generation. One kitten may unfortunately die or two or more kittens may be of such an extraordinarily high standard that the breeder desires to retain all of them for breeding. Could this have much of an impact on the movement towards homozygosis? If the numbers do not vary very much, the answer is no. This can be seen by the roughly similar values of the percentages given by adjacent entries in Fig. 5.1.

On the other hand, should the numbers of breeding cats in each generation fluctuate rather widely, then a significant impact must emerge. Over a series of generations, the smaller numbers have a more than proportionate influence over the larger.

The simplest method of demonstrating the problem would be to obtain the appropriate ratio for each generation and to multiply these together. This gives the approximate percentage of remaining heterozygosity. For example, suppose that over a period of seven generations, a cattery had consisted of a single male and the following number of females: three, four, five, six, 10, 12 and 15. The remaining proportion of heterozygosity would be approximately 39 per cent. The same reduction would also be achieved by a cattery made up of one male and a constant number of six females for each of the same number of generations.

The breeder must remember that the difference between repeated sib mating and the closed cattery is as follows:

- Sib mating leads to rapid fixation of all traits, sometimes so quickly as to block further progress by selective breeding.
- Closed cattery allows greater scope for selection to do its work, but also requires more generations for the cattery to begin to breed true.

On balance, the close inbreeding of sib mating appears to be too drastic in most cases.

Yet, there is another aspect of this form of inbreeding which has not been considered. Sib mating only requires two individuals per generation. This means that it may be possible to have more than one sib mating line in the cattery. The keeping of two or more sib mating lines has some advantages. The closed cattery system carries the breeding colony along as a whole, with each individual cat tending towards the general average. The situation is not the same for a series of sib mating lines. The rapid approach to complete homozygosis by such a process often induces a greater exposure of latent variation, which can then be seized on by selective breeding. The outcome of this blend of approaches is to have phenotypic divergence between the inbred lines, where some of them may be superior to the general average of the cattery. Some cats may even emerge as better than the results obtained by the closed stud system.

It is difficult to be certain of the outcomes, of course, but the point to be made is this: the full benefit of sib mating cannot be realized unless several lines are bred in parallel. Should one line fall behind the others in overall quality, that line should be closed down. It should then be replaced by a division of the best remaining line into two separate lines. In this manner, the number of lines is maintained at a workable level and selection can operate at two levels; between individuals within each line as well as between lines. While this may sound complex, it is not.

Grading-up and prepotency

The useful process of grading-up by the use of an outstanding stud male has two facets:

- Gaining the genes that make the stud male so outstanding.
- Raising the average quality of the cattery The likelihood of success is, however, dependent upon the degree of homozygosis of the male.

In a desire to obtain grading-up in this way, breeders often resort to repeated backcrossing of females. Repeated backcrossing of the females is a form of inbreeding, as the successive matings are that of daughter, grand-daughter, great-grand-daughter etc. The repeated backcrossings alone, however, are not sufficient. The decrease of heterozygosity brought about in this manner is rapid, but it does not lead to complete homozygosis unless the stud male is himself already highly inbred.

Take an example; assume that the stud male is descended from an inbred line and is, therefore, largely homozygous. The decrease in the heterozygosis of the average stock is 50 per cent for each generation. After only a few backcrosses, the offspring should take on some of the superior qualities of the foundation male. Furthermore, should the foundation male inadvertently die, another male (a son from the same line) could be substituted and the backcrossing continued.

The limit would be cats resembling the inbred line in many respects. As selection should also have been in progress at the same time, it is to be hoped the up-graded cats received most of the finer qualities of the line, but not the weaker or less desirable. At some stage, before the characteristics of the foundation male have become too fixed, it is useful to terminate the backcross while simultaneously maintaining or even intensifying the selection.

When the backcrossing is made to a foundation male that is not derived from an inbred line, the outcome will be different. In appearance, this foundation male may also be a fine specimen of his breed, but his heterozygous genotype means that he will not pass these qualities on to his offspring uniformly.

There will a decrease in heterozygosity as a result of the backcrossing's inbreeding, but the limit is 50 per cent of the proportion initially present. Even this level will not be attained until after a large number of generations. In the meantime, the male may have died of old age. There is no male of similar genotype to take his place because he was not from an inbred strain. At that point, the backcrossing comes to an end.

The value of an outstanding male of heterogeneous origin in this context thus lies in the genes he may be able to pass on to a few offspring by chance. It is usually worthwhile to try to capture these genes by selective breeding. However, this is far different from the general grading-up in quality which one might expect from the use of a superior foundation inbred male. So, the heterozygosis of the non-inbred male would be a severe stumbling-block to this type of program.

Because the nuances of inbreeding are difficult to fully understand, it is necessary to issue a warning against a breeding system that might trap the unwitting into thinking that it also represents grading-up. This is where a single backcross is made to a superior stud male. From the offspring, the breeder selects the best son who is used for breeding with the inferior stock. From among his offspring, still another son is selected, and so on. This is backcrossing in the wrong direction. Any good points that might have been gained from the first backcross are rapidly lost.

Prepotency

'Prepotency' is a term used to describe the situation when a male, or a female, possesses the property of producing offspring bearing a strong resemblance to himself or herself. Males are sometimes referred to in this way in error, by those who mistakenly think that the male, but not the female, has an innate propensity in this direction. That is not the situation; rather males appear to have the characteristic because they have greater opportunities to reveal this ability. A point that is too often overlooked is that bad, as well as good, features may be transmitted by such a cat.

The reason this happens is that the cat has become homozygous for a single gene, or group of genes, with dominant effects. This may be by chance, especially if both selection and inbreeding are being employed at the time. Should these characteristics be desirable, there is every likelihood that these may become fixed in the cattery's line as the cats bearing them are retained for further breeding.

The interesting fact is that the more inbred an individual cat may be, the more homozygous he or she will be, and the greater the chance that he or she will display prepotency. This is where the foundation male from an inbred strain scores over the stud male of heterozygous origin even should the latter be phenotypically superior. The prepotency may not be derived entirely from dominance in the case of an inbred male as he transmits a uniform set of genes in every gamete, whereas the queens will not. Hence, on average, the offspring will tend to resemble the male.

Mating like to like and the opposite

The breeding together of cats of similar phenotype is often advocated as an alternative to inbreeding, particularly with so-called minority breeds. This is known as breeding or mating 'like to like'. The usual reason for undertaking such breedings is a belief that this will lead to fixation of characters. They do not accomplish fixation. These matings are, however, valuable for perpetuating a character.

Inbreeding is the only key to character fixation. Inbreeding, coupled with breeding like to like, is the surest means of securing and then stabilizing a desired degree of intermediate expression. In other words, breeding of like to like is itself a form of selection. As a general policy, breeding like to like has much to recommend it. In fact, the total score method itself produces a high proportion of such breedings for the various characters that contribute towards the score.

The opposite of the like to like breeding is the breeding together of unlikes. This process is often advanced as a means of compensating for faults in one cat against those of another cat. It should be understood that **the breeding of cats with similar faults should be avoided at all costs, otherwise there is a danger of fixation**. While this may not necessarily occur in every case, when there is inbreeding, there is a risk. As some of the so-called minority breeds are already inbred, fixation is always a danger with them, regardless of the lack of apparent inbreeding on the pedigrees.

The total score method undoubtedly causes some breedings of unlikes but these can be tolerated, unless they recur frequently. If they do, the breeder should review both the composition of the score (from page 69) and the genetic behavior of the constituent characters. The latter is recommended as it may be that an inverse relationship (from pages 94 and 116) has been exposed, in which case improvement in one character can only be achieved at the expense of another.

The major drawback of breeding unlikes is that it tends to be a negative policy for breeding. While it may be useful to combat the chance fixation of faults, it does so at the expense of encouraging heterozygosity. Even if the bad features have disappeared or are ameliorated in the next generation, they could still reappear in those following generations. This is especially true if there has been over-compensation. In over-compensation, cats that are exceptionally good or bad in some points are appropriately matched with the intention of producing offspring with average all-round qualities. The result would then be an otherwise average cat, which still manifests an undesirable character.

Anyone who looks ahead to later generations should be able to appreciate the problems which breedings of unlikes to unlikes may entail. This form of breeding should not be viewed as a settled policy, but rather as an opportune way to handle a difficult situation that cannot be resolved by other methods.

Limits to selection

It is impossible to eliminate all variation among cats because a proportion of that variation is due to non-genetic causes. They are due to idiosyncrasies in the development of the individual cat and/or to environment. Little can be done about idiosyncrasies in the development of any individual cats but the impacts of the cat's environment can be minimized by providing as constant an environment as possible that is conducive to strong and continuous growth. However, even under optimum conditions, it is not always possible to remove all of the genetic variation nor to achieve a given objective at the first attempt.

The key to fixing an intermediate expression of a character is the removal of genetic variation. The mating of like to like can make some contribution to this end, but that method is relatively slow when compared with inbreeding. Close inbreeding can reduce the genetic proportion, provided it is maintained for sufficient generations. Sometimes, however, the progress is not as fast as might be expected or the variation still seems to be as great as before the inbreeding began. There may be several possible reasons for this:

- The genetic proportion of the variation is not the same for all characters. That means that it may be that the proportion is low for a particular character. Inbreeding reduces this, but the effect may be negligible if the genetic proportion was not making much of a contribution in the first place.
- The more heterozygous animals are the more healthy and thus these may be preferably chosen for breeding. That means that the genetic portion of the variation may persist. Choosing the less vigorous, but more homozygous, cats could lead to a reduction in variation, but only at the risk of the onset of inbreeding depression (from page 114). This is not a necessary consequence of all inbreeding but it is wise to be on the alert for it, and, as importantly, to be on the alert for those factors that can bring it into being.

One of the peculiarities of selection for extreme expression is that the extreme phenotypes of some traits may remain tantalizingly out of reach. A breeder may find that the breeding program produces the occasional cats that have the desired characters, but may also find that it is very difficult, if not impossible, to breed more cats of the same type. There are several reasons that could be behind this:

- The genetic proportion of the variation may be small. If this is the case, those few individuals that do turn up owe their appearance to non-genetic causes. Given this, it is not surprising that these cannot be reproduced by selective breeding.
- If the nature of the non-genetic factor is unknown, the appearance cannot be produced by manipulation of the environment.
- A rather similar situation can occur when the genetic proportion of the variation is small. Some progress may occur, but this soon stops and further selection is unable to produce progress.

Even when the variation is largely genetic, it may still be that the results fall short of a breeder's expectation because the genes present in a particular stock are incapable of producing the extreme phenotype. The cats actually lack the genetic potential, despite the fact that another line was able to reach the desired extreme. The solution is relatively straightforward: introduce genes from the successful line by means of crosses to that line.

It is also possible for a line to fail because, though it originally carried the necessary genes, some became homozygous and others were lost before they could become combined. Inbreeding can actually bring this situation into being. Once again, the solution is to outcross to another successful stud, either by taking a queen to the particular stud male or by purchase of a suitable cat for the breeding program. Both of these solutions are themselves forms of grading-up. The breeder takes advantage of the availability of cats that apparently have the necessary genes to produce the desired phenotype.

Another barrier to selection for extreme expression arises when an inverse relationship exists between the characters. This subtle phenomenon can occur, often unexpectedly, in a number of guises. It usually comes to light because progress with selection in one character can actually hold back progress in another and vice versa. A hypothetical example may help illustrate the problem. Suppose a breeder of longhairs is selecting simultaneously for very long hair fibers, especially in the undercoat and also for density of the fur coat. The breeder may find, over a period of time, that those cats with good long coats appear to lack density while those with dense coats usually appear to be lacking length. It does not seem possible to combine the two characters. Though such a situation may not exist, this example illustrates the principle of inversity between two separate characters.

Whenever any such inverse relationship is encountered, it usually means that a third character is mediating the other two. The breeder must first try to establish whether or not the inversity actually exists. In the above hypothetical example, the extra flexibility of the coat in the very long haired cats may produce the illusion of a lack of density. Or, the long hair fibers may only be produced at the expense of fiber thickness, which again results in the illusion of lack of density. In both cases, the number of fibers per square inch of skin, the usual measure of density, may actually be unaffected.

Assuming that the lack of density is not merely an illusion, the increase in hair length may only occur at the expense of number of hairs for a given skin area. This could happen if the supply of hair substance, a keratin precursor, for example, was limited. Fiber length could only then increase if there is a corresponding reduction in number of hairs. In these circumstances, an increase in hair length, with no reduction in number of hairs, could scarcely be accomplished except by a greater supply of hair building substance. This may not be easily achieved by breeding selection based on either hair fiber length or density. This is because changes in a key trait, the keratin substance, only subject to indirect selection (on both hair length and density simultaneously), are usually more intractable than if breeding selection can be applied directly. It should be noted that that the above example is fictitious.

Finally, limited progress may be made because the selective breeding is being sloppily or inconsistently applied. While half-hearted attempts at selection may produce positive results of a sort, in the long run, it is more probable that they do not. Or, the achievement of improvement in one generation may be frittered away in the next. Illogical changes in the emphasis on the selection of different characters could quickly undo years of careful selection. If the total score method is used, it may be that the score itself is badly constructed, either for the characters considered, their grading or their weighting. These items should be checked.

Technical appendices

A: Working ratios of declines in heterozygosis

Working ratios of declines in heterozygosis are as follows:

- Sib mating   81 per cent
- Offspring to younger parent   81 per cent
- Shift from A to B or B to A   84 per cent
- Male to two-half sisters   87 per cent

The ratio of decline of heterozygosis that has been calculated for various systems of inbreeding should not be taken too literally:

- The ratio is quite general in that it is independent of the initial proportion of heterozygosis and the total number of genes, for most practical purposes.
- The ratio applies most accurately to autosomal genes but less accurately to sex-linked genes. However, for some breeding systems, the ratio is similar for both sets of genes and, in others, the discrepancy is small. As sex-linked genes are in a minority, the error is negligible, unless the inbreeding is continued for a very long period. This is an unlikely prospect as it is also undesirable.
- A discrepancy could arise from selective breeding favoring the most vigorous and healthy animals as this may select out the more heterozygous individuals. As a result, the movement towards homozygosity may not be as rapid as the calculated ratio would indicate. However, only in rare and exceptional circumstances would a large difference emerge. The ratio may be regarded as a useful index to the amount of inbreeding which is taking place.
- The ratio states the degree of change from the original start of the breeding program. Thus, if the program began with pedigreed cats, it is starting with cats that are, to one degree or another, inbred already.

This same system can be used to evaluate how quickly any size cattery will lose a fixed percentage of its initial heterozygosis.

B: Calculating the decline in heterozygosity

Should the need arise to calculate the ratio of decline of heterozygosity more exactly than that given in figures or tables in this chapter, or for numbers of males and females not shown, the following formula should be used:

Ratio = $1\frac{1}{2}$ [1 − 2A + $\sqrt{(4A^2 + 1)}$]

where A = (M + F)/8MF and M = number of males and F = number of females. If the number of generations to reduce the initial heterozygosis by half is required for this ratio, the following should be used:

Number of generations = 0.301/log(ratio)−1

Chapter 6

Breeding practices

> * The meaning of lines
> * Gene pools
> * Elimination of anomalies
> * Persistence of anomalies
> * Technical appendices
>   A: Case study – head conformation and bite
>   B: Record keeping

The meaning of lines

Many breeders, at some time in their career, may feel that they would like
to have a line of their own. But what is a line (or strain)? In the Cat Fancy,
all breeders may register a cattery name. They then register all kittens that
are born to previously registered parents under that cattery name. The
registry process introduces a small degree of control and helps ensure that
a stud cat becomes widely known when its descendants are regular
winners. This is turn may generate a demand for kittens and for stud
service to queens from other catteries.

Over time, a certain amount of inbreeding may occur within the kittens
from the particular cattery, so that it may be legitimate to speak of a blood
line, the original source of the term 'line'. Eventually, the word may be
applied in a more general sense to all of the cats bred within the cattery
and/or from purchased cats not too many generations removed.

The result is that the terms 'line' or 'strain' are often used rather loosely
in cat breeding, most often to indicate a relationship rather than anything
else. This is particularly true for a line of ancestry tracing back to an
exceptional animal or lineage of exceptional cats. Collateral descent is an
important aspect of true blood lines, when breeders seek to show that
certain cats are related via a remote, but common, ancestor.

> *When planning a breeding program, breeders must realize that doubling
> on the good traits in a cat also results in doubling the defects.*
>
> Kitty Angell, Scottish Fold breeder and cat show judge,
> Angell (1996)

Some in the cat fancy hold blood lines in high regard, particularly when
outstanding cats feature prominently in the pedigree. However, good
blood lines are not the same as genetic worth. This is because cats of
championship or grand championship status may still produce mediocre
or downright inferior kittens. To the breeder, this means both that the
appearance of the cat should always be a primary consideration in acquir-
ing a cat and that care must always be taken to examine the pedigree of
such a cat with a critical eye. This is especially true when champions and

grand champions are absent from one side of the pedigree, or do not occur in the more recent generations. In the first case, this could indicate that some grading-up has been taking place. In the second case, it might mean that the cattery has not been faring very well recently in competition or has not been in active competition at all.

In cat breeding, therefore, the designation 'strain' or 'line' should not be lightly granted. Ideally, it should be limited to describing a stock of cats of distinctive, if not truly exceptional merit. It should represent a cattery of relatively true breeding cats that possess unique features that tend to make them stand out as a group. This reputation is not achieved overnight. Rather, it is the result of years of unremitting, selective breeding and resultant wins in competition. However, for the purposes of discussing breeding practices, a group of closely related cats that have been inbred for several generations, that is beyond five or six generations, would also qualify as a line or stain. This is true even if the cats are not of particular note in other respects.

The founding of a line or strain of elite, healthy cats should be the goal of all responsible breeders. Not every breeder may have the opportunity to do so, nor will every breeder who attempts to accomplish this be able to succeed.

Gene pools

A term often bandied about when cat breeders gather together is 'gene pool'. Some people probably wonder what that term precisely means. As one may probably guess, it has something to do with the genetic constitution of the individual cat. More exactly, it has to do with the genetic constitution of a group of individual cats.

To summarize Chapters 1–4, genes are minute entities on the chromosomes that determine the growth and eventual appearance of the cat. The chromosomes are present in pairs in the individual. As the genes are carried at specific points on the chromosomes, it follows that the individual cat has two of each specific gene. If a group of individual cats has, say, – in number, then the sum total of specific genes is $2n$. The term 'gene pool' denotes this number.

The concept of the gene pool is usually discussed in relation to specific cat breeds, particularly with respect to the numerically smaller breeds, known to breeders as 'minority breeds'. The implication is that too small a gene pool is undesirable, or even potentially worse, is actually detrimental. The reasoning behind the belief is that a small gene pool implies an absence of genetic variability that is essential for successful selective breeding.

Some breeders might think that if the breed has attained a high degree of perfection this is not necessarily bad. The individual cats are all of excellent quality. However, suppose the cats are not outstanding, but rather downright mediocre? What if they are of excellent type, but carry with them a hereditary disease or defect, such as polycystic kidney disease (PKD)? It will then be difficult, if not impossible, to bring about any improvement.

So the concept of the gene pool is rather abstract. It is useful, however, for focusing attention on the impact of a limited number of breeding cats. The effective breeding population is always less than the population at large. The effective breeding population is the number of individual cats that actually contribute descendants in the next generation. For example, a pair of cats may produce several litters of kittens over a number of years. But not all of these are necessarily added to the effective breeding population. Some may die before reaching breeding age and others may spend their lives as altered, and therefore non-reproductive, but well loved, pets.

To illustrate this concept, suppose a specific pair of cats has produced four litters of six kittens, for a total of 24 kittens. It only requires that the breeder retain two kittens for breeding, replacing the now-altered parents, for the breeding population to be stable. Any number beyond those two implies that the breeding population is increasing in size. While the total population for the new generation is 24, the effective breeding population (EF) is almost always less. For the population to be stationary, the EF is two; even if the EF doubled, the number only has to grow to four. However, in this case, doubling the size of the EF does not equate to enhanced genetic diversity. Breeders may not readily appreciate the relative smallness of these figures if the generation interval is spread over several years.

People concerned with the long term well-being of breeds that are small in effective population numbers have some justification for their concerns. The reason is that the limited number of whole cats brings about unavoidable increases in inbreeding. To have this occur, the inbreeding need not be close. Indeed, breeders may be carefully seeking to avoid close inbreeding. Inbreeding still arises because of the mating of collaterally related cats – cats that share common ancestors in the not too distant past.

The common practice of almost everyone rushing to breed to the currently popular male show champion [dog] is probably the most significant factor reducing whatever diversity remains [after working with small numbers of breeding animals].

John Armstrong, dog fancier

A little analysis of numbers proves this. For an individual cat to be truly non-inbred, all of the ancestors must be different. Yet this is essentially impossible, because the number of different ancestors double for each generation studied. The number of ancestors in each generation begins small enough – two, four, eight, 16 . . . for the first four generations – but the number soon becomes very large indeed. At the twelfth generation, for example this would require 4096 completely different ancestors to be able to say that the cat is not inbred that far back. Therefore, it can quickly be seen that for virtually every pedigreed cat, any individual cat must almost certainly have some common ancestors on both sides of the pedigree – if a breeder will just go back far enough. This occurs more quickly in so-called minority breeds.

This inbreeding is not necessarily detrimental. As discussed in Chapter 7, the negative impact of inbreeding depends on factors such as how many common ancestors there are and on how frequently these recur. The potentially ill-effects of inbreeding depend both on its intensity and on how long it continues. If a breed is small in total numbers, the inbreeding may be weak, but it will still be continuous. Therefore, the question arises: at what level can inbreeding be tolerated? There is no quick answer to this question as it is probable that some breeds can tolerate a little more than others. Please note here it is breeds, not lines. But if the breeders of a line of cats within a particular breed resist outcrossing, that line is also governed by the rules which impact minority breeds.

Another critical factor is the number and severity of the deleterious polygenes latent in the particular breed. It is these polygenes that are responsible for the decline in health and vigor commonly associated with inbreeding (see page 114).

The counter to inbreeding depression (as this decline is called) is persistent and consistent selection against weak cats. Weak cats are those that may carry with them any inheritable defect or disease, no matter how excellent they may be in other qualities. With most forms of selective breeding described in Chapter 5, the breeder has to balance the good and bad points against each other, but should never make a compromise for indifferent health. There is no merit in producing championship cats if these or their descendants tend to succumb to illness or be poor breeders, due to inbreeding depression.

Elimination of anomalies

While every breeder of pedigree cats agrees that undesirable genetic anomalies must be eliminated, they appear to persist tenaciously. The reason for this is twofold:

- First, the problem can be more complex than appears on the surface.
- Second, the remedy may demand more drastic action than is acceptable.

Different problems arise and different procedures should be followed according to the known or assumed mode of inheritance. That is, whether the anomaly displays dominant, recessive monogenic heredity or polygenic heredity.

> *Simply put, there are a vast number of things that kill us and our animals, and we do not know where they come from. We have a vague idea of how they work, or a good idea of how they do damage (not the same thing). Gene mapping is a start, but a small one. That we know how to identify the gene that causes a heritable problem does not mean that we'll wipe out that anomaly by testing and avoiding a breeding of two carriers.*
>
> Gene Rankin, Abyssinian breeder

Before trying to eliminate an evident anomaly, the responsible breeder should take time to be certain that the problem is in fact an anomaly. Some problems which are environmentally or nutritionally based can appear to be the result of anomalies. A good example of this is cardiomyopathy. An inheritable problem, not limited to any breed, it presents as significant physical damage to the heart. Breeders rightly fear its occurrence in their lines. But they and their veterinarians often forget to inquire into other causes which may present in a similar manner. Toxoplasmosis, a disease generally associated with eating infected raw meat containing an intracellular parasite, can also occasionally present in a manner similar to cardiomyopathy.

Dominant monogenic heredity

When an inherited disorder caused by a single dominant gene is passed on it is known as dominant monogenic heredity. When the disorder is obvious at birth or is constantly seen in the progeny of a particular breeding pair of cats there is no problem in eliminating it. However, it is not always that easy. For example, the affliction may not be evident until later in life when the cat has been breeding for some time.

Theoretically, all dominant monogenic anomalies could be eliminated if every descendant of every afflicted cat was prevented from breeding. This would be drastic action indeed when it is considered that about 50 per cent of the animal's descendants are free of the anomaly. Unfortunately, the price to be paid is that the other 50 per cent hand on the anomaly until they are eventually detected. An example of this type of anomaly in the cat is progressive retinal atrophy which ultimately results in blindness. The late onset of this affliction means that the animal may have bred before the first symptoms are noticed.

Recessive monogenic heredity

With recessive monogenic heredity, the problem is in the detection of the heterozygote or 'carrier'. The carrier cat is not evident by clinical signs but appears fully normal. The detection lies in either one of two ways. The older method of detecting carriers was that of test mating. Test mating is accomplished by actually breeding suspected carrier cats to known affected cats and checking the resulting litter. Obviously this can only be accomplished if the anomaly does not interfere with reproduction. If a sufficient number of normal kittens are produced, without the appearance of a single anomalous kitten, then the cat may be judged not to be a carrier. The number of kittens to be bred in each test depends upon the level of acceptable error. It may be that a carrier animal could produce entirely normal young by chance but the chance of this happening becomes smaller as the number of kittens increases.

Test mating of severely affected cats was practiced in the past but with the advent of more sophistication in testing, it is no longer necessary and is considered to be irresponsible. In all methods of test mating, the resulting kittens may well be affected by the genetic anomaly for which you are checking. This, obviously, results in ill kittens or in kittens who will grow to become ill cats. Breeders of pedigreed cats do not breed for cats who will be ill or affected by genetic anomalies. However, many ethical breeders find they are producing kittens who have genetic anomalies because they are practicing inbreeding. In fact, the first time a genetic anomaly may be discovered is when inbreeding is practiced.

Polygenic heredity

There are two main types of anomaly with polygenic heredity. The first is that where the severity of the anomaly is variable because of the effects of different numbers of genes. This implies that culling of the most affected animals will bring about a gradual improvement. The extent of the improvement and the rate at which it occurs depend upon the level of culling. In general, the more ruthless the culling, the greater the relative improvement. There are various complicating factors, of course, of which the most important is that certain of the mildly affected animals, which are not culled, are capable of producing severely affected offspring. Against this is the fact that the average level of severity should decline per generation of selection.

The second type of polygenic trait is where the anomaly is due to a threshold effect. Despite the underlying polygenic inheritance, the cats are either normal or abnormal. The degree of abnormality may vary and this may be polygenically determined but the normals are fully normal in appearance.

Persistence of anomalies

How does the odd genetic anomaly apparently persist in spite of proper, responsible breeding techniques and patient selection? The answer must be sought among a variety of causes, several of which may combine to reinforce one another. Genes producing anomalies cannot multiply throughout a breed on their own but they are opportunistic to the extreme in the sense that given favorable circumstances, they can spread surprisingly.

> As PKD is the result of an autosomal dominant gene, it is relatively easy to track and eliminate....The quickest way to eliminate the problem is to neuter or spay those individuals [who show the presence of cysts on the kidney].
> David Biller, DVM, DACVR, Stephen DiBartola, DVM DACVIM and Wilma J. Lagerwerf, RVJ, RLAT, AHT, veterinary researchers.
> Biller, DiBartola and Lagerwerf (1998)

A major factor in the spread of an anomaly is a relaxation of culling. This is more likely to occur when a breed becomes exceptionally popular. When this happens, breeding stock is scarce and the demand for kittens is high. The temptation is to breed from every animal, even from those which would normally not be used in the breeding program. This means that 'inferior' (from a show standards point of view) animals can pass on their less than perfect qualities, even if an effort is made to secure the services of a good sire. The practice of selling unneutered kittens to people who promise not to breed them is scarcely a sound long-term policy. Under pressure, the promise may be conveniently forgotten. US veterinarians have studied the effects of 'early' altering (spaying and neutering at three months of age) and have found no long lasting deleterious effects on the cats. Reassured by this study, many US breeders now refuse to release such an unaltered kitten from their cattery.

Instances are known where a much admired and widely used stud animal has subsequently been found to be a carrier of a recessive anomaly. This was, of course, unknown at the time he was siring but becomes only too apparent after his offspring have multiplied and spread throughout the breed. Inbreeding, however distantly, ultimately brings into being a rash of occurrences of the same anomaly. Breeders may suddenly find themselves confronted with the twin problems of preserving the reputation of the breed and of eliminating the gene causing the anomaly. This process is often behind the so-called mutant 'epidemics'.

> *But it is also true that none of this will do us any good unless we change our whole approach to breeding by stopping 'keyholing' practices of breeding most of a generation's females into just a handful of males each generation. The breeders who are in favor of the outcross proposal, are united in trying to keep the breed's diversity intact by utilizing many different pairings for their males and females. We are carefully mentoring new breeders to be aware of these problems and to use genetic conservation practices for breeding Havana Browns.*
>
> Candice Massey, Havana Brown breeder

A feature of this event is that the appearance of the first anomaly is usually delayed for several generations from the ancestral point of origin and that many years of effort are required to either eliminate the anomaly or to reduce it to such a low level that it is no longer a problem. Chance plays a major role in determining the type of defect which could be unwittingly spread in this manner, and the breed in which the process occurred. On the other hand, it may occur in any breed and at any time. These situations have taught us not to place too much reliance upon one or a few exemplary sires. The process is usually mediated via the male as the female cannot produce enough offspring to influence the course of events.

Even in more normal periods of breeding where supply of kittens is roughly geared to demand, a particular defect may seem to strangely persist. Two possibilities may account for this. One is that the amount of culling may be reduced to a minimum because of a deliberate policy of not breeding more kittens than necessary to cover replacements and sales. The other is that of heterosis or hybrid vigor. Generalizing, there is a correlation between healthy vigor and the amount of genetic heterozygosity. It may be that when the amount of heterozygosity falls below a certain level, so-called 'inbreeding depression' sets in. These animals appear sickly and weak and are culled. However, their more robust but heterozygous siblings are retained. Included among these may be carriers of a recessive anomaly.

Of course, should the gene producing the anomaly be associated with extra vigor when heterozygous, which is possible but not always likely, a ready answer is available for the persistence or even spread of the gene responsible.

A similar situation may arise in those circumstances where a breed standard encourages the breeding of a certain type of defective animal. The rise of the defect is inadvertent, of course, and may take many years to become a part of the way the breed looks. Even if the defect is condemned, and it generally is, it recurs because breeders are endeavoring to conform to the standard. A conflict situation may even come into being. As the breed moves closer to the standard, the incidence or severity of the defect may become greater. It has been suggested, for example, that the sinus ailment and running eyes of some Persian and Persian-type cats such as Himalayans and Exotic Shorthairs is a consequence of selective breeding for a short nose and flat face. In the Burmese breed, a preference for a distinct head type resulted in the perpetuation of a mutation known as the 'Burmese head fault'. Cats with this head structure were heterozygous for this defect (See Technical Appendix to Chapter 11).

Different registering bodies of the cat fancy will ultimately deal with the issue of health and breeding:

- In the US, the Cat Fanciers Association (CFA) has created an overall standard which every cat, no matter what breed, must meet. A cat or kitten at a CFA show must reach this standard in addition to the specific standard for its breed. This standard states:

    'Though individual breed standards sometimes describe unusual physical traits, the ideal show cat is free of any characteristics, exaggerated or otherwise, which cause discomfort or jeopardize health and well-being'.
- The major registering body in the UK, the Governing Council of the Cat Fancy (GCCF), has also taken steps to ensure that breed standards do not describe unfit animals. For instance, Longhairs (Persians) are not allowed to have nose leather higher than the bottom of the eye. This is an effort to prevent health problems that may be associated with 'overtyped' cats.
- In Europe, FIFe (Federation Internationale Féline), the primary registry, has taken a public position vis-à-vis breeding practices and a specific health problem, polycystic kidney disease (see Chapter 11). FiFe recommends that breeders should have their cats examined by ultrasound to find out if they have polycystic kidney disease. The position holds that generally speaking breeders should avoid breeding from those cats with the disease.

When such criteria, particularly those aimed at particular physical characteristics, are based on substantive research and experience, they can serve to advance the health and welfare of the breed(s) in question. However, there is always the danger that such pronouncements can be based more on speculation than on science. In such cases, they will fail to advance the health and well-being of pedigree cats.

Technical appendices

A: Case study — head conformation and bite

The conformation of the head is an important feature of the makeup of competition cats. So important is the shape of the head that the profile is a major characteristic of many breeds. The conformation is primarily determined by the dimensions of the individual bones making up the skull. These in turn are fashioned by the genetically controlled growth processes, initiated during fetal development and continuing right through to maturity.

That heredity is an important factor is shown by the fact that most breeds, by and large, reproduce kittens which mature to conform with the breed standard. One has only to compare the head shape of a Persian cat with that of the Siamese to appreciate the extent of the differences which exist. This comparison is significant because it probably represents the extremes of skull variation in the cat.

There is some variation between individuals, and this is to be expected, due to accidents of growth, diet and minor illness. However, the characteristic head conformation is primarily the outcome of many decades of selective breeding. The effects of selective breeding have resulted in modification of the individual skull bones, especially those nasal and frontal bones governing nose shape and the jaw. Breeding for an excessively short nose or a very prominent nasal depression (or 'stop') can interfere with normal breathing. The nasal passages could be partially obstructed which could induce labored breathing, particularly under stressful conditions. It is not uncommon for the tear ducts to become narrowed or blocked, resulting not only in an unsightly 'running' eye, but more seriously, in infection.

No one can realistically dispute that sound mouths are very important for the well-being of the cat. It only requires a small modification of growth processes to induce detrimental changes in the relative length of the jaws, positioning of the teeth and how these meet when the mouth is closed. Various degrees of bite may be recognized, depending on subtle changes in growth. If terms may be borrowed from the dog fancy, the bite may be said to be overshot, scissor, level, reverse scissor and undershot, depending upon the extent to which the upper jaw is longer, the same length or shorter than the lower.

The normal bite is where the prominent upper jaw incisor teeth are positioned, immediately behind the lower incisors when the mouth is closed. The frontal teeth should be scissor or level. When an obvious gap exists between the teeth, there is cause for concern. Both the overshot and undershot jaws are generally held to be undesirable. Bite is determined by the relative length of the upper and lower jaws. One can gain some idea of this by examining the general profile of the cat. For instance, selection for a short nose could easily upset the delicate balance of growth gradients and cause an undershot bite. On the other hand, selection for an elongated head could encourage the overshot bite.

Differences in bite is part of the usual variation of the bones of the skull and in that sense is not exceptional. It is possible that the jaw bones – the maxillae and the mandible – are more prone to variation than other bones, but it may be that bite has emerged as a problem because it is more detectable. It is doubtful if a major gene is involved in the production of either undershot or overshot bite. This is not to say that a mutant gene for a jaw anomaly could not arise at any time in any breed but that does not seem likely at this point. Generally, the genetic aspect is almost certainly polygenic. That is, numerous genes with minor effects are controlling the shape of the bones. As an abnormal bite is often a case of either being present or absent, the condition could be due to the threshold heredity which can mimic the assortment of a major gene but is still polygenic at root.

Abnormal bite, in the sense of an imperfect alignment of the teeth is just one of several mouth problems which may occur. In addition, mouth problems include narrow or twisted jaw and abnormal angulation of the incisors. Teeth which are underdeveloped or missing are also a concern. The only means of dealing with the problem of incorrect bite is by continuous selection of sound animals for breeding purposes. The occurrence of an odd individual with the incorrect bite could be due to vagaries of fetal development. If a number of cases recur, serious attention should be given to the diet and husbandry techniques. If the diet is nutritionally sound and the husbandry is acceptable, the breeder should remove the cats who have produced kittens with incorrect bites from the breeding program. Selective breeding for perfect mouths may be 'hard' or 'soft'. Hard selection is where any individual with poor bite is immediately rejected from breeding, regardless of the severity of the anomaly or any excellent compensating qualities the cat may possess. Soft selection is less stringent. With soft selection, the breeder takes into account the severity of the condition and this is then balanced against other qualities of the cat. But breeders must remember that if the anomaly is really severe, there can be no compensating factors. Even if the proposed partner in the mating is excellent and all of that cats' offspring have normal mouths, the partner could be a genetic carrier of mouth deformities and could transmit the defect to future generations.

If the breeder is using the recommended scoring method of selection, the mouth can be one of the aspects on that scoring. This means that the mouth will now be considered as a matter of course as the future breeding stock is assessed. If the condition is a problem, the breeder must treat it as important and allocate a high weight in the scoring system, perhaps even higher than the breed standard itself assigns to it.

Despite an avoidance of close inbreeding, many breeds of cats are inbred to some extent. Indeed it cannot be avoided if the breed is to be composed of a homogeneous group of animals of recognized breed conformation. In this sense, it is desirable. On the other hand, inbreeding is more conducive to bringing out the latent anomalies in comparison with a truly random breeding population. Therefore, while anomalies are likely to appear in both pedigree and random bred cats, their presence is more likely to be discovered by inbreeding.

It is extremely unwise to breed from animals with inherited defects which have been surgically corrected. Even if the defect is relatively minor, it could reappear in later generations in an aggravated form. This aspect is probably diminishing in importance as it becomes more widely appreciated that, while such surgical intervention may be desirable for the individual cat, the genes for the defect are still transmitted in the gametes, surgery or no surgery.

B: Record keeping

Purposes

A simple, but efficient system of record keeping is vital to advancing cat breeding. The art of successful cat breeding depends on the generation and retention of reliable records and then on the use to which these are put. Unfortunately, for many cat breeders, they often put off, to some future date, writing up of breeding results, including notes on the appearance of each kitten. While this is understandable, it cannot be justified in any responsible breeding program. Fortunately, the majority of cat breeders appreciate the value of record keeping. This is true even if the records being kept are the most basic, such as a log of past breedings and births as an aid to future breedings.

Record keeping in cat breeding fulfils three functions:

• It presents an accurate record of familial relationships.
• It provides information upon the phenotypical characteristics and breeding performance of each cat.
• It is a source of data that breeders can use to help make future decisions.

It is easier to outline the minimum of data that ought to be kept, but it is not as easy to set an upper limit. Clearly, if record keeping is not to be a burden, the chosen methods should be simple. On the other hand, the amount of information a breeder should collect depends on the nature of the breeding program that the cat breeder has set for himself or herself. It also depends on the breeder's temperament. Even among experienced cat breeders, opinions will differ on how relevant a particular piece of information is to a given task. As a rule, however, it is advisable to record as much data as possible, under two conditions:

• It appears to have potential value to the breeder.
• It does not make the whole process too burdensome.

Traditionally, only one place brought together all of this information: the stud book

At one time the stud book was quite literally that – a bound book, permanently recording all of the critical data concerning the breedings, the pedigrees and related matters. Even today, major registries publish stud books. However, the cat breeder can now consider other options for collecting critical data and maintaining it for future use, particularly computer programs. While computer programs for cattery management and pedigrees are increasingly a cat breeder's tool, they have several drawbacks:

• They are not all compatible, so that sharing information among breeders or between breeders and registries is not always easy.
• Unless the cat breeder is very careful about backing up computer files, a simple error can wipe out years of accumulated data.
• What data breeders record are driven by what the designers of the software have decided is useful. It is not easy, or even possible in some cases, for users to modify this software.

For simplicity, however, the cat breeder's records, in whatever form, are referred to here as the stud book.

Basic record-keeping principles

Identification
It is essential that each cat should be individually and readily identifiable once it has been entered in the stud book. When a cattery has only a few breeding queens and all of the queens are seen daily, many breeders might question whether or not a means of individual identification is really necessary. While it does not seem necessary, experience shows that you can never rule out a mistake. Remember, it is not always possible for the owner of the cats to be present to identify them. For example, what if a stud male gets loose while an assistant or cat sitter is cleaning a cage? Do we really expect the assistant to be able to identify the particular sable Burmese female whom the male mounted before being recaptured? What happens if the breeder becomes incapacitated and someone else must manage the cattery or even liquidate it without the breeder's assistance?

With a larger cattery where new litters of kittens may be frequently arriving during the peak of a breeding season, reliable methods of clear identification are clearly desirable. While the use of collars has been common in the past, there are good reasons why they are no longer desirable.

- First, if a collar comes off, there must be another way for someone to identify which cat was wearing it.
- Second, collars can be very dangerous. If they become loose, they can pose a danger to the cat wearing it. Collars can catch an open jaw and dislocate it, or worse, can quickly strangle a cat jumping down to the ground.
- Third, collars cannot be used for very young kittens, where identification may be critical.

What other options are available? There are many options. Basically, they fall into two groups: permanent and temporary.

Permanent identification is usually most effective in cases where a third party might have to have to identify the cat. The most common methods available are tattooing and chipping.

Tattooing involves placing a permanent identification name, number or code somewhere on the cat. The benefits are that this is permanent and that any efforts to change it will be clearly detected. However, because it is permanent, some registries do not permit cats being shown to have them. For breeders involved with these registries, tattooing is limited to cats not being shown, or to those no longer being shown. The custom is that the cat is tattooed on the inside of a leg. That means that, for longhaired breeds, the cat may have to be shaved to see the tattoo. That in turn means it is not useful for on-the-run identification in a cattery environment. Also, unless a registry sanctions tattoos and records them, an individual finding a cat tattoo may not be able to determine the proper owner.

Chipping entails the subcutaneous insertion of a microchip containing data on the cat and its owner. The goal is to provide the following:
- A permanent way in which a lost or stolen cat can be identified.

- A permanent way that its owner can also be identified.

This is accomplished by contacting a permanent registry with the data supplied by the chip.

As with tattoos, registry rules may preclude the use of chipping on cats being shown. As with chipping, it is really best used for protection against loss or theft, as it requires the use of a scanner to read the chip.

The second option, and the one best used for a working cattery's record-keeping, is some system of temporary identification, coupled with special record-keeping.

First, the cattery should have a separate record of every cat, whether in the working cattery or not. This would enable a third party to enter the cattery and take steps to protect the cats should something happen to the owner. Ideally, this record should contain information such as the following:

- The cat's registered name.
- The cat's call name.
- The cat's date of birth.
- A basic color/pattern description.
- A note of any distinguishing physical feature, e.g. the cat is odd-eyed, that is it has a blue eye on the right and a gold eye on the left.
- Reproductive status — male, female, spay or neuter.
- Blood type. This is important not only to avoid problems with fading kitten syndrome (neonatal isoerythrolysis), but also in case a cat needs a transfusion.
- A color photograph.
- Important information for a caretaker, e.g. the cat is a diabetic.

The breeder should make sure that this information is easily located. For that reason, it is wise to tell individuals who might have to gain access to the cattery where it is stored.

In terms of the cats within the cattery, then, identification becomes easier. For example, you can 'mark' queens of the same breed and color, such as Sable Burmese, by shaving spots on their bodies. Remember that this works as long as you both keep them shaved and have a written key to the marks. If you have your cattery physically divided, simply placing a card on the outside door, which lists the cats in the room by call name, may be sufficient. With young kittens, if the fur is not too dark, you can mark them with iodine. Again, record the marks and keep them refreshed. An alternative is to use nail polish. This should be used only on the claws and care must be taken to ensure the polish dries quickly so that the cat or others do not lick it.

Breeding

A day-to-day record on breeding queens can be kept as ordinary small index cards, filed in a closed box. Then you can use a separate card for each queen. Then, you can record the following:

- When you confine a queen with a stud cat.
- The name of the stud cat.
- The date and time of delivery.
- Details on the delivery.
- Preliminary details on the litter.

The queen's call and registered names and, or, reference number in the stud book (see below) should be written at the top of the card. It can be useful to use the queen's and sire's registry numbers in the stud book. The breeder should note every confinement with any male. This should be undertaken at the time it starts as well as when it ends, noting both the name and reference number of the male, as well as all relevant dates. Should the desired mating occur, the breeder should note the date(s) and approximate time(s). If a mating does not occur, the breeder should also note this; if a reason for the failure can be determined, this should be noted as well.

After the queen conceives, the date of birth of the litter and the number of kittens delivered should be recorded. If possible this should be undertaken at the time of the delivery. Brief notes can be kept on the same card, such as whether or not the kittens look healthy on delivery, their approximate birth weights and if the queen had an easy delivery. These cards then serve as way of checking the reproductive history of the queen. For example, whether or not she conceives readily and if she produces the average number of kittens per litter can be seen at a glance.

When the time arrives for the kittens to be examined and be entered separately in the stud book, the details of the litter can be transferred at the same time. The litter reference number in the stud book can be written on the card as a cross-reference. As with the numbers for the queen and sire, it is best to use the litter registration numbers assigned by your registry for this purpose. The breeder should preserve all of these cards, even after the queen has ceased to breed.

The stud book

The stud book is the permanent repository for all information and most systems of recording cattery information revolve around some sort of permanent record. The book may range from an ordinary permanent note book to a loose-leaf binder, and can even be done on a computer with a pedigree program.

A loose-leaf binder allows you to add extra pages that you can need surprisingly often when your breeding program is going well and you find new aspects of it that merit additional record-keeping.

One system of recording is based on the successive numbering of litters. Beginning with the first page of the stud book, the breeder prominently writes a number in the top right hand corner, beginning with 1, 2, 3,..., etc. It may be convenient to have the number at the top right-hand corner of the next available blank page, according to the amount of space required. This could be as little as a page or could extend over several pages depending on the amount of information to be entered. Each succeeding litter is then assigned the next unused number in the book. Alternatively, you can use the litter registration number assigned by your registry once you have registered the litter.

As certain details are the same for all litters, consider setting up the pages with standard headings already printed. Figure 6.1 shows a possible arrangement of these basic details. The figure shows an example for a litter designated as 42 (the number at top right). This litter is produced by a mating of a queen, with stud book reference 17d, with a male, with reference 9a. Note that their call names are also given in parentheses. The mating occurred on 12 February, and the queen gave birth to five live kittens on 18 April, after a normal parturition.

One of the kittens died at birth, but the other four were successfully reared. The kittens were weaned successfully. The record also shows both coat color and length. Two were shorthaired self black, one a shorthaired blue and the last a longhaired black. Each kitten is assigned one of the first few lower case letters of the alphabet. That means each kitten has now been precisely designated both by a litter number (42) and then a letter. The breeder may add notes, such as whether or not the queen nursed the litter satisfactorily. Finally, the breeder can leave space for information on the later history of the kittens. That is, if they were sold (if so, to whom), died from a disease or accident (if so, state the cause) or from old age (if so, give date). After a while, the procedure soon becomes a matter of routine.

The main genotype can usually be appended to the color description of the kittens as shown. However, it will also be highly desirable to record variations of polygenic characteristics, either by a description or by grading on a suitable scale. In Chapter 5, the advantage (if not the necessity) of employing such a breed-specific scale was emphasized. These were used for analyzing a polygenic character and for the calculation of a total score for a cat. If the total score method is being used in your cattery, there is no reason why this should not be used here. It can provide a concise method of describing the variation for kittens as well, with certain necessary adjustments. For example, it may be difficult or even impossible to grade coat texture or certain colors in kittens, while it is easy for an adult. Also, there are some features, such as head shape, that a breeder cannot grade at birth, but can only evaluate at later stages of growth and maturation, due to factors such as molding. There are even some physical characteristics, such as whisker break, which a breeder can more easily evaluate when a kitten is still wet, following its delivery.

The breeder can always make additional supplementary notes, though this ought not to be necessary, as every effort should be made to assure that the scoring is as accurate as possible.

Figure 6.1 shows how grading the four kittens can be based on the same system described for the construction of a total score (Chapter 5). Suppose, for example, that this breeder is interested in the self blacks. Though the blue SH and the black LH will be not be a part of this breeding program, the breeder should grade all of the other characteristics for these cats as conscientiously as possible. These will vary independently (with the possible exception of CC because of the long hair in kitten d could interfere with accurate grading) of each other. For that reason, no opportunity should be neglected to obtain data on the variation.

The nature and amount of data that a breeder records depends entirely on the interests of the breeder. For instance, it may be that the breeder is seeking to create a particular type of spotted tabby that cannot be easily graded. In that case, each kitten's pattern may have to be described in some detail if the breeder is to have an adequate permanent record. Photographs (kept with this record and identified on the back of each photograph) would be useful, particularly if the photographer can standardize the posture of each kitten to minimize distortion. Breeders should try to use sketches only if they can prepare outlines beforehand so that it is simply a matter of filling in a few simple details.

(Litter registration number)

Queen: 17d (Abigail)   Reg. No.: 1234-5678

Sire: 9a (Racine)   Reg. No.: 5678-1234

No. of Matings to Conceive: One

Date(s) of Matings: 12 Feb. 1998

Date of Birth: 18 April 1998

Parturition: Normal -- uneventful

No. of Kittens Born:

        Live   4

        Dead   1

Details of Litter:

        a   Male black SH   aaD-L-   2.75 oz.

        b   Female black SH   aaD-L-   3.00 oz.

        c   Male blue SH   aaddL-   3.25 oz.

        d   Female blue LH   aaddll   2.75 oz.

Condition at Weaning: Excellent

Grading of Characteristics

Kitten	H	CC	CT	BB	HS	F	T
a	10	9	9	6	6	4	4
b	10	8	8	7	4	5	4
c	10	-	7	6	5	6	4
d	5	5	-	5	6	3	3

Figure 6.1 A sample page from the stud book showing the basic data that should be recorded for each litter and a proposed layout of the entries

Numbering systems

The advantage of having a reference system based on consecutive numbering of litters is that it facilitates quick cross-references in the book itself. That way, all the information both on litters and on individual cats is in one book. If at any time a breeder has to check on any cat, it is only necessary to turn to the appropriate page number (which is the litter number) and then consult the appropriate letter. For example, in Fig. 6.1 the queen is 17d, indicating she is the fourth kitten from litter 17. The composition of this litter, number 42, might provide additional data on her genotype. Suppose she is a shorthaired black. The colors of the kittens is this litter show that she must be heterozygous for blue dilution and for long hair. If the heterozygosity was unknown (or only suspected) at the time the breeder wrote up litter 17, the record in the book can reflect this. All the breeder does is to turn back the pages and add the new, relevant, data to that already entered for kitten d there. Similarly, the breeder can add any new information on the male, 9a. If handled this way, the comprehensiveness of the stud book increases as the entries increase.

After a number of years, the stud book may come to consist of a number of volumes. However, if the principle of consecutive litter numbering still applies, the numbers would be carried on from one volume to the next. The numbers contained in a volume could then be written on the spine for easy reference.

There are two ways to handle the addition of cats acquired from outside the cattery.

- One is to treat the new cat as if it were a 'litter' and then assign a number to it at the time of purchase (while also recording that it had actually been purchased).
- The second is to designate those cats by simple numbers or capital letters. An alternative is to use a group of capital letters selected to act as a mnemonic for the origin of the cat. If the breeder uses this second option, a full page should be left for each cat to record any data that is or may become available.

The seller's pedigree should supply such basic details as date of birth and parentage. Other details, such as information on litter sibs should be easily obtained from the breeder of the acquired cat. These pages may be inserted in the stud book at any convenient position, such as in serial order before the cattery-bred litters.

Non-breeders may not understand the need to use somewhat impersonal litter numbers and lower case letters to identify kittens. The breeder should explain to them that the use of these identifiers in no manner replaces either call names or the more formal names under which pedigree cats are usually registered. These reference numbers are primarily to facilitate the quick and easy location of individual cats in the stud book and to allow for tracing parentages or ancestral lineages extending through successive generations. The stud book system has been proven to function very well in this respect. When this is linked with records on the reproduction of the individual cat and the quality of the kittens produced, it forms a serviceable system of permanently recording breeding data.

On the other hand, using the registration numbers assigned by a registry permits the breeder to track cats back and forth through other pedigrees.

It also allows a breeder to use a registry's own services (such as producing reverse pedigrees or multi-generation pedigrees) to supplement a cattery's own records.

If a breeder wishes to maintain a cattery's own stud book, the better practice would probably be to use a cattery's own stud book numbers, while also keeping the registry numbers in the records for quick reference.

Chapter 7

Inbreeding

In general

Inbreeding is an emotional topic for some people. One cause of this is that it brings forth disturbing visions of incest. Another cause for emotional responses is that some breeders may feel that they are incapable of managing it. Despite these reactions, inbreeding has a place in animal breeding. It can be quite important, being one of the two mainstays of improvement; the other being selective breeding (see Chapter 5).

The majority of cat breeders probably have some general idea of what is meant by inbreeding. If pressed, they would probably answer that inbreeding involves the breeding of close relatives, usually citing the breeding of brother to sister, father to daughter, or mother to son. These breedings do indeed constitute inbreeding. In fact, these are the closest possible types of inbreeding, but they are only three of a large number of possible breedings that all come under the heading of inbreeding.

Inbreeding is an inclusive term, covering many different breeding combinations and degrees of relationship. Generally speaking, the more distant is the relationship, the less is the intensity of inbreeding.

Some breeders use another term: line-breeding. By that, they mean the mating back to a particular stud or line, to impress the desirable qualities of that stud or line on the kittens. This may be done repeatedly; if so, it is actually a form of inbreeding. It is commonly viewed among many breeders as a more permitted form of inbreeding. In fact, line-breeding has been used incorrectly to denote lesser forms of inbreeding than those close ones described above.

Given the mathematical nature of the laws of heredity (see the technical appendices for this chapter), it is possible to calculate the intensity of inbreeding for any mating of related cats. It is important to have this information when merely considering whether or not to undertake inbreeding. The reason is that the intensity of inbreeding varies with the degree of familial relatedness of the cats and it is not always wise to use the more

Table 7.1 Table of breedings: a comparison of the amount of inbreeding which will follow from the mating of related individuals

Form of mating	Degree of inbreeding (%)
Father to daughter	25.00
Mother to son	25.00
Full brother to sister	25.00
Half brother to sister	12.50
Uncle to niece	12.50
Aunt to nephew	12.50
Grandparent to grandchild	12.50
Single first cousins	6.25
Single first cousin to second cousin	3.13
Single half first cousins	3.13
Single second cousin	1.56

intense forms of inbreeding. To be more accurate, it is not wise to use the more intense forms too often.

The closeness, or intensity, of inbreeding for the most commonly employed breedings between related cats is shown in Table 7.1. The usual convention is to designate the inbreeding as a percentage, so that the larger the percentage, the greater the degree of inbreeding. The amount of inbreeding decreases in steps of one half (Table 7.1). This ratio is not due to chance, but occurs from the heredity of the genes. (For the technically minded, the percentage actually measures the expected decrease in the number of heterozygous gene pairs in the offspring.)

Brother to sister and parent to offspring (father to daughter and mother to son) breedings represent the closest, that is highest percentage, inbreeding. What is surprising to many breeders is that these two variations of inbreeding are of equal strength.

The next in decreasing order of intensity is a group of six breeding combinations including the breeding of half-brother to sister. This ranks equally to grandparent to grandchild inbreeding.

The remaining eight breedings in the table involve those between less closely related individuals. As expected, the intensity of the resulting inbreeding declines steadily as the relationship between the stud and the queen becomes more remote. The determining factors here are both the number of generations separating the individuals and the number of related individuals in the particular breeding. For instance, looking at the table, consider the difference in inbreeding intensity between a mating of single first cousins and a mating between double first cousins. The latter breeding is twice as intensive as the former as the ancestry contains more related individuals.

Other breedings between more distantly related individuals are referred to in a general manner as cousin breedings, involving third, fourth etc. half cousins as well as full cousins. Cousins need not be in the same generation, such as the first to second cousin breedings shown. The intensity of inbreeding is low for most of these combinations, except for those cases where multiple cousins are involved.

Cat breeders sometimes refer to inbreeding as 'doubling up', or 'concentrating the heredity', of ancestors in the inbred cat. Technically, what actually occurs is an increase in the number of homozygous genes in the individual. That is, the closer the inbreeding, the greater the likelihood of pairs of genes becoming homozygous. This is desirable if the genes are those which result in an outstanding specimen of the breed. What if these same pairs produce undesirable features? Inbreeding, as a matter of fact, is quite impartial in this respect.

This is where selection must enter the picture. There is an important rule associated with any inbreeding: 'the more intense the inbreeding, the more careful and stringent must be the selection'.

Selection is important for all breeding programs, but it is doubly important when inbreeding is involved. In particular, the breeder should carefully monitor the health of the cats in the program. Inbreeding does not necessarily lead to a decline of health and vigor but it may. When it does, all of the good work of patient selection breeding will be of no benefit. It is far more desirable, and the mark of a responsible breeder, to work to prevent a possible decline in the first place.

Every breeder, at one time or another, has pondered on the effects of inbreeding. Should I try inbreeding? What exactly does it accomplish? Are the effects good or bad – or a bit of both? This is not a frivolous issue. Questions such as these should occupy the thoughts of all serious breeders.

In practice, inbreeding may arise at two levels:

• That which occurs in the hands of individual breeders.
• That which arises in the breed as a whole.

The former occurs when a breeder chooses to have breedings between related cats or affirmatively chooses to remain within the same lines (see below). The cats do not have to be closely related, because the mere fact that they are related implies inbreeding, even if it is weak inbreeding.

Inbreeding arises in a breed because of the fact that there is only a finite number of breeding animals for each generation. For a breeder to completely avoid inbreeding, he or she must be certain that every ancestor of every cat is different. However, this is impossible in practice.

To illustrate the point, take any one cat. The number of ancestors doubles for each succeeding generation. The number of different cats needed to fill out a pedigree start low enough but soon become astronomically large. After only a relatively small number of generations the numbers of cats needed will eventually exceed all cats that have ever been born. For example, to fill out the pedigrees of two cats for only 20 generations with unduplicated names would require 2 097 152 different cats.

If the above reads like a contradiction, as all cats have ancestors, the solution is that common ancestors recur for remote ancestors. It is quite clear that the further back you look in the ancestry, the greater will be the number of recurrences (that is, common ancestors) you will find. **Every cat in a breed is collaterally related via these ancestors.**

The presence of common ancestors is a sign of inbreeding, the actual amount depending on the number and how far back these occur in ancestry. The larger the breed in terms of numbers of breeding animals, the smaller the chance of finding common ancestors and, frequently, the more distant will these occur in the ancestry. It follows that breeds that are not numerically strong have the greater likelihood of being inbred.

This type of inbreeding may be 'background inbreeding' or 'long-term inbreeding' to distinguish it from inbreeding which breeders may affirmatively undertake. The background inbreeding would be influenced, to some extent, by that practiced by breeders but it is likely that this is small. The reason for thinking along these lines is that while some breeders may be doing a little inbreeding, others may be avoiding it. Furthermore, crosses between partly inbred strains can largely nullify the inbreeding of each.

Nonetheless, numerically small breeders cannot escape the background inbreeding imposed by limited numbers of breeding animals. It is possible to estimate the maximum number of sires and dams that a breed should have for the avoidance of the possible harmful effects of long-term inbreeding. This requires an assumption that a breed can tolerate a given level of inbreeding. Two proposals have been made in this respect:

- The breeding is carefully controlled by selective breeding.
- The loss of innate genetic variability is not too great.

The levels of long-term inbreeding should not exceed 5 per cent for the first proposal and not to exceed 1 per cent for the second (see Table 7.2). Because breeds are now expected to have an indefinite life, the problem of long-term inbreeding deserves to be approached from another viewpoint. As the generations progress, the total amount of inbreeding increases. This means that the total should be taken into account. Just as it is wise to set an upper limit to the rate, it is also wise to set an upper limit for the total.

The recommended limit for total inbreeding is 50 per cent and, ideally, this should not be exceeded. If the rate is known, it is possible to calculate the number of generations to reach the 50 per cent limit. For the rate of 5 per cent per generation, the limit is reached when 14 generations have passed and, for the rate of 1 per cent, the limit requires 69 generations.

Table 7.2 Table of the minimum number of individuals for two levels of inbreeding: (A) 5 per cent and (B) 1 per cent

(A) Cats	Queens	(B) Cats	Queens
3	15	13	329
4	7	14	117
5	5	15	75
		16	57
		17	47
		18	41
		19	37
		20	33
		21	31
		22	29
		23	27
		24	26
		25	25

These are 'cat generations' so if we express them, say, as an average of two years per generation, the time span will be in the region of 28 and 138 years, respectively.

A breeder, as an individual, may take notice of the 28 year limit if he or she is forward-looking but not, presumably, of the 138 year limit. On the other hand, a committee of a cat club may (or perhaps should) take notice. The committee should be taking the long view of the prospects of the breed. If it felt that the rate of inbreeding is excessive, steps should be taken to combat it.

The effect of inbreeding is to increase the homozygosity – the degree of pure breeding – of the cats. Unfortunately, inbreeding tends to uncover any minor deleterious genes that may be latent in the breed. Normally these are not particularly troublesome but if a number become progressively exposed, 'inbreeding depression' may make an unwelcome appearance. The depression may take a number of forms but typically impacted animals are sickly individuals.

If inbreeding is intense, these minor deleterious genes can be uncovered and fixed in the breed before selection has had the opportunity to weed them out. This is the aspect which has given inbreeding such a bad name. Yet, if the inbreeding is weak, the minor deleterious genes are exposed, but they are less likely to be fixed. Selection can then be used to eliminate them. The process is slow and ongoing. In this respect weak inbreeding is beneficial in that it is ridding the breed of minor deleterious genes.

To sum up: inbreeding can be good or bad. While even close inbreeding can be good in special situations, as a rule close inbreeding should be avoided. On the other hand, weak inbreeding can sometimes be useful applied so it should not be condemned out of hand.

Inbreeding and breeds

Most people instinctively appreciate that inbreeding is the mating of individual cats that are blood relations. They also grasp that the degree of inbreeding can vary, depending on the closeness of the relationship of the cats.

Inbreeding occurs at two levels. The first is inbreeding of the individual cat or within an individual cattery. A breeder may be concerned with selection and inbreeding for his or her own group of cats. The breeder's activities may be, in general, independent of other breeders. On the other hand, other breeders may be involved, e.g. in the buying of breeding stock or to acquire stud service.

In a majority of breeds it is now impossible to find two cats unrelated to each other because every pedigree is based on a few early founding cats.

Joan Miller, Vice President,
The Winn Feline Foundation and cat show judge
Miller (1998)

In any given breed, it is doubtful if any breeder can (or should) ever be fully independent of other breeders. The more common, and preferable, situation is where a number of prominent breeders are well established. Consequently, their cats are being diffused throughout the breed. Different strains and lines of cats may thus emerge, and a particular line may actually be in the hands of several breeders. In other words, a breed often operates like a loosely interconnected collection of strains or lines.

The second level of inbreeding is that for the breed as a whole. The concept is based on another definition of inbreeding. If the parents of an individual cat share common ancestors, there is inbreeding. If the common ancestors are merely a few generations removed from the particular cat, it should be possible to define the usual familial relationships, that is, grand-father, second cousin etc. If they are remote, this is usually not worth the effort. In such cases, the relationship is said to be collateral.

In the early days of the breed there was a major problem with infertility and the breed was almost lost. Careful outcrosses to other breeds solved this.

Carol Barbee, Cornish Rex breeder

It should be clearly understood that all individuals of any breed have collateral relations; that is, they all must share common ancestors at some stage. As the number of generations increases, the number of ancestors required to avoid duplication increases very rapidly. This continues until the numbers involved quickly exceed the total number of cats of that breed ever born. It thus follows that, at some point, the same stud cats or queens must recur somewhere in the ancestry, possibly frequently, for more popular stud cats or queens.

This recurrence of studs or queens represents inbreeding. The actual level of inbreeding depends on the numbers of individual breeding cats in each generation. If there are many, the frequency of repeats need not be large. On the other hand, if the number is small, the frequency of repeats may be substantial.

One consequence is that a numerically small breed is always subject to some measurable degree of inbreeding. The exact amount will depend on the average number of breeding studs and queens in each succeeding generation. If the breeder knows these figures, then he or she can calculate the average rate of inbreeding.

This leads to the question: is there some tolerable level of inbreeding?

It is reasonable to assume that there are at least two different levels of the inbreeding rate to be measured. These are:

- Control of breeding stock.
- Conserving genetic variation as much as possible.

In the first case, the breeder's control takes the form of careful selection of breeding individuals, not only of conformation for the breed, but particularly for health and fertility. These aspects should always have priority.

In the second case, the selection aspect still applies, but must be accompanied by a weaker degree of inbreeding. As inbreeding causes the loss of genetic variation, the more intense the inbreeding is, the greater the loss becomes. Therefore, the breeder must consider the rate of loss. It is a question of how much of a loss can be tolerated.

For the above cases, **it is advisable that the rate of inbreeding should always exceed 5 per cent for the first case and 1 per cent for the second case.** The minimum requirement to achieve the 5 per cent level is three studs and 15 queens. For four and five studs, the minimum number of queens can be lower, that is at seven and five, respectively. For six or more studs, provided the number of queens exceeds that of the number of studs, the level is 5 per cent in each case. Obviously, it is far better to have larger numbers of studs and queens than the bare minimum shown in Table 7.2.

The minimum number to achieve the 1 per cent level is 13 studs and 229 queens. For larger numbers of studs, smaller numbers of queens are permissible, as indicated by Table 7.2. For 25 studs, it is sufficient to have as few as 25 queens. But in practice, it is unlikely that every breeder has equal numbers of studs and queens. Again, the larger the number of unrelated breeding studs and queens the better will be the prospects for the breed.

Keep in mind that for both cases it is assumed that the studs and queens will be bred more or less at random. That means that each individual stud and queen contributes equally to the next generation. This restriction applies particularly to the stud cats – one or more studs must not sire an undue majority of kittens used later for breeding. As it may be difficult to achieve equality in breeding practice, the numbers of studs and queens per generation should be increased to allow for this limitation.

In genetic terms, the consequence of inbreeding is to increase the homozygosity of the genome. That is, with inbreeding, the genes become progressively more alike. Genes occur in pairs in the genome, such as AA, Aa and aa, where A and a are two unlike genes. With inbreeding, the Aa pair is slowly eliminated, leaving only AA and aa. As there are tens of thousands of gene pairs in the genome, the elimination does not occur all at once, but progressively as the inbreeding continues.

The rate of elimination of heterozygosity varies with the rate of inbreeding. The greater the rate of inbreeding is, the more rapid is the elimination. The effect of inbreeding here is to make the breed genetically more homogeneous. This is desirable in establishing a breed, as the cats will tend to conform to the standard of excellence. However, the inbreeding also uncovers both good and bad aspects of the genome. Some of the bad aspects are subtle and induce 'inbreeding depression' The animals produced are then below par in growth and health, as well as in breeding. This is why emphasis must be placed upon selection for growth and health.

The purpose is to prevent these tendencies from becoming established. Only unremitting selection is capable of doing this. By selection of the most vigorous cats, it is likely that the more heterogeneous are chosen. This, in turn, is likely to counter the potential inbreeding depression. The genes for the depression are likely to be recessive and the selection should favor the AA and Aa genotypes in preference to aa.

Elimination of the Aa pairs of genes is a formal way of saying that inbreeding brings about a progressive loss of variation. Unfortunately, this is a double-edged sword. On the one hand, it is desirable because the individual cats become more and more alike. On the other hand, it also brings to a halt additional progress. Both good and bad characters are 'fixed' with fine impartiality. That fixation may (and often does) occur before all of the good points have been realized and some of the bad points have been eliminated. The greater the inbreeding, the quicker the fixation occurs.

A breeder must make a compromise between the rate of inbreeding and the loss of variation. The 5 per cent level should be regarded as the absolute maximum, with the one per cent as the more desirable level, particularly with so-called minority breeds. Table 7.2 presents the numbers of cats and queens that a breed should have to maintain a rate below the recommended level. A numerically small breed could be at risk in the long term, but so could a numerically large breed if it is subdivided into separate lines. If the subdivision is not rigid, a trickle of inter-group mating may be sufficient to maintain the overall well-being of the breed.

As noted, the situation is more serious for those breeds with a small number of breeding animals. Several methods may be available to help improve the situation for minority breeds. One would be to popularize the breed to recruit new adherants. Another would be to encourage breeders to make their stud cats more freely available. For example, a group of breeders might agree among themselves that no stud cat can be the sire of more than a stated percentage of matings. Ideally, there should be as many breeding cats as queens and no queen to be mated more than once to the same stud.

Another alternative might be to actively discourage matings closer than a given familial relationship. For instance, a group of breeders might agree to avoid breedings unless they show no common ancestors until the third or fourth generation. Finally, new stud cats could be imported from abroad, although the breeders would have to minutely scrutinize their pedigrees to assure that these are as unrelated as possible.

The problem of long-term inbreeding in breeds with limited numbers of breeding animals in each generation is complex. Although the general principles are easily stated, these vary from breed to breed and are complicated by other factors. What breeders must keep in mind is that **for all practical purposes breeding pedigree cats always involves some degree of inbreeding, even if it is not immediately evident on the pedigree itself**.

Inbreeding depression and hybrid vigor

Inbreeding can bring about a decline in vigor or general weakness. This is usually called 'inbreeding depression'. Loss of vigor is associated with the homozygosity of an increasing number of genes, with harmful effects. These are polygenes, in as much that the effect of any one in isolation is small. However, the cumulative effect can mount up and eventually become noticeable.

In the ordinary randomly bred population, most of these genes are present as heterozygotes so that their existence may be unsuspected until exposed by the inbreeding. This is not to suggest that all cats carry these genes, or that inbreeding must inevitably produce weakly stock. On the contrary, the inbreeding of inherently healthy stock is usually quite safe. On the other hand, some cats do carry deleterious genes and these deleterious genes may make their presence felt due to inbreeding. For this reason, inbreeding depression should watched for in any inbreeding situation.

In cases of inbreeding depression almost any feature of the normal cat may be affected:

- There may be a decline in birth weight or vigor, as shown by small, thin or lethargic kittens.
- There may be developmental problems, such as poor growth in later life and below standard adult individuals.
- There may be a fall in average litter size, an increase in the number of stillborn or abnormal kittens in litters.
- There may be problems in reproductive performance. This may be shown by a reluctance of the male to copulate, the female to come into heat or by partial sterility in either sex.
- There may be a greater proneness to illness at any stage of development, such as the regular appearance of cancer in younger animals. Alternatively, there may be significant losses of cats or kittens to the same disease, due to the loss of immunological diversity.
- There may be physical indications such as asymmetry, crooked noses, misaligned jaws, uneven eye size or alignment.

It is impossible to predict what form inbreeding depression may take in each case. For example, only one of these problems may be present, but be may be manifested in extreme examples. On the other hand, several may show small yet detectable deteriorations. In addition, inbreeding depression usually comes on gradually, affecting some individuals and not others.

[Cat breeders] must be careful not to 'fix' immunodeficiency when we are trying to 'fix' type.
                    Heather Lorimer, PhD, Oriental Shorthair breeder
                                                    Lorimer (1998)

This means inbreeding depression can be countered by breeding **only** from the most healthy cats in the program. This should be true at all times, but it is particularly important whenever any inbreeding is practiced.

Should inbreeding depression become established in spite of efforts to prevent it, there is virtually no option but to outcross to wholly unrelated stock. If the outcross is made wisely, the breeder should still be able to preserve many of the better qualities of the line or, at least, not to lose too many of these qualities.

It may also be desirable to intercross two inbred strains which are displaying early signs of inbreeding depression. This could happen when several inbred lines are being bred in parallel. Should this be done, the first-cross offspring may turn out to be exceptionally healthy and fertile. This phenomenon is known as hybrid vigor or 'heterosis'. It does not always occur, of course, but it occurs often enough that most breeders have at least heard of the phenomenon. Random bred cats rarely show heterosis because much of their taken-for-granted vigor is in fact heterosis of a less obvious kind.

Some breeds or lines of pedigreed cats show ongoing mild signs of inbreeding depression as a result of generations of selection and their somewhat inbred ancestry. This is often the case with breeds which are described as delicate, temperamental or hard to breed. This may be tolerated, provided it is not too severe, because to outcross would destroy their unique characteristics.

Inbreeding depression can be particularly insidious and pervade many individuals of a particular breed, particularly when a majority of cats are related in one way or another. Weak inbreeding is then very difficult to avoid. In such cases, every effort should be made to breed only from the most healthy cats to prevent the worsening of the situation.

Inbreeding and the appearance of anomalies

On occasion, breeders may express concern because it is felt that inbreeding can cause anomalies. While this concern is somewhat justified, it is not precisely the situation. In the first place, inbreeding itself cannot induce anomalies, but it can bring to light genetic defects which may be latent in the cats. In contrast, true random breeding tends to keep defects completely hidden or at least prevents their recurrence except for the odd cat here and there.

It is, therefore, possible for a recessive anomaly to be brought into the breeding program, persist for a few generations, and then be bred out without anyone being aware that it was there in the first instance. Those heterozygotes which may carry the defect are likely to be fully healthy, so there would have been no reason why anyone should be suspicious.

The chances of discovery of such a recessive defect vary with the amount of inbreeding. The chances of discovering it are small for weak (low percentages) inbreeding and not very great for moderate inbreeding. However, the chances of discovering it increase rather sharply for close inbreeding. This is the reason why inbreeding and the appearance of anomalies are associated.

If only a minority of studs possibly carry a recessive anomaly, then in most cases inbreeding does not produce anything abnormal. Of course, no one would be exactly pleased to discover an inherited anomaly. However, it is much better to know about it and then take immediate, active steps to eliminate it.

Fortunately, many recessive defects can be removed and several methods are described in this book. Thus, in some respects, inbreeding can be regarded as a cleansing operation, for it has a propensity to bring recessive defects to light. That, in turn, means it also leads to their eradication far more quickly than might occur through random mating. It should be emphasized that the chance occurrence of anomalies is not the same as inbreeding depression. It is a more troublesome and difficult problem to control.

Maximum avoidance of inbreeding

The occasion may arise where it is necessary to maintain a small group of animals with the minimum loss of heterozygosis. Such a case could be where a stud has attained a high level of perfection but signs of inbreeding depression have become evident. An outcross would be the obvious remedy but this is judged undesirable.

For practical or sentimental reasons, the owner may not wish to break-up the blood line or it may be that no outside stock is available of comparable quality. In this event, the decision whether to outcross or not may not be easy. One solution would be to increase the size of the stud so that larger numbers are available from which to select the most vigorous animals. However, if the selection is intense, as it should be in the circumstances, the number of parents is reduced and the stud will be exposed to inbreeding which may lead to further deterioration. The position is aggravated if it is only possible to keep a small number of animals.

A possible alternative would be to adopt a system of breeding in which the loss of heterozygosis is minimized. These take the form of groups of animals equally divided into males and females and are forms of cousin matings. Two of the simplest will be described, requiring only four and eight individuals per generation as shown by Figs 7.1 and 7.2, respectively. In the first, two males and two females are so paired that the resulting two litters (or two series of litters) provide either both the males or females for the next generation. It is important that the sexes be chosen from litters with different parents otherwise the system reverts to sib mating which it is expressly designed to avoid. The ratio of decrease of heterozygosity is 92 per cent, a value which cannot be bettered by any

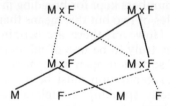

Figure 7.1 Diagram of pairings for a group of four cousins. Two different males (M) and two different females (F) form the group in each succeeding generation. These must be paired as shown by the lines of descent. The pairings repeat for each generation

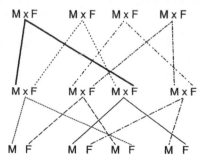

Figure 7.2 Diagram of parings for a group of eight cousins. Four different males (M) and four different females (F) form the group in each succeeding generation. These must be paired as shown by the lines of descent. The pairings repeat for each generation

other breeding system consisting of so few parents in each generation.

The second system requires four males and four females. The arrangement of pairing is more complicated and is best understood by reference to Fig. 7.2. Each of the four litters must provide two offspring for the next generation, a male and female. In the diagram, the letter M represents a male and the letter F a female, the lines of descent showing how the eight offspring must be paired for the next round of litters. Then, the whole process is repeated. In practice, both for the previous system and the present one, it is advisable to make out a sketch-plan showing the lines of descent but filling in the names of the animals in the cattery instead of the M and F symbols. The sketch-plan should be completed for two generations so that the pairing of the kittens is definitely fixed. Later, it will only be necessary to add a row of names for the next generation. This prevents unnecessary mistakes.

The ratio for the second system is 97 per cent which is again larger than other systems for a similar number of parents per generation The last two entries in Table 7.1 reveal how the two cousin groups preserve the amount of heterozygosis compared with other systems.

It is possible to propose a somewhat more flexible system of pairing than that outlined above for people who find it difficult to follow a set pattern. However, there are rules attached even to this system. The main one is that each pairing must contribute two offspring to the new generation. This is the same as before, of course, except that now there is no insistence that the pairs of offspring must be consistently of the same or unlike sex. Nor is there any need for the number of animals to be invariably four or eight. The numbers kept for breeding in each generation must necessarily be in multiples of two but this means that it is possible to have, for example, six or 10. However, there are certain rules which must be observed if the system is truly to be one of minimized inbreeding.

Though the choice of sex is left open as regards individual pairings, the total number of cats per generation must be equally divided into males and females. Thus, strictly speaking, complete freedom of choice only exists for the initial animals. Later selection of animals must take into account that the sexes should balance.

The advantages of the present system is the greater freedom of choice for at least half of the animals and that the pairing between the selected individuals need not follow a defined pattern. This is true, provided there is no inadvertent brother-to-sister pairing for too many consecutive generations. In fact, for the system to function as minimized inbreeding, it may be necessary to arrange that some brother-to-sister pairings are deliberately interspersed among more distant pairings. This policy implies that pairing within the system is not entirely at random but ought to be planned to some extent. At least, the pairings in successive generations have to be watched so as to avoid prolonged inbreeding, inadvertent as this may be.

Similarly, care must be taken that a group of eight breeding animals, for instance, are truly interbreeding and are not by mischance actually divided into two lines of four. The two cousin systems described above, on the other hand, obviate these worries because all of the pairings are fixed beforehand.

Once inbreeding depression has set in, sooner or later it is difficult to avoid making an outcross if the strain is to be saved. It is possible that one of the present breeding systems may defer the event and it is just possible that ruthless selection within the system might counter the depression. It is a hope, if the avoidance of outcrossing is that important. The usefulness of the two systems is that of a holding operation until suitable animals become available to which an outcross may be made.

Synopsis

The effects of selection versus inbreeding can be contrasted as follows:

Selection	Inbreeding
Small decline of heterozygosis	Steady decline of heterozygosis
Perpetuation of certain genes	Steady fixation of all genes
Increasing phenotypic similarity	Increasing genotypic similarity

A first reading of the tendencies induced by either selection of inbreeding might cause one to consider that the two processes are complementary and all one has to do is select the right animals and inbreed them. In very favorable circumstances, this might be feasible. The outcome would be a low level of heterozygosis, perpetuation of the desired phenotype and both phenotypic and genotypic fixation. Unfortunately, in practice, it is usually impossible to obtain animals correct in all of the characters which should be considered and too much inbreeding could bring about fixation of bad points before these can be eliminated.

A compromise has to be found and, generally, this will have the form of selective breeding (using any method which seems best for the problem in hand) in conjunction with moderate inbreeding. The rationale is that this program should bring together desirable combinations of genes and hold them until the inbreeding has led to the appropriate fixation. It must be emphasized that this is a general compromise. In special circumstances selection with the barest inbreeding may be the correct policy or selection with intense inbreeding may be more fitting. In essence, the degree of inbreeding is the factor which cannot be decided without knowledge of the problems to be overcome or the ultimate goal of the breeder.

Technical appendices

A: Calculating inbreeding from pedigrees

Inbreeding may be easily seen on the standard four or five generation pedigree. The pedigree should be visualized as being divided into two halves or 'sides'. Each side consists of those ancestors behind one of the parents. So the first side are the ancestors behind the sire and the second are those behind the dam. Inbreeding of some degree is present whenever an ancestor is present in both the sire's and the dam's sides, regardless of the generation in which it appears.

The impact of the inbreeding in a pedigree for an individual cat X can be revealed by two indicators:

- The number of different ancestors common to both sides of the pedigree.
- The number of times a common ancestor is repeated.

A third factor, which is often not revealed by a pedigree, is the degree of inbreeding for the common ancestor(s). That too impacts overall inbreeding.

A four generation pedigree for an individual cat consists of 30 ancestors, plus the cat. If all of the 30 ancestors are different, inbreeding is absent. If one or more ancestors are repeated, whether on one side or on both, then there is inbreeding present. However, if the repeat occurs in either the sire's or dam's side of the pedigree, there is inbreeding for the sire or for dam, but not for the individual cat. For the individual to be inbred, the repeated ancestor must be found on both the sire's and dam's sides of the pedigree.

Without any calculation it can be seen that the more remote the common ancestor, the less inbreeding is present. However, the exact degree, or closeness, of the inbreeding can be calculated by using the pedigree.

Taking the standard four generation pedigree with 30 ancestors of cat X, it shows 15 ancestors on the sire's side (indicated by the prefix S) and 15 on the dam's side (indicated by the prefix D) of the pedigree. The numbers in the pedigree represent the positions of ancestors for the two groups. For instance, the sire and dam of X are S1 and D1, respectively, while the four grandparents are S2 and S3 and D2 and D3, respectively, and so forth (see Fig. 7.3).

There is inbreeding whenever one or more common ancestors occur on both sire's and dam's sides of the pedigree. For example, a mating between a half brother and sister (that is cats having the same sire but different dams) will be shown in pedigree as an identical male at positions S2 and D2. If individual cat X is the offspring of a full brother and sister mating, not only would the same male be shown at positions S2 and D2, but the same female would be at positions S3 and D3.

The calculation is easy to do for the simplest cases of inbreeding. The procedure involves straightforward counting. Consider the half brother to sister breeding. Starting with the sire's side of the pedigree, count the number of generations forward from S2 to X, that is 2. Then count backwards on the dam's side, that is 1 step. Add these two figures, namely, 2 plus 1 to give 3. Take that number and multiplying 1/2 by itself that many times, or $1/2 \times 1/2 \times 1/2 = 0.125$. The final value is the amount of inbreeding for a half brother to sister mating, which is usually stated as a percentage or 12.5 per cent.

The full brother to sister mating is calculated in a similar manner, except now there are two common ancestors to be considered. The second common ancestor occurs at positions S3 and D3. The number of generations will be 2 from S3 to X and 1 back to D3, namely, 3. Multiplying 1/2 by itself three times gives 0.125 or, as a percentage, 12.5 per cent. Note that the results are exactly the same as the previous calculation. This is because the repeated ancestors S2 and S3 occupied similar positions in the pedigree.

Clearly, as both the common ancestors are contributing to the inbreeding, the values for each are added to give 25 per cent as the total inbreeding for X. As might be anticipated, the amount of inbreeding is thus twice that for half brother to sister mating (25 versus 12.5 per cent).

The full brother to sister mating is one of the closest forms of inbreeding. There is only one other as close – this is the mating of a parent to an offspring, either father to daughter or the less common mother to son. Take the more common example for a moment. The father will occupy positions S1 and D2 in the pedigree for such a mating. Counting in the usual manner gives forward from S1 to X, namely, 1, and back from X to D2, namely, 1. The total is 2. Multiplying 1/2 by itself gives 0.25 or 25 per cent. This is the identical percentage as found for brother sister mating. A similar count for the mother to son mating will reveal the same degree of inbreeding – 25 per cent.

A frequently encountered pairing is between first cousins. In a pedigree, this would appear as ancestors S2 and D3 having the same sire and dam, S4 and S5, and D6 and D7, respectively. Counting the generations for the sire gives 3 from S4 to X and 2 from X to S5, making 5 in all. The usual calculation produces 3.125 per cent as his contribution to the inbreeding. A similar count for the dam also gives 3.125. Adding the two values gives 6.25 per cent as the total inbreeding for a mating of what are sometimes called single first cousins.

It is always important to remember that the common ancestor is not counted when calculating the amount of inbreeding. That is because it is the number of generations (or individuals) separating the common ancestors which is important, a number which includes the individual cat X itself. Beginners frequently include the common ancestor in the calculations, because they feel that it must be involved in some manner. To do so always results in a significant underestimation of the amount of inbreeding.

Extending the analysis of inbreeding for many generations eventually becomes quite onerous, at the level of pencil and paper. However, the analysis can be greatly extended by the use of special computer programs which are incorporated with some pedigree software packages.

B: Complex inbreeding

It is superfluous to say that inbreeding can take many forms. It is obvious that the degree of inbreeding can vary from the intense (say, brother to sister or parent to offspring matings) to the very weak (where the familial relationship is not so distant that it may not even be regarded as inbreeding). Yet, if a collateral relationship can be shown between the parents, the offspring are inbred to some extent.

However, this is only the beginning of the story. An individual is inbred to some degree if it has an ancestor in common in both the sire's and dam's halves of the pedigree. Now, two situations arise: the common ancestor may occur but once, or it may recur a number of times. Several examples

Pedigree positions

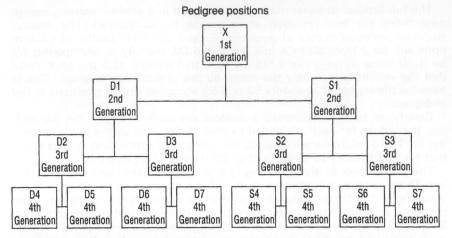

Figure 7.3 An example of a pedigree showing 3 generations of ancestors plus the individual cat (4 generation pedigree)

have been described previously for either situation.

The above may be cited as the simplest instances of inbreeding. More complicated cases are where two or more different common ancestors recur in the pedigree. It is easy to imagine that the inbreeding could vary from the slight to quite complicated cases. Within a four-generation pedigree there is not a great deal of scope for really complex inbreeding. However, if a pedigree is extended to include six, seven or more generations, the inbreeding could easily become complex.

There is yet another dimension of inbreeding which must be considered. This is where a common ancestor is inbred itself. The effect of this is to intensify the amount of inbreeding. That is to say, the amount is increased over and above that expected if the ancestor was not inbred. The increase reflects the presence of the remote common ancestors which contribute to the inbreeding.

An example will show how allowance is made for the effect of the inbreeding within a common ancestor. The allowance precedes in two stages. First of all, the inbreeding of the common ancestor must be calculated. Suppose that the ancestor is S2 shown on Fig. 7.3 who is the progeny of a half-brother to half-sister mating in generation four (not shown), namely S8 and S10 are the same male. The amount of inbreeding for half-brother to sister has been worked out previously and is 12.5 per cent.

If the male S2 occurs only in the male side of the pedigree for X, the inbreeding would not have any effect on X. This is because the ancestor must occur in both sides of the pedigree. Imagine now that S2 does occur on both sides of the pedigree, namely, additionally in position D2. Individual X is now the product of a half-brother to sister mating in the fourth generation, namely the DS and D10 is the same male as SS and S10. All other ancestors are assumed to be different.

If the inbreeding for X is a simple half-brother to sister mating, the amount will be 12.5 per cent. The path value in these circumstances would be (S2)-S1-X-D1-(D2). However, the present case is not simple, for the common ancestor for this inbreeding at positions S2 and D2 is inbred to the extent of 12.5 per cent. To allow for this inbreeding, a special term must be added to the path value. The term may be defined as the 'inbreeding term' and is found by multiplying the path value by the inbreeding of the common ancestor, namely 0.125. This will give 0.125 3 0.125 = 0.0156. Or 1.56 per cent The inbreeding term is added to the path inbreeding of 12.5 per cent to give 14.06 per cent as the final amount of inbreeding for the path.

When a pedigree under study has common ancestors, which are inbred themselves, the procedure is to calculate the amount of the inbreeding for each of the ancestors before proceeding to calculate that for X. Derive and make a note of the inbreeding term for each inbred ancestor. The method of paths should be used for analyzing the pedigree as a whole. The reason for this will become apparent later.

When each path for X has been calculated and, should the common ancestor be inbred, add the relevant inbreeding term to the path. The result will be the final value for the path. Sum these final values over all paths to obtain the amount of inbreeding for X.

Unfortunately, inbred common ancestors introduce a complication. The most important thing to keep in mind is this principle: the rule for a valid path is that all of the connecting ancestors must be different. Or, to reverse the rule, the invalid path is one where a connecting ancestor is present twice.

Unless the pedigree covers merely a few generations and the indicated inbreeding is simple, novices are forced to use paths for their inbreeding study. The method does have several advantages for large pedigrees. The most important is that this process could reveal unsuspected paths which otherwise might be overlooked. Remember, valid paths are those where all the connecting ancestors are different. However, even invalid paths have a function in such a study: these could easily reveal inbreeding of a common ancestor.

This analysis can be tedious and time consuming. Fortunately, computer programs are now available which can cope with quite large pedigrees with complex inbreeding determinations.

C: Law of descent

It should be apparent that the pedigree of an individual cat can yield valuable information on its constitutional background. The breeder who has most to gain from a study of a pedigree is someone who is familiar with the ancestors featured in it. Knowledge of the ancestral cats can be a useful guide to the breeding potential of the individual.

It is useful to yield some idea of the relative contributions of the ancestors making up the pedigree of an individual cat (say X). Is one more important than the others? If so, it would be desirable to know which ones. There is also the evergreen question of the amount of inbreeding.

To keep matters simple, only four or five generation pedigrees will be considered but the principles outlined can be extended to any number of generations. Consider first, the number of individuals involved per generation. These may be showed in Table 7.3 where X is the individual of the pedigree, 1 is the parental generation, 2 is the grandparental and so on. As is well known, the number of ancestors doubles for each successive ancestral generation.

Now, it may be stated that the parents contribute equally to the individual. Therefore, each contributes one half to the heredity of the individual. Each of the four grandparents contribute one quarter, and the great-grandparents each contributes one eighth, and so on. This is Francis Galton's

Table 7.3 Number of generations and number of cats in each in a five generation pedigree

Number of generations	X	1	2	3	4	5
Number of cats in each	1	2	4	8	16	32

'Ancestral Law of Inheritance' which was formulated in the late nineteenth century. The concept seems plausible and affords a useful mental picture but it should not be taken too literally because it fails to take account of the segregation of the genes.

The genes, whether considered singly or in total are present twice in the individual but once in the germ cells. Obviously, the fusion of germ cells at fertilization restores the double representation of the genes for each generation. This means that the chance of a particular gene being passed on from one parent to the next is one half. As this occurs for each generation, the probability of a particular gene being passed on from a grandparent is 1/2 times 1/2 equaling 1/4.

For the great-grand-parental generation, the probability is halved again as 1/2 3 1/2 3 1/2 = 1/8. Generalizing, the probability is 1/2 multiplied by the number of generations (n) removed from the individual or the reciprocal of the number of ancestors in the 'nth' generation.

Suppose now, that one particular ancestor occurs more than once in the pedigree. The probability of genes descended from that ancestor is increased. The above calculation is made for each occurrence and the results are summed. Note, that the recurrence need not be in the same generation. For instance, a common ancestor in the third and fourth generation has a probability of 1/8 plus 1/16 equaling 3/16 or 18.75 per cent. Had it also recurred twice in the fourth generation, this would have added another 1/16 to the probability, namely a total of 15 per cent. The result is in keeping with commonsense because the more an ancestor recurs, the greater is its contribution. These calculations show how it is possible to place a value on the probability for the contribution.

The above discussion has focused on ordinary descent, that which is unconnected with sex. In general, descent through the female is similar to the above and does not require special mention. However, the situation is different for the male. Genes carried by and exclusive to the male, i.e. those on the Y chromosome, are transmitted directly from father to son. These are very rare and are usually ignored unless special circumstances demand their attention.

What is happening at the level of the genes? The genes are present twice in the individual but once in the gene cells. Imagine that an individual A with the genes *AA*, is mated to an individual B, with has the genes *BB*. The offspring will have the constitution *AB*, receiving one gene from each parent. The offspring can pass on one only of the genes, either *A* or *B* at a probability of one half. This must be so because there are only two alternatives. It gene *A* is passed on, individual A's contribution is passed on but, if gene *B* is passed on, individual A's contribution is lost. This event will occur for each generation, with the equal possibility of 1/2 of either being passed on or being lost.

Under the law of compound probability, each single probability must be multiplied together to give the final probability. If individual A occurs in the third ancestral generation, the final probability will be 1/2 3 1/3 3 1/2 = 1/8 or 12.5 per cent. This is the value derived previously with a genetic meaning. It is the probability of the genetic contribution of progenitor A – the probability that some of its genes have survived the passage over the

Table 7.4 Probability of genes surviving over successive generations

Number of generations	1	2	3	4
Probability (%)	50	25	12.5	6.25

generations.

To calculate the probability of a single descent, it is only necessary to know the number of generations a progenitor is removed from X in the pedigree of X, whence a table of probabilities can be prepared once and for all (see Table 7.4).

The number of generations removed is the same as the position of the ancestor in the pedigree. This principle may be termed 'Law of Descent'. The total probability is the sum of probabilities for the number of recurrences of the ancestor.

The following is an interesting situation. The third generation consists of eight individuals, four males and four females, each with the probability of 12.5 of contributing genes to the individual X. Now, it is possible that each male and each female could be the same two cats, respectively. This means that, for each sex, there are four chances of the genes being passed on and that these must be added as stated earlier, to give a total probability of 12.5 + 12.5 + 12.5 + 12.5 = 50 per cent. There are only two different ancestral cats in the third generation and each contributes 50 per cent which, when added, gives the complete determination of the individual.

The sum of probabilities for individual X cannot exceed 100 per cent as in the case just considered where the two ancestors have contributed 50 per cent. The complete determination for X, in terms of probabilities for any generation, may be found as follows. Each line of descent must be considered and, for any ancestral generation, these will equal the number of ancestors. This is shown explicitly by the example just considered, where eight lines correspond to the eight ancestors of generation three.

Tracing lines of descent back to ancestors in different generations may raise a point which could be a source of confusion. Each successive generation opens up two additional lines. If one of these ancestors has been previously found to be the terminating ancestor of a line, the tracing must stop at this point and the probability computed for each line to derive the total probability. When a repeated ancestor occurs in different generations, some lines may be left 'dangling', as it were. These will be the partners to the ancestor. To complete the analysis of the pedigree, probabilities must be calculated for these even if they are 'loners'; occurring only once in the pedigree. Adding these will be a check on the calculations as the total probability must sum up to 100 per cent.

Should it be desirable to consider the particular contribution of a remote ancestor, it is possible that an earlier repeated ancestor may stand in the way. To perform the calculation in this case, the earlier ancestor should be ignored. However, if an ancestor is bypassed in this manner, all occurrences of the ancestor must be similarly bypassed. The calculations should proceed as if the ancestor represents two different individuals.

The contributions of recent ancestors are of greater importance than those of earlier generations and should be given preference. The contribution of a remote ancestor can be very small and, at some stage, can be considered to be negotiable. Two commonly adopted 'cut out' levels are when the contribution is less than 1 and 0.1 per cent. These levels will be when a repeated ancestor first appears at the seventh and 10th generation, respectively. The only exception is where the ancestor recurs as, even at these distant generations, the contribution may not be negligible. However, few breeders feel the need to trouble themselves with generations so far removed from the present. Indeed, a genealogical computer program may be required to handle the very large number of ancestors involved and to perform the arithmetic.

Although the contributions for various ancestors can only be expressed as probabilities and should not be taken as absolute determinants of the total genetic constitution of individual X, they should, however, be regarded as useful guides. The derived probabilities are open to two different interpretations depending on the adopted view point; whether that of descent of a particular gene or that of the genetic constitution as a whole.

At the level of an individual gene, the probability is that of a given gene being descended from a given ancestor. A gene commences its transmission at 100 per cent but has a finite probability of being lost at each generation. At the level of the total number of genes, which for a cat may be in the region of between 50 000 to 100 000, the probability may be regarded as the percentage of this number which has descended from a given ancestor.

D: Pedigrees

Breeders and geneticists both need the information provided by accurate pedigrees. However, over time, they have slightly diverged on how they label these:

- When breeders and registries refer to an 'n' generation pedigree, they usually include the cat whose pedigree they have in counting. Thus, for a breeder or cat registry, a four generation pedigree includes the individual cat plus *three* generations of ancestors (see Fig. 7.3).
- When a geneticist refers to a pedigree with four generations, he is usually referring to one with the individual cat plus *four* generations of ancestors (see Table 7.3).

Chapter 8

Coat inheritance

Coat composition

Before discussing the distinctive features of the various coat texture genes, the different hair fibers that make up the normal coat need to be described. Three main types are recognized:

- Guard hairs.
- Bristle or awn hairs.
- Down or wool hairs.

The guard and awn hairs are sometimes called, collectively, the top-coat, and the down hairs, the undercoat. All of the hair types serve a function in the animal:

- The down hairs serve mainly as an insulating barrier against excessive heat loss.
- The guard and awn hairs serve as a protective covering to the soft undercoat and provide sensory functions.
- The vibrissae or facial whiskers are extra stout hairs devoted primarily to a tactile function.

The three hair types are distinct and their unique appearance may be differentiated with the aid of a good lens. The guard hairs are normally straight and taper evenly to a very fine point. The awn hairs are thinner than the guard hairs and have a characteristic thickening in diameter (subapical swelling) near the tip of the hair before tapering to a fine point. The down hairs are the thinnest of the three types. They are of similar diameter throughout their length and are more or less evenly undulated or 'crimped'. The appearance of the awn hairs tends to be the most variable. Some may approach the guard hairs in thickness and form; while others may approach the down hairs in thinness, even to the extent of becoming crimped and showing a barely perceptible subapical swelling. The latter have been called awn–down hairs. If necessary, it is possible to distinguish three categories of awn hairs, but it must be emphasized that all three categories can overlap in appearance. The guard hairs are slightly longer than the other two types and the awn hairs are longer than the down hairs. This difference may result, in part, from the crimping.

All three hair types display a rather abrupt constriction in diameter at the point of entry into the skin. But they thicken again subcutaneously to form a slightly elongated club. This constriction probably enables the skin follicle surrounding the hair to grip and hold the hair. The hair lies in a sheath of flexible and probably contractile tissue that is of smaller diameter than the club. The club functions as an anchor, working in conjunction with cell adhesion at the base of the thickened region, to hold the hair in place. The adult cat has a diffuse molt. New hairs are produced throughout the year while old hairs are being shed. This is combined with a seasonal molt in late summer where replacement of new hairs reaches a peak, then gradually slowing to its lowest point in mid-winter. This cycle is similar for both sexes, except that the male begins to molt his coat about two months in advance of the female. Neutering of males appears to have no effect on the amount of molting nor on the cycle. The hairs of the winter coat are slightly longer than those of the summer coat, possibly as a result of an extended growth period.

The coat of the longhaired cat contains all three types of hair fiber. Their form appears to be unaltered except for length. The remarkable difference in length between the random-bred cat and the exhibition long hair is due to modifying genes. Long hair is a result of an extension in the period of hair growth. However, the ultra short coat of the Cornish Rex, for example (see later), is most likely caused by a slower rate of growth. The period of growth remains the same or similar between the normal and rex animal.

Rex hair

It is a common fallacy that the rex genes completely eliminate guard and awn hairs. This is a very over-simplified picture of the changes that take place. The typical soft rex coat is produced by abundant down hairs that are more or less normal. However, all of the various hair fibers are reduced in length and thickness, with the guard and awn hairs affected to a greater extent than the down hairs. In some individuals, the guard hairs may indeed be largely suppressed but, in most, the guard hairs persist. However, they so closely resemble the down hairs that a microscopic examination is necessary to distinguish them from one another. In some animals, the guard hairs can be seen above the undercoat as mere shadows of their normal selves. The length of the rex coat is variable and this probably parallels to a great extent the variation found in normal coats. The nature and degree of wave or curliness varies between different animals. It is related to the length of the hair fibers, the presence of an exaggerated curvature to the rex hair and the tendency for the individual fibers to 'lay' in a similar direction. This can cause a streaming effect and brings about a marcelled type of wave in contrast to a more randomized pattern of tight curls. Rex cats with these two extremes of curliness appear very different. They also differ markedly from the rex with a smooth coat having a minimum of wave or curl.

Five of the various rex coats have been examined in detail. In three rexes (Cornish, German and Oregon) the guard hairs appear to be lacking or, if not lacking, reduced to the appearance of awn hairs. This is in contrast to the Devon and Selkirk Rex that have all three hair types. The number of guard hairs vary from cat to cat; many display the subapical swelling that is characteristic of the hair type. The relative thickening, however, does not seem to be as great as that shown by the normal awn hair. In fact, it is not unusual for the distal swelling to be absent or barely perceptible. In this event, the hairs have the appearance of extra thick down hairs. It is not uncommon for a graduation in thickness to occur between the down hairs and the presumptive awn type hairs. This aspect may not have special significance, as awn hairs can also be highly variable in normal coats.

The German Rex coat contains awn hairs more persistently and more obviously than in the other rex breeds. In fact, no individual has yet to be found without them. The difference in thickness between the down fibers and the awn hairs is more marked and the subapical swelling is a little more pronounced than that found in the awn hairs of the Cornish Rex. The awn hairs in the German Rex would seem to reach a higher level of development than the Cornish. Not only are the awn hairs more well formed, but they seem to be more abundantly distributed in comparison with those present in the Cornish Rex coat. It is of interest that, while the awn hairs vary in thickness, there is no real evidence for the presence of a third type that could be labeled a guard hair. As the Cornish and German rexes have been shown to be mutations at the same locus, the variation in number of awn hairs probably reflects a difference of genetic background between the West of England and East German cat populations. That difference would be that the German population contained polygenes that encouraged the formation of numerous awn hairs.

The awn hairs are just slightly more well formed in the German Rex compared with those of the Cornish; however, the awn hairs of the Oregon Rex are even more well formed and thicker than those of the German. In the Oregon Rex, awn hairs are abundant in all fur samples examined and show unmistakable subapical swelling. The awn hairs also seemed to project a little more above the general coat level provided by the down hairs. This is supported by the impression that the Oregon awn hairs are noticeably less bent and curved over than those of the Cornish and German rexes. Once again, though the Oregon awn hairs show variation, there is no indication that a guard hair type is present.

The coat of the Devon Rex, in contrast, appears to have three types of hair. Both guard and awn hairs seem to be represented by stouter hairs of two grades of thickness. These hairs, however, are more grossly abnormal than the awn hairs of the other rexes. Instead of being of even or smoothly changing diameter, they are strikingly uneven and given to excessive constrictions in places. They also terminate abruptly in many instances, as if growth never began as a fine point or as if distal portions have been broken off. This latter possibility is supported by the observation of broken, but unparted, hairs on several occasions. This has not been observed in hair samples of any of the other rexes. The Devon Rex guard or awn hair could be more brittle than the ordinary hair or the irregularities of diameter noted earlier could produce weak points along its length. The constant grooming by the rough tongue of the cat could be responsible for the breakage. The Devon Rex rarely has a full complement of whiskers, not even as a young kitten. As older kittens or as adults, it is quite common for the whiskers to be absent or merely represented by a few bent stubs. This is a trait the breed shares with the Selkirk Rex. The Devon Rex also experiences a rapid loss of hair before the growth of a new coat, a feature unique to the breed. The coarse hairs present in the Devon Rex can be identified by a sensitive hand. It is these which set it apart from the other rex breeds.

The Selkirk Rex, like the Devon, exhibits all three types of hairs. Microscopic examination of the coat reveals that the hairs are shorter and thinner than normal. The coat on the body has sparse guard and awn hairs, a finding that would account for the softness. However, long thin guard or awn hairs were more prevalent on the tail. The whiskers and brow hairs are short and crooked and easily broken off.

The question that now arises is how much of the observed differences is due to the action of the rex genes themselves and how much is due to the genetic background? Only extensive intercrossing of the various rexes could provide a positive answer to this question. Unfortunately such intercrossing is not likely to occur. On the other hand, a little speculation may be in order. As will be discussed later, simple crosses between the Cornish, Devon and Oregon rexes have determined that each one is caused by a distinct, recessive mutation. The Selkirk Rex is unique in that it is caused by a dominant gene. Because of this, it is improbable that each gene will produce exactly the same biochemical effect, implying that differences due to the type of rex gene may well occur.

Long hair

The longhaired cat owes its unusually profuse coat to a recessive gene with the symbol l. This trait is most likely caused by a mutation in a gene responsible for producing a factor that defines the period of the growth cycle of the hair. Without a proper chemical signal to end the growth cycle, the period (known as the anagen phase) is abnormally extended. The length of coat is variable in the normal cat and these differences are more pronounced in the long hairs. The random-bred long hair has a shorter and coarser coat than that of the exhibition animal. In the latter, the coat is not merely longer but also feels more silky. This could result solely from the increase in length, but it seems possible that there has been a greater proportional increase in the length of the down hairs. The effect of this would be to produce a 'fuller' coat of exquisite texture. These differences of length and texture are due to polygenic factors and are the consequence of decades of patient selective breeding. Cats heterozygous for this factor may have identifiably different coats from a homozygous shorthair.

Genes and rexing

Cornish Rex

The first of the mutants to become popularly known was discovered in 1950 and is the Cornish Rex (or rex-1, as it was formerly known). This mutation is inherited as a recessive trait and has the symbol r. The rex coat is very different from the normal coated cat and, once seen, can never be forgotten. The coat is soft to the touch, mole-like, with an apparent absence of projecting guard and awn hairs. There is a definite tendency towards waviness in many individuals, which produces either a marcelled effect or that of waves of tight curls. The whiskers are shorter than normal, more curved and often bent. This latter feature provides a ready means of identification of rex homozygotes from an early age. The coat density varies from a thin, limp covering to one in which the hairs form a thick even pelage.

A longhaired Cornish Rex has been produced. The resulting animal is clearly rex as evidenced by its bent whiskers. The coat fibers are longer than normal but shorter and seemingly thinner than those of the ordinary long hair. The coat, therefore, has features of both hair types. This shows that the action of each gene is independent of each other and can function in combination.

Devon Rex

A second rex mutant was found in Devonshire in 1960. Crosses between it and the Cornish Rex soon revealed that the two are unrelated. The Devon Rex gene behaves as a recessive trait and has been symbolized by *re*. The new form was known as rex-2 for a period, but this ungainly designation has been discarded in favor of the more appropriate title of Devon Rex. In appearance, this rex is very similar to the Cornish. The coat is short and even in length, with a spurious lack of guard hairs by ordinary inspection. Again, there is a tendency towards waviness. There is a greater propensity for the Devon Rex to lose its coat and to have bare areas, especially on the belly, which persist until the next molt. The amount of hair loss varies between different individuals and is seemingly due to genes inherited independently of the rex gene.

A notable and probably a distinctive feature of the Devon Rex relates to its whiskers. The whiskers of the majority of animals are lost at an early age and many animals never seem able to retain more than a few stubs for any length of time. The existence of these stubs is suggestive that the whiskers are lost by breakage, rather than by a falling out of the hairs. Even at the best of times, the Devon Rex cat never, or rarely, has such a full complement of whiskers as carried by other rex mutants. The effect is enhanced by the relatively greater crookedness of those which do remain.

It is not entirely certain if the homozygous 'double rex' of genotype *rrrere* has been produced but, if it has, it will be a rex cat possessing the main features of each mutant. The coat would be expected to be softer in texture than the coat produced by either mutant by itself. The coat would lack guard hairs (due to the effect of *r*) and have hairs with constrictions along their length (due to *re*). The whiskers would be sparse or mere stubs, due again to *re*. There may be bare areas. One such rex has been identified by microscopic examination, but not confirmed by breeding tests.

German Rex

A third rex has appeared in East Germany, in East Berlin to be precise, in 1951. There is circumstantial evidence that the animal, a female, was born several years previously and could be the first of the recognized rex cats, chronologically speaking. The coat is typical, being smooth and soft, with a tendency to wave. There is an apparent absence of guard hairs and the whiskers are bent. Experiments soon disclosed that the German Rex was inherited as a recessive trait. The most interesting finding was not made until many years later. A few animals had been exported to the USA. There crosses between Cornish and German rexes produced rex kittens. This revealed that the two rexes genes are mutations at the same locus.

Oregon Rex

One of the most interesting of the various American rex mutants is that known as 'Oregon Rex' after its place of origin. The symbol *ro* is used to represent this gene. This rex was found in 1959 and was being bred by a group of enthusiasts for a while. Now, it appears to no longer be a viable breed. It is inherited as a recessive to the normal coat as in the case of all of the previous rex forms. Crosses between the Oregon Rex and both the Cornish and Devon rexes have produced kittens with normal coats. Thus, it would appear that multiple independent rex mutations are known for the cat.

Selkirk Rex

A new type of rex was discovered in Montana, USA, in 1987. The Selkirk Rex gene is inherited as a dominant trait, unlike the other rex genes. It is symbolized by the designation *Se*. At birth and as kittens, the coat is soft and wavy. By approximately two months of age the coat is at a phase where it is less curly. It then gives way in the adult cat to a dense, exceptionally soft and wavy coat. The combination of the Selkirk Rex gene with long hair results in a longer coat that is soft to the touch although the waviness can be less evident. The homozygous animal appears to have an identifiable appearance, with tighter curl, but a less dense coat. Like the Devon, whiskers appear to be very brittle, and break off easily.

Other rexoid mutants

It is of interest to record that even instances of rex mutants have been observed. One occurred in Italy about 1951. Little is known of the Italian rex except that three rex kittens were born by a normal mother. Without placing undue emphasis on this evidence, it could be surmised that the form is due to a recessive gene. The Oregon Rex of the USA has already been described, but it is worth mentioning that other cases have been reported from the USA. By all accounts, these have occurred at widely separated points. A form from Ohio was observed as early as 1952 but was treated very casually and was allowed to die out. Several rex animals were bred from the same normal coated parents. This would suggest that a single recessive gene has been observed.

Another instance occurred in California in 1960, apparently combined with long hair. Interbreeding with normal coated animals indicated that the rex type was inherited as a recessive. Hearsay evidence has it that crosses between the Californian rex and the Cornish Rex produced normal kittens. Rexed kittens, with a recessive mechanism of inheritance, have also been reported in the Maine Coon and colorpoint longhair (Himalayan) breeds.

All of the early occurrences of rexoid mutants have been, or are surmised to be, inherited as recessive to normal coat. This is not obligatory, of course. More recently, two cases of rex type coats have found to be inherited as dominant to normal coat. The first occurred in Holland; and there was some indication that the gene was not fully dominant, the homozygote appearing to have a more sparse coat than the heterozygote. The second case is the Selkirk Rex that was discovered in the USA and described above.

Wire-hair

The wire hair coat mutation occurred in the USA. It seems to be inherited as a simple monogenic trait with incomplete penetrance, dominant to normal coat. The mutation is designated by the symbol *Wh*. In appearance, the coat is rough and unruly in contrast to the smooth even coat of the normal animal. All three hair types are present but are abnormal. The guard hairs appear thinner than normal and are curved rather than straight. The awn hairs seem to be characteristically abnormal. These are thin but have the typical subapical swelling. Most of them show exaggerated undulation and a 'shepherd's crook' type of configuration in the region of the subapical swelling. The down hairs also display exaggerated and irregular curvature; unlike the more regular undulation of the normal hair. The overall effect is a sparse, wiry coat, coarse to the touch.

Chapter 9

Color inheritance

Introductory note

In this section colors and patterns are described in a technical sense only. The various registries around the world use some of these terms in very defined ways. For example, Siamese refers to the point-restricted color. Registries themselves differ on what colors are allowed to be shown under that breed name. The same is true for terms describing color placement and distribution. Here, references to black and white encompass everything from the van pattern to harlequin through bicolor to particolor, to use just a few of the terms in registry color descriptions.

It should be kept clearly in mind that genetics and registry terms are linked but not necessarily equivalent. It is best to keep in mind the registries' place in the breeder's litany: just because you can breed it does not mean you have a right to register it; and just because you can register it does not mean you have the right to show it.

A standard of comparison

In order to clearly describe variations in phenotype seen in a particular species, it is important to have a standard against which each individual can be compared. By convention, this standard is the phenotype seen in the natural, original state of the species. For instance, in domestic animals this standard describes the original, non-domesticated ancestor. In cats, this phenotype is that of the short coated, mackerel striped tabby as found in the European wild cat (*Felis silvestris*). Specimens of this type of tabby may be seen in almost all mongrel cat populations throughout the world. The genetic basis for this coloration has been passed down from primordial wild ancestors and persists more or less unchanged to the present day.

Eye color

Eye color in cats displays a remarkable degree of variation. The iris color may represent shades from chartreuse to emerald green, from gray-green to gold, from yellow to deep copper, or from pale gray to sapphire blue, depending on the breed. The more vivid, striking colors often belong to exhibition animals, while the more intermediate colors belong to random bred animals. Despite claims to the contrary, there appears to be no reliable evidence for monogenic control of eye color. The variation from yellow to orange is particularly distinctive and every graduation in-between can be seen. It may be assumed that the inheritance of this feature is polygenic.

A few of the color genes have an influence on eye color and, to this extent, it is possible to speak of monogenic mechanisms. The most obvious effect is the blue or bluish eye color produced by the genes for dominant white, Siamese, and blue-eyed albino and the unique aqua eye created in the Tonkinese c^s/c^b heterozygote. It seems feasible that the brown and dilution genes could have some effect on eye color. If this is so, however, this effect appears to be masked by the general degree of variability seen in the shade of eye color. The cat appears to be remarkable among mammals in having such variation of iris color.

The range of eye color occurring in a population of cats can be influenced by selective breeding. The spectrum of possible eye colors starts with blue eyes and continues through green eyes, yellow eyes, gold eyes, copper eyes and concludes with brown eyes, in order of increasing amounts of eye pigmentation. The deepest blue eyes in pointed cats are a result of the pigment reducing effects of the albinism allele combined with a low inherent amount of pigmentation. Thus, full colored cats from lines producing exceptionally deep blue eyes in pointed offspring, are more likely to have green eyes. Pointed cats from lines producing deep copper eyes in full-colored offspring, are more likely to have paler blue eyes than those from lines producing green or yellow eyed full-colored offspring.

Tabby and non-agouti

Tabby striping – A-

The wild type tabby pattern consists of black pigment (eumelanin) against a yellowish ground color (phaeomelanin). The gene that controls the deposition of color in this manner is highly conserved among all mammalian species and produces a molecule called the agouti protein. As a hair grows within its follicle, eumelanin is produced by cells within the follicle called melanocytes and deposited into the growing hair. As the amount of agouti protein increases within the melanocyte, eumelanin production is inhibited, resulting in a shift to production of phaeomelanin that is then deposited into the hair (Bultman, 1994). The agouti protein also inhibits phaeomelanin, but not as thoroughly as eumelanin. This results in a hair that is black at the tip, but yellow at the base. This occurs for each hair as it grows, resulting in the characteristic ticked, agouti coloration. The color is most commonly recognized as the natural color of the wild mouse or rabbit.

The cat, however, possesses a second system of pigmentation that these other species lack, through a mechanism that produces dark stripes interspersed through this agouti coat. This striping is caused by a marked reduction in the amount of agouti protein receptors or agouti protein itself in certain areas of the skin, eliminating the eumelanin to phaeomelanin shift. Hairs within these regions incorporate the eumelanin pigment from base to tip. The effect creates the impression of one pattern imposed upon another; a coexistence of camouflage colors which appears to be standard to most members of the cat family.

The mackerel tabby pattern can be seen in almost any mongrel population. It is characterized by the presence of vertical, gently curving stripes on the sides of the body. These may be continuous or broken into bars and spots, particularly on the flanks and on the stomach.

A second type of tabby is also found in most mongrel populations. This is the blotched or classic tabby. The head markings of this form are similar to those of the mackerel but the body pattern is very different. The even, vertical striping is replaced by broader bands which form whorls and spiral arrangements. The legs and tail are more heavily barred. The blotched pattern is variable with respect to the width of the bands and the amount of fusion they may display. Where the coalescence is extensive, a very dark tabby is produced.

A third type of tabby is found in the Abyssinian breed and has been passed to the Somali, Singapura, Asian and Oriental breeds (including Siamese). In this form, the tabby striping is minimized leaving only the underlying agouti coloration. Little or no evidence of striping is normally present on the body, though some may be observed on the face, legs and tail. Usually, the barring is finer than that displayed in the mackerel pattern, although this is not always so. In the best specimens of the Abyssinian breed, the legs and tail are devoid of barring or, at least, can only be seen with careful scrutiny. The depth of color in the phaeomelanin band may vary from yellowish-gray to a ruddy-brown but this variation is independent of the gene for the Abyssinian tabby pattern. Thus, while the striping is usually regarded as an integral part of 'tabby' coloration (certainly with the general public), not all genetic forms of tabby express themselves as stripes.

It had been believed for many years that the three forms of tabby pattern were inherited as an allelic series; however, it now appears as if at least two, and probably three, different loci are responsible for the various tabby patterns (Lorimer, 1995). At one locus is the Abyssinian or ticked tabby pattern, which is epistatic to both mackerel and to blotched tabby patterns. At another locus are the alleles for mackerel and blotched tabby patterns, with mackerel dominant to blotched. At another locus there appears to be a modifying gene for either the classic or mackerel patterns, resulting in the spotted tabby pattern. Other modifying factors are undoubtedly present, resulting in the wide variety of striped and spotted patterns seen in our various cat breeds.

The symbols for the three patterns have traditionally been: Abyssinian, t^a; mackerel, T; and blotched, t^b. However, as recent evidence has demonstrated that these forms are not allelic, a different nomenclature, by convention, should be used. It has been proposed to use the letters *Mc* to represent the dominant mackerel tabby pattern, while *mc* will represent the recessive classic, blotched tabby pattern. The letter *T*, therefore, would indicate the ticked tabby locus. Thus *T* would represent the Abyssinian form of tabby pattern and *t* would represent the absence of this pattern.

Expression of the Abyssinian pattern may manifests itself in two ways:

- As weak striping on the legs and rings on the tail for the heterozygote $T^a t^a Mc$ – or $T^a t^a mcmc$.
- As the absence or reduction of these markings for the homozygote $T^a T^a Mc$ – or $T^a T^a mcmc$.

There is variation in the expression of the markings and it is not impossible for some homozygotes to have faint markings. However, the two forms usually can be distinguished.

There appears to be at least two forms of the spotted tabby pattern. The first is a modification of the mackerel or blotched tabby in which the vertical stripes are discontinuous and take the form of short bars or spots. Modification of the blotched tabby pattern is seemingly responsible for the attractive round 'ocicat' type spots. Breeding data suggest a dominant modifying gene (provisionally symbolized as *Sp*) responsible for the spotted tabby phenotype. This change in the appearance of the stripes is almost certainly refined by polygenic factors. At one time, it was thought that the spotted tabby could be yet another allele of the *T/tb* tabby series. Breeding evidence suggests that this is not the case, as litters have been produced with all three patterns in a manner inconsistent with a single locus theory (Lorimer, private communication).

The second form of spotting expresses itself in more distinctive, rounded spots in a more random pattern. The case for a separate genetic allele, is much stronger for this form. Hybrids between domestic and non-domestic cats, such as in the Bengal breed, demonstrate that distinct spotting patterns can result from genetic factors obtained through such crosses. A unique recessive 'marble' pattern is seen in offspring of Bengal cats that are heterozygous for the spotting factor.

Non-agouti – *aa*

The gene responsible for the agouti pattern of the tabby has produced a mutant allele known as non-agouti. When this mutation is present, a defective agouti protein is produced that does not have the same strong inhibitory effect on eumelanin production as the normal protein. Eumelanin-containing granules are then deposited throughout the hair shaft in all stages of its growth. The resultant phenotype is the self black cat. Though the animal is uniformly black in appearance, it carries one of the tabby alleles in its genotype. The underlying tabby pattern is often revealed in the coat of young kittens and sometimes in the adult under certain circumstances because of the small remaining inhibitory power of the mutant agouti protein. Either the mackerel or blotched pattern is often discernible in young cats held up to reflected light. If no pattern is observed, this could mean that the Abyssinian genotype is present, but not necessarily. The non-agouti gene is inherited as a recessive and is represented by the symbol *a*.

In both agouti and non-agouti cats, phaeomelanin production is inhibited as the growth cycle of the hair advances. The inhibitory effects of the mutated agouti protein have nearly the same effect on phaeomelanin production as the non-mutant form. This results in similar phenotypes between agouti and non-agouti cats that are red or cream in color. Distinct 'solid' red cats or strongly marked red tabby cats can be produced through selective breeding for the desired appearance, as modifying polygenes are undoubtedly responsible for the degree of striping in all cats.

Wide band

A gene has been hypothesized as being responsible for changing ordinary tabby coloration into the more brightly colored golden tabby. The presumed effect of the gene is to widen the agouti band on the hairs. In addition, the gene is said to make the tabby pattern less distinct or blurred. The overall effect is a tabby of a rich golden hue. Longhaired cats expose more of the agouti band and do not have such an obvious tabby pattern as do shorthaired cats. This may be responsible for many cases of this phenomenon. Examination of hairs from golden tabbies reveals that they are nearly completely yellow with a black tip, with a suggestion of pale blue at the base. This is just as would be expected for a wide band phenotype. The golden tabby, shaded golden and chinchilla golden were developed from chinchilla longhairs. This may explain the difference between the silver tabby and chinchilla silver phenotypes. The breeding data to substantiate the existence of the wide band gene are slim; but the gene has been theorized as a dominant (either complete or incomplete) and has been provisionally symbolized by *Wb* (Robinson, unpublished observations).

However, the apparent difference between silver tabbies and chinchilla silvers, and thus brown tabbies and goldens, could be easily explained by polygenetic effects on the quantitative expression of the agouti and inhibitory proteins. As the level of these inhibitory proteins increases, pigment production is reduced. A chinchilla golden is simply a brown tabby with such high amounts of agouti protein production that the agouti shift occurs very early during hair growth. This inhibitory effect is so strong that it causes the shade of yellow pigment seen in the agouti band to change to a lighter color characteristic of golden cats. This maximization of agouti protein production has resulted from generation upon generation of selective breeding for the extreme inhibition of pigment production seen in the chinchilla silver.

Brown alleles – *B*, *b*, *b^l*

This site on a chromosome, commonly referred to as the brown locus, results in a change in the shape of eumelanin pigment granules. They change from the normal round, almost spherical shape to either oval in the case of bb (chocolate) cats or to a rod shape in $b^l b^l$ (cinnamon) cats. It is hypothesized that a lower degree of polymerization (chaining) exists in the eumelanin produced in the melanocytes of these cats (Ozeki, 1995). The two mutant brown alleles change the normal black appearance created by normal granules into different intensities of chocolate or brown. The color change is most obvious when combined with non-agouti to produce the solid, dark chocolate brown of the Havana ($aabb$) or the lighter cinnamon brown ($aab^l b^l$) that can be seen in the Oriental breed. Wild type allele B is dominant to both b and b^l, and b is dominant to b^l. Therefore both the heterozygote bb^l and the homozygote bb have the phenotype of chocolate brown.

The brown alleles do not appear to modify yellow (phaeomelanin) pigment-containing granules or, if they do, they seem to have the effect of producing a 'brighter' shade of these colors. It seems probable that b^l has a greater effect than b. However, this difference may not be evident given the variety of shades normally seen in red and cream cats.

Albino alleles

The albino series of alleles in the cat are particularly noteworthy because, between them, they are responsible for several of the cat fancy's most popular breeds. An essential enzyme for pigment production is manufactured at the albinism locus. This enzyme is called tyrosinase. The aromatic ring of the amino acid tyrosine gives eumelanin and phaeomelanin their unique color producing properties. The tyrosinase enzyme is responsible for incorporating tyrosine into these pigments.

In cats, there are five known albinism alleles: full color (C), Burmese (c^b), Siamese (c^s), blue-eyed albino (c^a) and pink-eyed albino (c). All four of the mutant alleles are recessive to full color but not necessarily to each other (Table 3.1). The c^b allele is incompletely dominant to c^s, resulting in an intermediate phenotype between Siamese and Burmese coloration in these heterozygotes. There is not enough information available to determine the interrelationships of c^b to c^a or c. Incomplete dominance is almost certain according to preliminary observations.

The normal gene C results in the production of black and orange pigment at full strength (hence the designation 'full color'). Biochemically, the various alleles cause a progressive reduction of pigment. With the c^b homozygote, the black eumelanin pigment is changed to a dark sepia or seal brown, while the orange appearing phaeomelanin is reduced to yellow. The black form of this color is referred to as 'Burmese brown', 'sable', or 'seal sepia'. It should not be confused with the recessive chocolate brown color created by the b allele at another locus. Color at the points (nose, ears, feet and tail) is usually darker than on the body, a feature that is obvious in kittens but less apparent in adults. The irises of the eyes appear to be less deeply pigmented than normal. They display a tendency towards yellowish-gray, or yellowish-green color and only rarely rich gold.

With the c^s homozygote, the dark sepia color is restricted to the points. This results in a body fur color of off-white or pale sepia, varying in shade.

The eyes are even more deficient in pigment resulting in blue color. In the c^a homozygote, no pigment develops in the coat (not even on the points) and the eyes are a pale blue. Finally, in cats homozygous for the c allele, pigment is totally absent. The fur is white and the eyes are pink because the blood is illuminated by light rays passing through the translucent tissue of the eye structures.

The albino cat reported in the USA and continental Europe does not appear to be true albinism seen in other species. The coat is white and the pupils of the eyes are a ruby red, but the irises are a pale milky-blue instead of being pink. This coloration could indicate either the presence of a small amount of pigment (less than in the eyes of the Siamese) or that the iris of the cat is bluish because of its structure. The former appears to be the more likely explanation. The few genetic studies that have been completed indicate that the blue-eyed albino is inherited as a recessive to full color and to Siamese. Tentatively, it is assumed that a mutation has occurred to an allele (c^a) just short of true albinism and positioned between Siamese and pink-eyed albino.

The existence of the complete pink-eyed albino has been described in the 1930s. However, the complete form has been discovered in the USA the 1980s. The albino allele is inherited as a recessive to full color (C) and, by implication, to all the other albino alleles.

The difference in depth of pigmentation of the extremities and body for the Burmese and Siamese is caused by temperature gradients over the surface of the body. The mutant tyrosinase enzymes are moderately temperature sensitive and the mutant enzyme is increasingly sensitive between the c^b and c^s forms. Heat loss from the skin and circulation differences cause this temperature gradient in the skin. In one experiment, the cat was left in a cold environment during a period of molt. The cat's body became covered with light sepia fur and new sites of intense pigmentation appeared on the shoulders and hips where the skin was stretched more tightly across the underlying bones. In another case, a bandage applied to a small area of shaven skin caused the growing hair to be white. Siamese and Burmese kittens are born a very light color, due to the high temperature they experience in the uterus, as compared to the colder environment they live in after birth. As cats age, their overall body temperature declines, resulting in darker coloration in older Burmese and Siamese cats.

The eye of the Siamese is deficient in pigment, especially the choroid tissues, but a small quantity remains in the iris, resulting in a characteristic blue color. A tapetum is present, a finding that contrasts with the blue eye of dominant white that regularly lacks a tapetum.

Dilutions

Dilution – *dd*

The dilute or maltese locus produces a factor essential for even distribution of pigment granules throughout the hair. In the mutant form, pigment granules are enlarged and deposited unevenly in the hair shaft. This results in clumps of varying size along the length of the hair shaft. Segments of the hair may be very sparsely pigmented or even lack pigment altogether. To the human eye, this impairment causes the coat to appear 'diluted' as this effect modifies the color to a lighter shade by allowing more light to pass through the hair. In cats homozygous for this allele, black becomes blue, chocolate becomes lilac, cinnamon becomes fawn and red becomes cream. The clumping of the granules does not occur in the tissue of the eye. Consequently, eye color is not paler in cats with dilute coloration, contrary to what may be expected. The dilute gene is inherited as a recessive and is symbolized by *d*.

Dilute modifier – *Dm*-

The dilute modifier is a dominant gene *Dm* that affects the coat color of dilute (*dd*) cats. The gene is considered a modifier because it has no effect on dense colored animals. Blue under the influence of this mutation takes on a brownish cast, but does not become as light in tone as the lilac. This color is known as caramel. With dilute chocolate (lilac), the coloration becomes a little paler and is known as taupe. The cream is also paler than usual and has been called apricot (Patricia Turner, personal communication).

The colors and their respective genotypes can be represented as follows:

Black	*aaBBDD* (*DM*- or *dmdm*)
Brown (chocolate)	*aabbDD* (*Dm*- or *dmdm*)
Blue	*aaBBdd dmdm*
Lilac	*aabbdd dmdm*
Caramel	*aaBBddDm*-
Taupe	*aabbddDm*-
Red	*D-OO* (*Dm* or *dm*)
Cream	*ddOOdmdm*
Apricot	*ddOODm*-

Pink-eyed dilution

In addition to blue dilution, a second type of dilution occurs commonly in mammals. This is known as pink-eyed dilution because it imparts a characteristic pink or ruby glimmer to the eye. The coat color is often a bluish-fawn. The genes responsible for this color are usually inherited as recessives. A female cat of this general description was reported in 1961. The eye is said to be pink and the coat a light tan in color. Mated with a chocolate pointed Siamese, this unique animal gave birth to three kittens, 10 days premature, which were not viable. However, it was possible to see that all three were typical tabbies. The implication is that the color is inherited as a recessive trait and is independent of the albino alleles. This would be expected if the color is due to pink-eyed dilution. Examination of the pigment granules of the hairs revealed that these were smaller and yellowish brown in color, when compared with the normal brown-black granules. This change is responsible for the unique coat color.

Inhibitor of melanin – *I*-

The dominant inhibitor gene *I* suppresses pigment fed into the growing hair. This results in the typical expression of white hairs with colored tips. Its similarity to the actions of the agouti gene suggest that an inhibitory protein is created at this locus as well. This gene appears to have a greater ability to suppress phaeomelanin pigment than eumelanin pigment, resulting in the prevention of the eumelanin to phaeomelanin shift. A feature of the gene is the wide variation of expression. That expression ranges from a barely perceptible white band at the base of the hairs next to the skin, to an almost completely white animal with the pigment restricted to the extreme hair tips. Because the melanin inhibitor gene is extremely variable in its expression, it can exhibit impenetrance, resulting in occasional cats with no visible white undercoat that nonetheless breed as smokes.

The silver tabby (*A-I-*) exhibits a fairly low level of expression of this gene, while the chinchilla silver (also *A-I-*) is a fine example of extreme phenotype created through selective breeding. The smoke is the non-agouti form (*aaI-*). The white undercoat is evident but each hair contains appreciably more pigment due to the lack of the additive inhibitory properties of the agouti factor. The restriction of the pigment granules to the distal portion of the hairs has been confirmed by microscopic examination in 1980.

Occasional break-through production of phaeomelanin pigment can occur in silver cats, resulting in a phenomenon commonly referred to as 'tarnishing'. In rare cases, this break-through can be so extensive as to result in a 'golden' appearing cat. This appears to solely occur in cats heterozygous for the *I* allele. Rare cases of extensive phaeomelanin production have also occurred where each hair is banded with a eumelanin tip, followed by a narrow phaeomelanin band, concluding with a white undercoat.

Dominant black

The existence of a gene for dominant non-agouti black coloration is something of an enigma. Tjebbes in 1924 published a report on crosses between a Siamese and a tabby that indicated that the Siamese transmitted an epistatic gene that obscured the tabby pattern. The F_1 offspring were black but the tabby re-appeared in the F_2. Attentive reading of the report revealed that the black F_1 were probably the offspring of a single female Siamese. Only two Siamese cats are described and only the female was used in the cross-breeding. The two Siamese were stated to be descendants of a pair of Siamese originally imported from Bangkok by a Dutch breeder about 10 years before. Historically, the Siamese strain has always bred true to type. In view of the apparent absence of the dominant black gene from the general population, the gene is not considered in Chapter 10, on breed genotypes. Should the gene be rediscovered, the inheritance of this gene can be reassessed.

Orange

Until recently, the gene responsible for the ginger or marmalade colored cat was known as yellow. The standard designation is now orange. This gene is unique because it is sex-linked. This means that the gene is carried on one of the sex chromosomes. Two examples of the inheritance of this color factor, located on the X chromosome, are illustrated in Figs 4.1 and 4.2. A complete list of possible matings and expectations is provided by Table 4.1. The recognized symbol for this gene is *O*.

The action of the *O* gene is to eliminate all eumelanistic pigment (black, chocolate, blue, etc.) from the hair fibers. This is accomplished by a biochemical diversion of those substances destined to become dark eumelanin into the alternate compound, phaeomelanin. The result is a lighter pigment granule, with different optical properties. Phaeomelanin is sensitive to both the normal and mutant form of the agouti protein, resulting in identical phenotypes between the *A-OO* and *aaOO* genotypes. In the tabby tortoiseshell (also called patched tabby or torbie), the deeper tabby striping pattern is carried through from the brown tabby areas into the yellow areas. There the barring appears as a rich orange color. The evidence of striping in the red areas of a tortoiseshell cat, especially one with large areas of red patching, also demonstrates that the *a* gene masks the presence of striping in eumelanistic areas. All tabby patterns can be found in red and cream cats. The mackerel and blotched forms can be readily identified but the Abyssinian is a subtle variation. The contrast between the yellow ground color and black ticking is lost in the orange form of the ticked tabby pattern. This results in a surprisingly uniform color throughout the coat. This sex-linked red ticked tabby color is not to be confused with the 'red' abyssinian color of some registries, which is actually cinnamon ticked tabby.

An interesting aspect of the genetics of the orange mutation is that the heterozygous (*Oo*) female is the tortoiseshell cat. The mosaic of orange and black is very striking and has led to considerable speculation upon its origin. Recall that male cats have only one X chromosome in their cells, while females have two. Thus, each of a female's cells must inactivate one X chromosome to avoid the overproduction of factors produced by genes on the X chromosome. This inactivation occurs at an early stage of development and all cells descending from these progenitor cells have the same functioning X chromosome. Ordinarily, this characteristic of the X chromosome would not be noticed. However, because the sex-linked *O* gene results in an obvious coat color change, the effects of this phenomenon can be observed visually. All melanocyte cells with the functional X bearing the *O* allele will be produce phaeomelanin. On the other hand, those pigment producing cells with the functional X bearing the *o* allele produce eumelanin. The outcome, as the embryonic cat develops, is a female with a mosaic coat of orange and black.

Tortoiseshell and white cats have a clearer segregation of orange and black than ordinary tortoiseshells, as demonstrated by the studies in the mid 1960s. Cats without white spotting tend to be brindled, having highly intermingled small areas of yellow and black hairs. As the amount of white increases, so does the extent of patching, until cats with a primarily white coat exhibit colored spots of only one color. Whether the yellow and black colors of the coat are brindled as opposed to patched is determined by the size of the population of melanocyte precursor cells. Each precursor cell in the brindled coat develops into relatively few melanocytes. In the patched coat, however, a single cell has reproduced to cover a wider area of skin surface. The greater the effect of the white spotting gene, the fewer precursor cells survive to develop into melanocytes (as described in the section on white spotting below). Thus the coat consists of large clonal patches of a single color.

It is not uncommon for yellow pigmented mammals to exhibit wide variation in depth of color. The cat is no different in this respect. The orange cat may vary in color from a sandy yellow to a rich mahogany red and include every shade in between. This variation is almost certainly due to polygenes that enrich the color independently of the O gene. This deepening of the color has been termed rufism, meaning to redden. The variation is most noticeable in all-yellow phenotypes but is definitely not limited to these. The auburn coloration of the exhibition brown tabby, the ruddiness of the Abyssinian and the variable tarnishing that occurs in many silvers are all manifestations of rufus polygenes.

Tortoiseshell males

A mention must be made of the tortoiseshell male cat. Theoretically, it would seem that these curious animals could not occur but they do, at a very low frequency (one in every 3000 male births). The fact that they occur only rarely is an indication that they must arise from a rather exceptional event. Four possibilities for the occurrence of the tortoiseshell male will be outlined.

Somatic mutation

Orange animals occasionally have small spots of tabby or black hair on their bodies. These animals are not considered tortoiseshells, whether they are male or female. However, it is occasionally possible for the black markings to be more extensive and to simulate a tortoiseshell coloration, albeit one that is predominantly orange. Little notice would probably be taken if the animal is a female but it would attract attention if it was a male. Such an animal would be fertile and would breed as an ordinary orange male. The cause of this is a mutation (from O to o) occurring in only a few of the body cells of this orange cat. The result is that these cells now produce black pigment instead of yellow. The size of the area would depend upon the developmental stage at which the mutation occurred. The earlier in development, the larger the anomalous area would be expected to be. Somatic mutations of this kind can be considered mistakes in development. The germ cells are almost invariably not involved.

XXY genotype

The second explanation revolves around the fact that only one of the X chromosomes is functional in body cells. Most tortoiseshell males have extra X chromosomes in their body cells, resulting in the genotype XXY, instead of the XY genotype of the normal male. As the cells inactivate the extra X chromosome, as in a female cat's cells, the effective constitution in each cell is XY; the same as a normal male. This causes the animal to develop into a male adult cat. However, the cat's tissues consist of two different forms of XY, depending upon which of the two Xs is disabled. If one X carries O and the other carries o, one tissue (O) produces orange pigment and the other (o) produces black. Although the XXY cat develops into a male, this abnormal constitution has the characteristic effect of rendering the cat sterile.

XX and XY mosaics

The third explanation is developed from microscopic studies that have revealed that the tortoiseshell male may result from quite a variety of unusual chromosome constitutions. Their tissues may be comprised of mixtures of XX and XY cells, XX and XXY cells or XY and XXY cells, for example, or of even more exotic combinations of cell configurations. This phenomenon is known as mosaicism. For tortoiseshell coloration to occur, the male must carry at least two X chromosomes in a number of skin cells and have X chromosomes with the O allele and those with the o allele. The extremely rare case of the fertile tortoiseshell male may be explained by the presence of only normal XY cells in the germ cell tissue, but abnormal chromosome configurations in other tissues, including the skin. While the XXY configuration is abnormal for testis tissue, if this organ contains XY cells, functional sperms can be produced. The male may be fully or only partially fertile. This depends on a number of factors, including how much of the testicular tissue is capable of producing viable germ cells. This topic is covered in greater detail in the Technical Appendix to this chapter.

Chimeric cats

Chimeric cats are known to exist, demonstrating a fourth mechanism for the existence of tortoiseshell males. In chimeric males, dissimilar XY cells could arise from the fusion of two different fertilized eggs. The difference between the two cells is that the X in one could carry O while the X in the other could carry o. Paradoxically, the animals would appear to be uniformly XY under the microscope and would be fully fertile.

Sterile, black females

In addition to the rare occurrence of tortoiseshell males, exceptional black females may occur. These are exceptional because they arise from matings in which the color is not expected (Table 9.1). These animals do not usually attract attention because they do not represent such a unique phenotype as the tortoiseshell male but, nevertheless, they are of genetic interest. Many of them could be tortoiseshells that have failed to manifest any orange or yellow hairs. However, there is reason to believe that some of these female cats lack a second X chromosome. Karyotyping, where the

Table 9.1 Reported observations on the inheritance of yellow and tortoiseshell and the occurrence of male and female tortoiseshells and black females

Mating		Offspring					
Dam	Sire	Males			Females		
		Yellow	Tortoiseshell	Black	Yellow	Tortoiseshell	Black
Black	Yellow	–	1*	58	–	53	13*
Tortoiseshell	Yellow	63	1*	44	58	46	6*
Tortoiseshell	Black	45	1*	43	–	29	–
Yellow	Black	23	–	–	–	19	–

Note: Black is used as a euphemism for non-yellow colors (black, tabby, blue, etc.) and yellow covers red and cream.
*Exceptional or unexpected colors

chromosomes in cells taken from an animal are examined, would determine if a suspected black female has the chromosomal configuration XO. This phenomenon is referred to as Turner's syndrome. These cats are usually undersized and sterile.

Occurrence of exceptional colors

The breeding data of Table 9.1 present an interesting picture of the inheritance of yellow and tortoiseshell and of the occurrence of the exceptional colors. The frequency of tortoiseshell males would appear to be about 0.6 per cent, while the black females would be about 3.6 per cent. These figures should be accepted with caution. It has been reported that the frequency of tortoiseshell males is less than this, while the frequency of black females may be much overestimated. Some of the black females could be tortoiseshell females in which the yellow areas are so small as to be undetected. Although no exceptional yellow females were recorded, these would conceivably be expected to occur as frequently as the exceptional blacks.

White and white spotted cats

Breeds of cat exhibit several forms of white markings in the coat. In all, there are four kinds of white spotting that may be genetically defined in the following manner:

- Dominant white – the coat is completely white. The irises of the eyes are one of the following three types: blue, non-blue (including shades of deep copper, golden yellow or green depending on the breed) or odd-eyed where one eye is blue and the other non-blue. In the case of odd-eyes, one or both eyes may be partly blue and partly non-blue.
- Piebald spotting – the coat is tricolored or bicolored. The coat is colored except for a variable amount of white. Typically, the head has a white blaze in the form of an inverted V extending between the eyes. The chest and stomach may be largely white. The lower parts of the legs are often white and the body shows various amounts of white. The

body may be very white, to the extent that the colored areas are broken up into several patches or spots. In extremely white animals the color persists only as small spots on the head and on the rump, although the tail usually remains colored for the larger part of its length.

- Gloving – the white is confined to the paws of the feet. The paws are usually white with limited, but some, extension further up the feet. On occasion there may be a little white on the face, belly and chest. This is most likely to be simply a form of expression of the piebald phenomenon.
- Brisket spots and lockets – this involves small white spots or streaks on the throat, chest and stomach. These are rarely large except, perhaps, for the streak on the stomach. Some breeds exhibit white toes as a form of this phenomenon.

Dominant white

The completely white cat, either with blue, non-blue or odd eyes, is due to a dominant gene symbolized by W. As the coat color is pure white, it is impossible to ascertain by inspection which other genes are present in the genotype. In other words, W is epistatic to all other color mutants, masking the effect of all other color genes. The only possible exceptions are those which influence eye color and there may be uncertainty even for these. The results of crosses between white and self colored cats, as reported in the literature, indicate that dominant white is inherited as a simple, autosomal entity. This disproves previous theories that the all-white cat is simply the result of the accumulative presence of several piebald genes. It has also been suggested that the dominant white gene is not independent of the main piebald gene but is an allele of it. Breedings between white and bicolored cats have established that this is not the case and that the W gene is present at a separate locus from the piebald spotting gene (Shelton, 1995).

The W gene has multiple potential effects on coat and eye color. It is also associated with deafness. The production of a white coat is the most regular expression of the gene, because of the lack of melanocytes in the skin. A proportion of kittens may possess a spot or smudge of colored fur on the head, due to a few surviving pigment-producing cells, but this rarely persists into adulthood. The eye color is transformed to blue in a large proportion of cats, either bilaterally (both eyes) or unilaterally (the odd-eyed white). A lack of the tapetum structure of the eye is associated with the color change. Deafness is more likely to occur with blue-eyed animals but the association is not consistent. A survey of 185 white cats reported the following results:

- Twenty-five per cent had yellow eyes and normal hearing.
- Thirty-one per cent had blue eyes and normal hearing.
- Seven per cent had yellow eyes and were deaf.
- Thirty-seven per cent had blue eyes and were deaf.

The deafness is due to degenerative changes in the succule and cochlea. This appears to be caused by the lack of migration and viability of the necessary precursor cells from the neural crest. As with eye color, the deafness may be either bilateral or unilateral.

Cats with white coats are significantly more liable to skin cancer through the absorption of solar ultraviolet rays. The study focused on white cats, including very white piebald individuals. Breeders who reside in semi-tropical or tropical countries should ensure that their cats have the opportunity to rest in areas shaded from strong sunlight.

Piebald white spotting

Piebald, or white spotted, cats are exceedingly common. The spotting may occur in conjunction with any color as an independent entity. The manifestation of the spotting can vary between two extremes. It may be limited to small tufts of white hair on the breast or belly. The other extreme is an almost completely white cat with the pigment areas confined to the tail and to small spots on the head or body. The increase in amount of white is variable but is not without a certain logical progression. As the belly becomes largely white, the neck and chin becoming increasingly involved, together with the front paws. As the amount of white increases, the white extends up the sides and appears on the head and hind paws. From this point onwards, white is spreading all over the animal, breaking up the remaining colored areas on the back into spots of decreasing size.

Figure 9.1 is one attempt to portray the progression of white. When the amount of white is small, this is commonly referred to as low-grade spotting. When it is extensive, this is referred to as high-grade spotting. In low grade spotting, the face shows an inverted blaze combined with white paws or legs and a white stomach. In medium grade spotting, the body is patterned with white, with the amount of white varying from 40 to 60 per cent. In high grade spotting, the body is almost all white with the color restricted to a few colored patches or spots, usually on the head and hindquarters. The tail frequently remains colored.

The medium grade level of spotting is the typical bicolor of many breeds, while the high grade is a breed characteristic of the Turkish Van. Piebald spotting is inherited as a semi-dominant, with the gene symbol S. In general, it can be assumed that all low grade, and some medium grade, spotted cats are heterozygotes Ss, while some medium and all high graded spotted cats are homozygotes SS. It is impossible to state that a cat with a certain degree of white is either Ss or SS, due to the extreme variability in expression of this trait. As this is a dominant character, to breed bicolored kittens at least one parent must be a bicolor. Self colored kittens bred from a bicolor can not carry this gene recessively, although in rare instances the amount of white spotting can be so minimal as to be undetected.

From research in other mammals, it can be assumed that the white spotting gene, represented as the symbol S, causes a defect in special embryonic cells, called melanoblasts. The melanoblasts are destined to become the melanocyte cells that produce melanic pigment granules for the hairs. These defective cells are reduced in number and fail to reach all parts of the body. The melanoblast cells arise from the neural crest along the back of the embryo and migrate from there all over the body during embryonic growth of the skin. However, if they fail to reach their

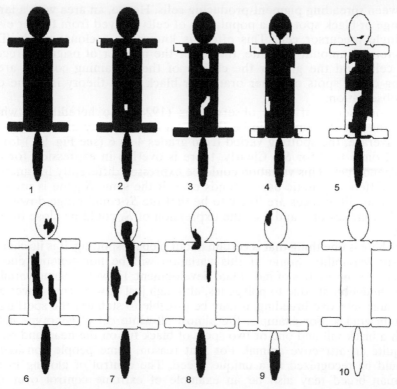

Figure 9.1 Variety of expression of piebald white spotting. Grades 2 and 3 show the typical location on the stomach, while grade 4 through 9 show the progressive increase in the amount of white and the break-up of coloured areas. Grade 10 represents an all-white cat

allotted positions before the skin is fully formed, the skin is then deficient in these cells. This results in a lack of pigment production for the hairs in that area. The outcome is a white spot.

The central line of the chest and stomach are the most distant from the neural crest and, therefore, the most likely parts of the body to reflect a tardy migration. The slower the migration, the larger the spots will be. In the 'van' colored animal, very few melanocytes are present and they are in the areas closest to the originating neural crest, on the head and spine line. Rarely, very white piebald cats may have a partial or completely blue eye, associated with a lack of tapetum, as is seen in the blue eyes of dominant white cats.

Tortoiseshell cats without white have an intermingled mosaic of orange (O) and black (o) colored fur, with a few patches of solid color. This indicates that the spread of both O and o cells occurs at equal speed and probably competitively. The presence of white causes the orange and black to form patches. And the greater the amount of white, the larger are the patches, as a rule. Reduction of the number of original precursor cells produces white areas and decreases competition between spreading pigment-producing cells. Hence, an area with a large orange or black spot has a population of cells derived from few or even a single precursor cell. This effect is known as a clonal patch. The greater the amount of white, the fewer the number of original precursor cells, and the greater the chance of the remaining colored areas being clonal spots of either orange or black. This theory is borne out by observation.

In one series of early observations (1928), the heredity of white spotting was determined to be that of an incompletely dominant gene. On average, the spotting varied from grades 4 to 6 (see Fig. 9.1) for Ss and from 5 to 8 for SS. Clearly, there is overlap in expression for the two genotypes. This variation could be expressed differently for animals with different genetic backgrounds even if the same S gene is present. The main differences are likely to be that the Ss could range down into the low grades of 2 and 3 or the expression of Ss could be close to that of SS.

If there is one thing that is certain about piebald spotting, it is its characteristic variability. Some of this variation will be non-genetic, due to random eccentricities of individual development. However, some variability is undoubtedly due to polygenes, although just how much is uncertain. Through selective breeding, it may be possible to stabilize the spotting at certain grades. For example, the almost all-white cat of genotype $aaSS$, with a black tail and one or two spots of black fur on the head and body, is quite an attractive animal. For that reason, some people consider it should be recognized as a unique breed. The control of gloving in the Birman breed may also be an example of extreme control over this variable trait.

It may be that the postulation of a single gene for piebald spotting is a genetic oversimplification. Multiple genes, such as one controlling low-level white spotting, may be present. It also seems possible that some cats may exhibit such low levels of white spotting as to be imperceptible. The presence of other genes, interacting with S, could be partly responsible for the wide variation in spotting.

Gloving

Gloving is the name given to a trait that is expressed as a limited amount of distal white on the feet. It had been previously hypothesized to be the result of a recessive gene, but breedings between self colored cats and gloved cats reveal that it is a dominant gene with incomplete penetrance. Thus, a low level, undetected amount of white can be seen in cats with this gene, although they are capable of producing kittens with more substantial gloving. There is a degree of variation in the expression of this trait. The paws are usually white 'gloves', but the lower portions of the legs can be more extensively white. This creates the 'stockings' or 'laces'. This trait has been highly refined in the Birman breed. The Snowshoe breed in the USA also displays another form of low grade of piebald spotting, with limited white markings on the forehead and breast. It is unclear at this point whether gloving is due to (a) a separate allele at the piebald locus, (b) an allele at another dominant gene locus, or (c) is simply a level of expression of the common piebald gene controlled through extensive selective breeding.

Lockets

Brisket spotting, or lockets, is a term given to minor white spots that occur on the underside of the body – the throat, chest, stomach and groin. They are irregular in occurrence, where a chest spot in one generation may turn up as a chest or groin spot in another. These spots are variable in size and may occur as streaks, particularly on the stomach. In rare cases, chest and stomach spots may be connected.

The irregular expression of brisket spotting makes it very difficult to decide if a single gene is responsible. It is likely that the manner of inheritance is polygenic. The trait can be eliminated through selective breeding. The presumed polygenic inheritance and the irregular expression can appear to mimic dominant or recessive inheritance in different matings. In the USA, Havana Brown, a form of white spotting limited to the feet was established as a recessive trait. Bicolored cats can carry brisket spotting, masked by the piebald spotting, which can be revealed when crosses with self colored cats result in the unsuspected appearance of this trait.

The exact cause of brisket spotting is unknown, but the mechanism is probably similar to the phenomenon that results in piebald spotting. The pointed pattern exhibited by the Siamese is not a form of white spotting, despite the blue eyes and whitish coat. This pattern is produced by a completely different gene, one in the albino series.

Rufism

Rufism is a term given to denote the wide variation in the expression of yellow pigmentation, especially the deepening of the color to create the shade of red found in the sow (exhibition) cat. It is the opposite of the lighter 'ginger' shade most common in non-pedigree animals. The variation appears to be continuous from the lightest to the darkest shades and the mode of inheritance is almost certainly polygenic.

The range of variation is most obvious in the contrast between the ginger alley cat and the rich red of the exhibition red tabby. However, the same polygenes are doubtless involved in producing the warm ruddy-brown color of the Abyssinian and the warm ground color of the exhibition brown tabby. Without this enhancement, the Abyssinian would be a drab and nondescript animal. The tarnishing seen in some silver cats probably owes its mechanism to a similar group of polygenes. The show silver and chinchilla are found in breeds where selective breeding has minimized or eliminated the influence of these polygenes. The result is a phenotype exceptionally devoid of yellow pigment. It must be remembered that any polygenic complex has both up-regulating and down-regulating polygenes. Diligent breeding results in accumulations of either one or the other in an effort to achieve the standard of perfection for that breed or color.

Technical appendix

A: Black-yellow mosaics

All of the numerous coat colors of mammals are produced by genetic modification of two basic pigments:

- Eumelanin (commonly called black or brown).
- Phaeomelanin (commonly called red, orange or yellow).

Black and brown do not vary a great deal although the brown can be so dark as to be called chocolate. On the other hand, the red to yellow series is subject to notable variation as indicated by their descriptions. However, genetically, all of these are termed yellow as the differences are merely due to the depth of color.

Domestic animals

All of the usual domestic animals sport the above colors, sometimes in more than one form. The two pigments are probably derived from the same precursor substance, but a gene controlled switch early in the embryonic biochemical pathway causes either black or yellow to be produced. The normal pathway is the production of black pigment and the production of yellow pigment is caused by a mutant allele of the normal gene. The result is a completely yellow individual – a red tabby in the case of the cat. Another way of viewing the change of coat color is to say that it is devoid of black pigment. For this reason, 'yellowing' alleles were designated as 'non-extension of black' or, simply, as 'yellow'. The symbols for these genes and alleles are F for the production of black pigment and e for the production of yellow pigment.

Typically, such alleles are inherited as recessive to black pigmentation. For example, the familiar yellow varieties of the guinea pig, hamster and rabbit are all caused by recessive alleles. In the cat, the genetic situation is different. There the mutant allele for yellow is borne on one of the sex chromosomes, the X. The cat was, for many decades, unique in having a sex-linked yellow. Now, a similar mutant has now been found in the Syrian hamster. The inheritance of sex-linked yellow is not as straightforward as recessive yellow but the expected outcomes can easily be worked out. They are usually presented as a table of matings and of any expected progeny. The interesting aspect is that the allele can create a distinctive color pattern in the female in certain matings. This result is the well-known black and yellow tortoiseshell.

Normal gene

Denote the normal gene by the symbol O and the sex-linked yellow allele by o. Using this convention, the tortoiseshell has the genotype Oo. That is, the color is heterozygous for the genes O and o. The pattern is engendered as if some of the body cells are producing black pigment while others are producing yellow. There is little order in the production so that the pattern is extremely irregular. The above supposition is correct and is a peculiarity of sex-linked genes. In each cell, one of the X chromosomes ceases to function. In the case of the tortoiseshell, with its heterozygous genotype Oo, if the X carrying O is inactivated, the cell will produce black pigment due to the active *o* gene. But, if the X carrying *o* is inactivated, the cell will produce yellow pigment, due to the active *O* allele.

Initially, which of the two chromosomes ceases to function is a matter of chance. Once one of the chromosomes has become inactivated in a cell, the same chromosome in all of the cell's daughter cells remains inactivated. As the cat develops, the cell lineages intermingle, resulting in the mixed up pattern of the typical black and yellow tortoiseshell. As a consequence of the sex-linked inheritance, it would be expected that all tortoiseshell cats are female. In the normal course of breeding this expectation is borne out. Rarely, however, tortoiseshell males make an appearance. Usually, the tortoiseshell color on a male is caused by abnormal sex chromosome constitutions (from pages 144). Typically, they possess more than one X chromosome. Most are sterile; only a small minority are fertile.

The majority of breeders and veterinarians are probably familiar with mutation in the germ cell tract as this is how all of the colors of cats originated. However, mutation can occur in the cells that make up the body. Most of the time, these would pass unnoticed but they can become noticeable under certain circumstances. One of these circumstances is that of the uncommon tortoiseshell male. That mutations can occur in the body cells may seem novel. However, each cell of the body contains a full set of genes although not all are functional at a given stage of development. However, most genes are functional during the active phases of embryonic growth and this is where the effect of a mutation is most like to be seen.

On rare occasions, yellow colored varieties of animals may have variable sized patches of black. This is due to a mutation for *e* to *F* in an embryonic body cell. Or, in the particular case of the cat, it is due to a mutation from *O* to *o*. Now, the group of cells carrying the *o* gene will produce black pigment, as opposed to all of the other cells carrying *O* that will produce yellow pigment. The size of the black patch depends on the stage of embryonic development at which the mutation occurred, the earlier the occurrence, the larger the patch. Mosaics with small spots would be expected to be the more frequent, as the older the embryo, the more cells there are in which a mutation could occur.

Mosaics

These curious black and yellow animals are known as mosaics, a black/yellow mosaic to be precise. A female mosaic cat would not excite much curiosity as it is likely to be taken as an ordinary tortoiseshell. On the other hand, a male mosaic is likely to be a focus of comment, the more so because he would be behaving as a fertile male tortoiseshell. The mosaics could occur in a litter from any mating in which yellow offspring are to be expected. However, one mating in particular would distinguish the mosaic from the tortoiseshell. This is the pairing of two red tabbies. All of the kittens would be expected to be red tabby. Hence, if an apparent tortoiseshell is produced, it is almost certain to be a mosaic, even if the individual is a female. Both sexes will be fertile and probably breed as red tabby because the mosaic condition is a property of the body cells and is rarely heritable as such.

A number of probable cases of mosaicism in pedigree cats have been found in The Netherlands recently. This has generated a certain amount of discussion as to whether or not these should be registered as tortoiseshell. These are red tabby with small spots of black on various parts of the body. They are almost certainly black/yellow mosaics. In addition, the small size of black areas would indicate that the mutation occurred late in embryonic development. A proposal to register these cats as 'red with black spots' to distinguish them from ordinary reds and tortoiseshells is being discussed in one registry. The smallness of the black spots indicates that they will breed as ordinary red tabbies.

Chapter 10

Genetics of color variation and breeds

- Introduction
- Conformation and type
- Color variations
- Breeds
- Technical appendices:
  A: Color likelihood from matings involving chocolate and dilute alleles
  B: List of color and coat mutant genes and symbols
  C: Blood types
  D: Breeds and outcrosses

Introduction

Whether they are the revered bobtailed cats of Japan, the tailless cats of the Isle of Man, or the shaggy, longhaired cats native to the state of Maine, the groups of cats identified as 'breeds' share a common history. They have undergone an evolutionary process that has made them unique representations of the same species, *Felis domesticus*. For unique breeds to be created, a number of prerequisites must be met. The germinal incident in the creation of a breed is often a gene mutation. Such mutations can include changes in coat color, fur length/quality or even skeletal malformations. For a breed to be established, the mutation must be compatible with life to such an extent that the cat must be able to reproduce. The next step in the creation of a breed is that of isolation, where the trait is allowed to establish itself and become reinforced in a number of cats. This isolation can be geographical, where a group of interbreeding cats is physically separated from the rest of the species, such as on an island or behind a range of mountains. But this isolation can also be artificial, a result of the interference of humans on the mating habits of cats.

Historically, such interference has occurred when people have selectively chosen as pets those cats that were particularly aesthetically pleasing to them. When, for instance, a blue or pointed cat was born in a group of more common black or tabby cats, it would be prized for its rarity and kept as a pet. The unexpected appearance of a recessive trait has also been attributed in some cultures as a sign from the gods, with the consequence that most 'temple' or 'royal' cats have exhibited recessive traits: the blue Korat, the sable Burmese, the blue longhair and the pointed Siamese.

This chapter contains a detailed discussion of the genetic mutations that have come to be recognized as characteristics of cat breeds. Much of what is known about the nature of the genetics behind the different breeds is the result of careful observation by breeders. Scientific research into the precise mechanisms of these traits is still in its infancy. The field should not be considered static, and as new information becomes available, many of the present hypotheses will be challenged.

Conformation and type

An established breed may be considered to have three components: general conformation (consisting of various components such as body structure and stance, head shape and ear carriage), coat type and coat/eye color. Although color and coat type can sometimes define a breed, conformation is by far the most important feature that determines the uniqueness of a breed. While the longhair and rex breeds have their origin in simple coat mutations, body conformation must still be regarded as an important characteristic. The fact that coat characteristics play a subordinate role to body confirmation is evidenced by the recognition of several colors, and even both coat lengths, within the same breed. Breeds usually exhibit a characteristic body type that is recognizable regardless of coat color or length. Color differences within a breed are properly termed varieties.

Two rather distinctive body conformations tend to be evident in the cat breeds. One is a compact, powerfully built frame, with a round head and the other is a sinuous, more lightly built frame, with a 'wedge-shaped' head. These tend to divide the breeds into the 'British' or 'Persian' type versus the 'Foreign' or 'Oriental' type. There are, of course, numerous variations within these two broad categories. Cats of intermediate conformation can be seen, implying that the two types represent the extremes of a range of expression. Body build is under polygenic control and is also influenced by diet and general care. On the assumption that the last two items are adequate, conformation is primarily influenced by selective breeding. Polygenes responsible for determining the size and shape of individual bones that make up the skeleton frame and the size and shape of the musculature are the determinants of conformation. These are the underlying elements which breeders manipulate in their efforts to improve and maintain 'type', as it is termed.

The establishment of distinct body conformations in various cat breeds comes at a price. In order to create a consistent, identifiable type, a degree of inbreeding is necessary. Frequently, a single male fitting the desired conformation of a breed is bred to a large number of females during his lifetime. In order to further cement the traits of this sire, his offspring and/or their progeny are bred back to that exceptional male. This can create a 'founder effect' whereby all members of a breed are related to the same cat. The policy of some cat registries to reward prolific cats with such titles as 'distinguished merit' or 'outstanding sire' further reinforces this breeding practice. This is fine if the breed is popular and the number of stud males is reasonably large. Should the breed have a limited gene pool, inbreeding depression could occur, causing such problems as small litter size, small size of offspring, infertility and suppressed resistance to disease. Any attempt to counteract this inbreeding by outcrossing to other breeds presents the challenge of finding another breed whose traits will not counter the carefully nurtured distinctive body type. As a compromise, it may be advisable to build up certain broad categories of body type and establish breeding policies within the registries which will deter but not inhibit absolutely the occasional judicious outcross.

In the domestic dog, selective breeding for distinct body conformation has been carried to extraordinary lengths. It is doubtful whether the cat should be manipulated in this manner or even whether it is possible to do so. Cats may not have the inherent genetic plasticity to produce, for instance, either miniature or excessively massive breeds. However, the existence of several breeds with distinctive body types indicates that skeletal structures such as skull shape, length and thickness of the leg bones, spine and rib cage, as well as tail thickness and length, can be influenced by the process of selective breeding.

Color variations

The selfs

The self (or 'solid') colored breeds are found in six basic colors: black, blue, chocolate, lilac, cinnamon and fawn. These exist as the uncomplicated non-agouti, self phenotype. All self colored cats possess the non-agouti (*aa*) genotype. White is excluded because this is not a 'color' in the sense defined here. Sex-linked red is discussed later.

The black cat is produced by a combination of the alleles *a* (non-agouti), *B* (black pigment) and *D* (dense coloration), giving the genotype *aaB-D-*. In depicting the genotypes throughout this chapter, a capital letter indicates a dominant allele, while its lower case counterpart represents a recessive allele at the same locus. A dash indicates the presence of either the dominant or recessive allele. Thus, *B-* should be taken to represent either *BB*, *Bb* or *Bb^l*. A black cat could be genetically either *aaBBDD*, *aaBbDD*, *aaBBDd* or *aaBbDd*, depending on its ancestry.

The most beautiful expression of the black phenotype is that of a solid jet black color, as absolute as possible, with no sign of rustiness. Any animal which has a persistently brownish tinge or fading of the undercoat as an adult should not be used for breeding unless it is positively outstanding in other respects. Outside of genetic influences, the biggest enemy of a rich black coat is sunlight. Sunlight combines with saliva deposited on the cat's coat in an oxidative chemical reaction that results in a 'rusting' of the fur. All of the self colors, in fact, can be adversely affected by sunlight, some to a greater degree than others. Possible environmental influences should be considered at all times, as not all coat color is solely a result of inherent genetics.

Gray color, termed 'blue' in the cat fancy, is produced at the dilution or maltese gene locus, by the allele *d* in the formula *aaB-dd*. The color is chemically black pigment (eumelanin), but with a dilution of the apparent color, caused by the clumping of melanin granules in the hair shaft. This results in colorless areas of the hair shaft, allowing more light to pass through the hair and thus lightening the color. The depth of color is variable and can be manipulated to some extent by selective breeding. Cats approaching most closely to the ideal breed color should always have preference for breeding, provided other important features are considered. Four breeds have the basic *aaB-dd* genotype as a breed characteristic. These are the Chartreux, British Blue, Russian Blue and Korat. The continental breed of Chartreux may be regarded as approximately equal to the British Blue, although in the USA it has been developed into a unique breed. The more subtle differences between the breeds lies in the shade of blue, their coat texture and in their body type. These characteristics which are undoubtedly polygenetic and do not lend themselves to simple genetic representation.

The third self color is chocolate. This mutation of black coloration has been distributed to a diverse variety of breeds. The Havana (also known as the Chestnut Brown) is the self chocolate foreign type cat of genotype *aabbD-*. In the USA, brown cats of Siamese based heritage have been isolated into the breed Havana Brown. These cats are dense-colored animals, also of eumelanin pigmentation, but with oval, chocolate pigment granules replacing the spherical black granules. Exceptional richness and soundness of color will only be maintained by careful selective breeding of those individuals which approach the ideal color. This also applies just as cogently to body type and other characteristics of the breed.

The fourth self color is the lilac of genotype *aabbdd*. As indicated by the genetic constitution, the lilac is dilute brown; bearing the same relationship to brown as does blue to black. The lilac color is stunningly attractive, being a 'softer' and often rosier shade of blue. This color has been developed in many breeds, including the Persian (longhair), Oriental and Rex breeds.

The above colors have been known in the cat for 50 to 100 years, probably much longer for the black. Cinnamon is a comparative newcomer. The shade is a pleasing medium, warm brown as opposed to the dark chocolate of the Havana. The color is produced by a second recessive allele of *B*, denoted by the symbol b^l, causing a further elongation of the pigment granule. The genotype is $aab^l b^l D$-.

Fawn, the sixth and final basic color, is the dilute version of the cinnamon, possessing the genotype $aab^l b^l dd$. The color has a resemblance to lilac but is a lighter shade. The cinnamon and fawn colors are seen in the Oriental/Foreign breeds in its non-agouti form. It is most commonly found, however, in the agouti form where this color creates unique varieties of the Abyssinian and Somali breeds.

Red and tortoiseshell

All of the ginger, marmalade and red tabby cats display the sex-linked orange gene *O*. The gene is carried by the X chromosome and this means that the inheritance of the gene is a little more complicated than with many other traits. The sex of the parent introducing the *O* gene into any cross has to be taken into consideration (Table 4.1). Males have only one X chromosome while females have two (XX). Therefore, male cats have only one *O* (red) or *o* (non-red) allele while the female has two: *OO* (red), *Oo* (tortoiseshell) or *oo* (non-red). Tortoiseshell cats are heterozygous, as implied by their brindled or patchwork phenotype and are always female (with the exception of males with certain chromosomal abnormalities, as discussed in the previous chapter).

The action of the O allele is to convert the production of black pigment (eumelanin) into orange (phaeomelanin). If no black pigment is present in the coat, one cannot discern if it is solid black or has been changed to chocolate or cinnamon by the actions of b or b^l. Therefore, an orange cat may have the genotypes BB, Bb, Bb^l, bb, b^lb or b^lb^l. Any gene which acts only on black pigment cannot be detected in orange animals.

The rich red of exhibition cats is caused by the selection of rufus type polygenes. The intensity is enhanced by the presence of blotched tabby in the genotype $O(O)mcmc$ as opposed to mackerel (OMc-) or ticked tabby (OT^a-) as the deep red markings are more pronounced.

The tortoiseshell is a remarkable cat in a number of respects. Tortoiseshells are a mosaic of orange and non-orange areas. The orange areas are orange regardless of the type of tortoiseshell, whereas the non-orange areas show the effects of genes A, a, B, b, or b^l. In these cats, it is easily apparent that O masks the effects of these genes. The equivalency of tabby striping in the eumelanistic and pheomelanistic areas is shown by the behavior of the pattern in the tabby tortoiseshell. The pattern carries through from the tabby to the orange areas without a break except for a change of color.

As all tortoiseshells are obligate heterozygotes, the color cannot be true breeding. Being females, they have to be mated to either orange or non-orange males to give the results shown in Table 4.1. There is no reason to prefer one sort of mating to the other. The actual tortoiseshell pattern, brindled vs patched, is due largely to non-genetic or polygenetic causes affecting embryonic development and are largely beyond the control of the breeder. The wide variety of expression of tortoiseshell can sometimes produce unexpected breeding results. These arise where the tortoiseshell female appears to be non-tortoiseshell (due to an absence or apparent absence of orange areas) or completely orange (due to an absence or apparent absence of non-orange areas). These rare cats breed as tortoiseshells although they do not seem to be tortoiseshell in appearance.

The tortoiseshell and white (also known as calico) has the genotype $aaOoS$-, the white areas being produced by the dominant S allele. In most respects, and in breeding behavior, the tortie and white is identical to the ordinary tortoiseshell. There is a tendency for the variety to be less brindled, with clearer and larger patches of orange and non-orange, as discussed in the previous chapter. Often, the greater the amount of white, the larger the patches of single color are. However, there is tremendous variation and even the best tortie and white often shows some brindling.

The cream and blue-cream are dilute variations of the red and tortoiseshell, respectively. The color change follows from the incorporation of d into the genotype: cream male ddO, cream female $ddOO$ and blue-cream $aaddOo$. A pale, rather than a rich, cream is preferable for exhibition and these are the animals favored for breeding purposes. In the UK, the colors of the blue-cream should be softly intermingled whereas, in the USA preference is given to those cats with segregated patches of blue and cream.

The chocolate (*aabbD-Oo*) and cinnamon (*aab^lb^lD-Oo*) are rather fascinating tortoiseshell varieties, despite the relative lack of contrast between the orange and non-orange areas. The lilac (*aabbddOo*) and fawn (*aab^lb^lddOo*) with cream coloration in place of orange, complete the range of self-colored varieties.

A comparable range of tabby tortoiseshells can be bred. Their genotypes are identical to those discussed above, with the substitution of the agouti gene *A* for *a*. These cats are often referred to as Torbies. Finally, the addition of the inhibitor gene extends the spectrum of colors into the silver and smoke varieties. Each of these can be found in the usual six standard colors. It should be apparent how the number of varieties can multiply with each addition of a mutant allele to the genotype.

Tabbies

Everyone is familiar with the tabby cat. They abound in mongrel populations throughout the world. The common tabby is gray or yellow in color with characteristic darker patterns which differ from cat to cat but are consistent enough to fall into four generally recognizable forms. These are the mackerel striped, the blotched or classic 'bulls-eye' pattern, the spotted tabby and the ticked or abyssinian form of tabby.

The black-based mackerel tabby is the wild type, as defined earlier and has the genotype *A-B-D-Mc-*. In exhibition cats the vertical striping should be well defined, evenly spaced and as unbroken as possible. The ground color (the color of the agouti band) of this form of tabby, should not be drab or 'cold' in tone but more auburn or 'warm'. Exceptional richness of ground color is due to enrichment by rufus modifiers.

The exhibition brown classic tabby is the blotched tabby of genetics. The genotype is *A-B-D-mcmc*, differing from the mackerel in the possession of the *mc* allele. The tabby pattern can be very variable but brown tabby breeders have managed to bring about some degree of stabilization. The tabby markings must be well defined, as black as possible and symmetrical. The agouti ground color should be a rich warm color, not dull and lifeless. There is a tendency for the tabby pattern to be invaded by excessive agouti ticking and a continuous watch must be kept on this, otherwise the pattern becomes ill-defined and loses its solid appearance. Some of the most spectacular examples of this color exist in the American Shorthair breed, where ideal color consists of such components as a butterfly between the shoulders, double vertical rows of buttons on the chest and stomach, bracelets and unbroken necklaces.

The third form of tabby is the spotted. The genetics of this tabby is not precisely known and in some breeds it appears to be caused by a distinct mutation. In others it may merely be the effect of a modifier gene on the mackerel tabby pattern. The striping of the mackerel has an inherent tendency to break up into short bars or spots. It is fairly easy to take advantage of the tendency and to develop a spotted tabby by selective breeding of broken mackerel tabby cats. The almost continuous variation from mackerel to clearly spotted in some breeds is indicative that the difference between the two is most likely polygenic. Breeders would be wise to breed only from those spotted cats which come closest to their concept of the ideal animal. In some breeds, the spotted tabby pattern appears to behave as a simple dominant allele (*Sp*). The dominant modifier of the blotched tabby pattern seems to have reached the peak of perfection in the Ocicat, a superbly spotted cat. Exceptional spotting is also seen in the Bengal breed, a hybrid between Asian leopard cats and domestic cats. These cats also display a dominant form of the spotted pattern, but with an underlying blotched tabby pattern that appears to have been inherited from the non-domestic cross. This pattern is inherited as a recessive to the spotted form and is referred to as 'marble'.

Some of the most striking spotted tabbies are not the ordinary brown tabby color but are, instead, silver tabbies. This is not a coincidence as the inhibitor gene eliminates pigment from the agouti band and thus between and under the spots. A distinctively spotted tabby is the result. Superb chocolate spotted tabbies with distinct, rounded spots have also been produced and the same principle could apply to them. As the tabby pattern consists of darker (intensely tipped) and lighter (slightly tipped) hairs, the chocolate tipped hairs between the spots would blend into the reddish/yellowish background, allowing the spots to stand out more strongly.

The last tabby pattern is actually the lack of pattern; the ticked tabby or Abyssinian tabby. Breeding experience with the Oriental Shorthair, a breed in which all tabby patterns can be seen, has demonstrated that this gene is not an allele at the same locus as the mackerel and blotched tabby patterns, but is a separate gene entirely (Lorimer, 1997). It appears to act as a simple dominant to the other tabby patterns. In the ticked tabby, deeply tipped hairs are uncommon, usually seen only on the legs, face, at the neck and in circles around the tail. This pattern will be discussed more later.

To avoid unnecessary repetition in the following discussion of the various colored tabbies, these will be assumed to be blotched (*mm*). This is the pattern most commonly found in exhibition cats. In general, all of the remarks apply equally to all tabby patterns. However, there is one difference to be remembered. The mackerel and ticked tabbies are less heavily pigmented than the blotched. The contrast between the tabby pattern and the agouti background is, therefore, less distinct. This difference can make the recognition of certain phenotypes easier for one variety of tabby over the other.

Blue tabby color results from the substitution of *d* for *D* in the genotype, namely *A-B-dd*. The tabby markings are a slate blue and the agouti areas are cream to oatmeal colored. The chocolate tabby has the genotype *A-bbD-*. Here, the tabby markings are rich chocolate in color, contrasting with a yellowish agouti band. The cinnamon tabby (*A-b'b'D-*) is brighter in color. It must be noted that the genetically 'brown' tabby is not the same color as seen in the breed variety that carries this name. The exhibition brown tabby is a black tabby genetically because it has the dominant *B* allele for black pigmentation. To avoid confusion, the genetically 'brown' tabbies should be called either chocolate or cinnamon tabby, as the case may be. The lilac tabby (*A-bbdd*) and the fawn tabby (*aab'b'dd*) complete the sextet of basic tabby varieties. The last two colors possess a lilac-fawn coat with a cream undercoat, the lilac being darker than the fawn on average. However, there may be too much overlap of apparent color for reliable differentiation.

All tabby cats are agouti, i.e. have the dominant agouti allele A. The uniformly dark coat of non-agouti coloration is epistatic to the expression of tabby pattern. It is difficult for a dark pattern to be observed in a coat which is already dark. This is not wholly true, of course, as a 'ghost' tabby pattern can frequently be seen in kittens revealing the underlying tabby pattern that exists in all cats. This disappears later with the growth of the more deeply pigmented mature coat.

A point of genetic terminology may be commented upon at this stage. In discussing the various non-agouti cats, the tabby alleles were omitted from the genotypes. It is true that a tabby allele must be present but, as the a gene effectively 'covers them up', there is no point in including them. Another practical aspect is that the actual tabby allele present is often unknown. However, the underlying tabby pattern may have a subtle influence on the color of the cat. An underlying blotched tabby pattern in a pointed cat, for example, may spoil the color as the cat matures and the body color darkens. But if this cat has an underlying ticked tabby pattern, the body color may remain clearer as the cat ages.

There is an important exception to the rule that all tabbies are agouti. This is the orange or red tabby. These need not necessarily be agouti. The reason for this is that a different sort of epistasis is involved in their case.

Red and cream tabby

Because a red or cream tabby pattern is shown against a lighter orange or yellow background, in a similar manner to the other tabbies, the view is often held that the red or cream tabby cat must be agouti, A-. The expressed pattern may be either mackerel, blotched, spotted or ticked tabby. It is a easy to understand why this misunderstanding occurs. All black, blue, or brown tabby cats are agouti. The recessive alternative to agouti is self black, a uniform color against which the tabby pattern is almost invisible.

As discussed in the previous chapter, the hairs of the coat are colored by minute pigment granules which are deposited in the shaft of the growing hair. A particular color is determined by the nature of the granules and how these are distributed in the hair The granules are colored by two sorts of pigment, black (eumelanin) and yellow (phaeomelanin), just before the eruption of the hairs. The ground color, the yellow band underlying the tabby pattern, is called the agouti band because it occurs on all agouti hairs regardless of animal species. Agouti coloration is seen on many species, including the mouse, hamster or cat. The purpose of the tabby pattern in the wild is to camouflage the animal against predators or to avoid being seen when stalking prey.

The agouti ground color is produced in a curious fashion. The hairs of a normal tabby cat are not uniformly colored from top to the tip. They start as black at the tip, then change to yellow for a short distance, before changing back to black. This may be seen by examining the secondary guard hairs under a strong magnifying lens. It may be argued that the black tip and the yellow band are easily seen but the basal part of the hair is blue, not black. This is an optical effect. The granules are black but these become more sparse towards the root of the hair To human eyes the reflected color becomes diluted or bluish.

In the tabby cat, the dominant agouti allele causes an inhibition of pigment production. During the hair's growth cycle, the level of inhibitory agouti protein in the cell increases. In the black/brown tabby, black pigment production stopped shortly after the hair started to grow, is replaced by yellow pigment production. But yellow pigment is not produced at full, however, as it is also inhibited by the agouti allele, although to a lesser extent than black pigment. In the red tabby, black pigment is not produced at all. Strong yellow pigment is produced, until it begins to be inhibited by the agouti protein. The red tabby pattern can therefore be described as an overlap of extra yellow pigment at the tips of the hairs which is so intense that it appears as red. The actual tabby pattern is not changed, hence the cat is a red tabby. The pattern results from areas of less pigment inhibition, where the agouti effect is not as strong.

What will be the outcome of substituting the non-agouti allele for the agouti allele? One might suppose that a solid red or cream cat would result. However, this is not the case. The outcome is a red or cream tabby indistinguishable from the agouti red or cream tabby. Red/cream tabby can exist in two forms: as an agouti and as a non-agouti. The mutated form of the wild-type agouti gene, the non-agouti allele, produces an agouti protein that does not inhibit black pigment (resulting in self colored cats), but still is able to inhibit yellow pigment. Thus, the tabby pattern is produced in red and cream cats, despite the non-agouti mutation. This is known as 'masking', where one gene (here, yellow) masks the presence of other alleles (here, agouti vs non-agouti).

The above model can be demonstrated by comparison of the tabby tortoise shell with the black tortoiseshell. The tabby areas of the former are clearly agouti/tabby while the black areas of the latter are just as clearly non-agouti (i.e. black). However, examination of the yellow areas of the two tortoiseshells reveals that both have the lighter and darker red areas of the red tabby.

Another proof of the existence of two forms of red tabby is the existence of red tabby male kittens from the mating of a black stud to a black tortoiseshell queen. These can be typical red tabbies in appearance and yet must be non-agouti because both parents are non-agouti. Agouti is dominant to non-agouti and it is impossible to breed a dominant form from two recessive parents.

Despite this, a solidly red or cream appearing cat can be created. The Abyssinian ticked tabby gene restricts the pattern to the head, limbs and tail. By producing red cats that are genetically ticked tabbies, a solid appearing red cat can be created. Selectively breeding for a less distinct pattern, even in cats of other tabby patterns, can also result in a solid appearing red or cream cat.

A breed which has taken advantage of the uniform body pattern of the Abyssinian gene is the Burmese. The red Burmese is a self red in appearance, due not only to the presence of the Abyssinian gene but also to the Burmese gene which is a general lightening gene. The pale red color which is produced is quite acceptable for the breed. Vestigial markings on the head, limbs and tail are barely detectable.

Smoke

Smoke is formed by the combination of the inhibitor gene with non-agouti (*aaI-*). The action of *I* in producing white undercolor is clearly seen in this variety. 'Ghost' tabby marking of dark and light pigmentation may be observed in most kittens if one searches carefully enough. It may persist in adults. The extent of the white undercolor is variable and the overall color may be described as dark, medium or light, depending upon the amount of top color or tipping. The white undercolor itself is not always stark white in the smoke. The color may vary from off-white to bluish, barely distinguishable from the blue undercolor of ordinary black. Very dark smoke can be confused with black, producing the apparently paradoxical situation of a smoke kitten being bred from black parents. In these cases one of the parents may be a smoke in genotype but not in appearance. The great variation in undercolor is comparable to that which distinguishes shaded silver from chinchilla and is presumably due to the same modifying genes.

The exhibition smoke may be short- or longhaired (*aaB-D-I-*) but it is the latter which is most well known. The combination of the *I* allele with other mutant alleles at other loci produces smokes of various colors. For instance, the blue smoke (*aaB-ddI-*), chocolate smoke (*aabbD-I-*) and the lilac smoke (*aabbddI-*) have been developed. The light undercolor is more apparent when combined with a long coat and its beauty enhanced. The corresponding shorthaired smokes can be attractive animals but cannot compare with the sheer magnificence of these colors in the longhaired cat.

Silver tabby

The silver tabby owes its name to an absence of yellow pigment from the agouti areas of the coat. Consequently, the black tabby pattern stands out against a white background. The exhibition cat is very striking, especially in the shorthaired cat. Careful selective breeding results in the complex pattern characteristics mentioned previously with the brown tabby. The silver looks its best when devoid of any suggestion of a tawny or yellow suffusion, known among breeders as 'tarnishing'. This fault often appears in cross-bred silvers, indicating how successful breeders have been in eliminating this blemish through selective breeding.

Early studies to discover the nature of this gene, published in 1928, led to the conclusion that this was a recessive trait, potentially another form of albinism. A Siamese cat was bred to a silver longhair, resulting in only black kittens. When these kittens were bred together, cats with white undercoat were again produced (along with pointed long- and shorthaired cats). Investigations in the 1970s into the inheritance of silver demonstrated that the color is, however, produced by a dominant gene. An explanation for the misleading results of the first study could be that the 'black' kittens produced were not in actuality true blacks, but were cats with such a low amount of white undercoat as to appear solid in color. Genetically, some of these black kittens were black smokes. The white undercoat became more apparent in the next generation. The variability of expression of the inhibitor gene, represented as I, results in cats with varying degrees of tipping: heavy tipping where cats have a narrow, or even almost invisible, white base to the hairs or light tipping where cats have an almost completely white coat with only a subtle overlying cast of their underlying color.

The dominant inhibitor allele I suppresses the development of pigment in its deposition in the growing hairs. The smoke cat is the non-agouti expression of this allele, while the silver is the agouti form. The inhibitory qualities of the agouti protein increase the effect of this form of pigment inhibition – silver cats have more white undercoat than smokes. Unlike the agouti protein which has a greater effect on eumelanin than on phaeomelanin, the l allele appears to have a greater inhibitory affect on yellow pigment than on black pigment. It completely eliminates the yellow pigment of the agouti band. The first silvers showed some yellow in the coat, but breeders have selected against this and eventually the silver became devoid of yellow. Tarnishing is the breakthrough of phaeomelanin production.

The most commonly known exhibition silver has the genotype A-B-I-$mcmc$. It is possible to have a mackerel-striped silver of genotype A-B-D-I-Mc-. Other colors may occasionally be seen. The blue silver of genotype A-B-ddI- is an interesting, subtle, color. It has a bluish tabby pattern against an off-white background. The chocolate silver (A-bbI-), lilac silver (A-$bbddI$-), and the rarer cinnamon (A-b^lb^lD-I-) and fawn silvers (A-b^lb^lddI-) complete the series.

Chinchilla/shaded silver

Basically, the genotype of the chinchilla or shaded silver (A-D-I-Mc- or A-D-I-$mcmc$) is identical to that of the silver tabby. In fact, in kittens, until the hairs grow long enough to show the pronounced white undercolor, the chinchilla looks like a silver tabby, exhibiting its underlying tabby pattern.

The majority of longhaired chinchillas seem to begin as blotched or classic tabby. Later, as the hair becomes longer, the pattern is dissipated. Only the extreme distal tips of the hairs are pigmented. During the kitten phase when just the tips of the hairs are protruding through the skin, the tabby pattern is apparent because it is this portion of the hairs which is tipped with pigment.

Two factors define the superb chinchilla Persian: highly successful selection for extreme phenotype combined with long hair. The absence of pigment has been achieved by increasing the extent of the white undercoat through selective breeding. The long hair adds to the overall effect by exposing and emphasizing the undercolor and preventing the pigmented hair tips from forming any sort of pattern.

Non-silver agouti cats (ii) bred from heterozygous chinchilla cats (Ii) are not identical to other tabbies, as would be expected, but are much brighter in color. They have been given the name of golden tabby, Chinchilla golden or shaded golden. In goldens, the agouti band of the tabby pattern is widened. Examination of hairs from goldens reveals that these are nearly all yellow with a dark tip and a slight gray undercolor at the base.

It has been proposed that the chinchilla and goldens owe their unique phenotype to the presence of a wide band gene provisionally denoted by *Wb*. However, breeding studies appear to contradict this in favor of a more polygenetic model that possibly acts by increasing the amount of agouti protein produced in the melanocytes. As the wide banded tabby is less heavily pigmented than the ordinary tabby, combination with the *I* allele produces the phenotype of the chinchilla as opposed to that of the typical silver tabby. Other modifying polygenes are undoubtedly involved in dispersing the pattern and weakening pigmentation of eye color to the characteristic blue-green or emerald green. These modifiers put the finishing touches on the chinchilla phenotype.

The standard chinchilla has black-tipped hairs with the genotype *A-B-D-I-*. However, chinchillas with blue-tipped hairs are not unknown, with the genotype *A-B-ddI-* presumably arising from an out-cross to a longhaired blue in past generations. These cats are not easy to detect as adults but are obviously blue as young kittens. The chocolate chinchilla (*A-bbD-I-*) appears ticked with dusky brown or off-colored black as adults although it is more readily detectable as baby kittens. Lilac (*A-bbddI-*), cinnamon (*A-b^{l}b^{l}D-I-*) and fawn (*A-b^{l}b^{l}ddI-*) varieties are also theoretically possible.

Cameo/red smoke

The combination of the genes *I* and *O* results in the cameo and red smoke. These cats are very delightful creatures with the appearance of orange-yellow tipping or veiling over a whitish background. The genotype is *A-I-O* or *aaI-O* for the male and *A-I-OO* or *aaI-OO* for the female. Note that because the non-agouti allele has no effect on red cats, the difference between smoke and shaded cameos, unlike that between black smokes and shaded silvers, is not due to the genotype at the agouti locus. The parti-color or tortoiseshell cameo has the genotype *aaI-Oo*, if the non-red areas of the coat are smoke or *A-I-Oo*, if these areas are silver tabby or chinchilla. The tabby patterns are relatively unimportant in the cameo. The *m* allele could be involved in producing the darker-shaded forms while the *M* allele is probably involved with the lighter. However, this must not be regarded as a hard and fast rule.

A property of the cameo is the considerable variation in the amount of orange veiling. This is recognized by the general acceptance of three grades of tipping. The most heavily shaded is the red smoke or smoke cameo, with rather dense tipping, followed by the shaded cameo, with noticeably less intense veiling, and the shell cameo, the lightest of all. In very light animals, only the extreme distal tips of the hairs are orange. The major difference between the shaded silver and chinchilla vs the cameo is the conversion of black pigment to orange by the *O* gene. The fundamental gene in the creation of these two series of varieties is the inhibitor gene *I* and similar polygenes are obvious shared between the shell cameo and the chinchilla silver.

The various cream cameos have genotypes identical with the corresponding red cameo with the addition of the *d* gene. The two fundamental constitutions, therefore, are *I-ddO* (male) and *I-ddOO* (female). These occur in the three intensities of veiling discussed above. The dilute parti-color may be either *aaddI-Oo* if the non-cream cameo areas of the coat are blue smoke or *A-ddI-Oo*, if the areas are blue silver tabby or chinchilla.

Breeds

Abyssinian

The Abyssinian is an interesting cat genetically. Fundamentally, the breed owes its appearance to a unique mutant of the usual tabby pattern of the cat. The Abyssinian, or ticked tabby, allele produces a restricted form of tabby, the pattern occurring on the head, limbs and tail, but only faintly on the rest of the body. Breeders of exhibition Abyssinians have further restricted the pattern but the ancestral form often reappears. The body fur is agouti, as shown by the evenly ticked appearance. The early Abyssinians were, in fact, affectionately known as 'bunny cats' because of their resemblance to the agouti rabbit.

The usual (black) or ruddy Abyssinian is produced by homozygosity at the ticked gene (T^aT^a) and the agouti gene (AA). The full genotype may be written as $AAB-D-T^aT^a$. The most dominant color of the Abyssinian, 'usual' or 'ruddy', is a handsome cat and first class specimens show minimal traces of tabby pattern. The ground color has been intensified to a warm, almost mahogany, red. This increase in depth of color is on a par with the change from the mongrel ginger cat to the richly colored red tabby. It is probably, if not certain, that the same polygenes are concerned. All Abyssinian colors are AAT^aT^a and this must he added to the above genotypes given in Table 10.1. The color described as usual/ruddy is the normal or black and has no mutant color genes. The Somali colors have identical genotypes to the above with the addition of $llAAT^aT^a$, that is, the breed is a longhaired Abyssinian.

Table 10.1 Genotypes of Abyssinian colors

Color	Genotype	Color	Genotype
Usual/ruddy		Tortie	*Oo*
Chocolate	*bb*	Chocolate tortie	*bbOo*
Blue	*dd*	Blue tortie	*ddOo*
Lilac	*bbdd*	Lilac tortie	*bbddOo*
Sorrel	b^lb^l	Sorrel tortie	b^lb^lOo
Fawn	b^lb^ldd	Fawn tortie	b^lb^lddOo
Silver	*I-*	Silver tortie	*I-Oo*
Chocolate silver	*bbI-*	Chocolate silver tortie	*bbI-Oo*
Blue silver	*ddI-*	Blue silver tortie	*ddI-Oo*
Lilac silver	*bbddI-*	Lilac silver tortie	*bbddI-Oo*
Sorrel silver	b^lb^lI-	Sorrel silver tortie	b^lb^lI-Oo
Fawn silver	b^lb^lddI-	Fawn silver tortie	$b^lb^lddI-Oo$
Red	*O(O)*	Red silver	*I-O(O)*
Cream	*O(O)dd*	Cream silver	*ddI-O(O)*

The sorrel Abyssinian was known as the red before its true genetic nature was discovered and the color was renamed. This color is still known as 'red' in some registries of the USA. This color is, genetically, cinnamon tabby. The genotype is AAb^lb^lD-T^aT^a, differing from the usual/ruddy by the substitution of the b^l allele for B. The color is a distinctive and attractive reddish brown, fully justifying its popularity. The chocolate Abyssinian ($AAbbD$-T^aT^a) is a somewhat darker colored version of the sorrel Abyssinian, resulting from the replacement of the b^l allele by b. The two forms are usually distinctive in general appearance but, if difficulty is experienced, the solid colored tail tip is a ready means of differentiation. The color of the tip is light brown for the sorrel but deeper chocolate brown for the chocolate.

The blue Abyssinian has the genotype AAB-ddT^aT^a, with bluish ticking over a cream to oatmeal ground color. The lilac has the genotype $AAbbddT^aT^a$, with lilac ticking over the cream ground color. It is fairly easy to distinguish the two dilute forms with experience. Again, the color of the solid tail tip helps decide matters. The fawn Abyssinian is the dilute of the sorrel, with the genotype $AAb^lb^lddT^aT^a$. The ticking is lighter than that shown by the lilac and the coat is more cream in appearance. Unfortunately, taking into account the color variation of the lilac and fawn, it is often difficult to separate the two varieties.

The true red Abyssinian results from the orange O gene to give the genotypes AAB-D-OT^aT^a for the male and AAB-D-OOT^aT^a for the female. The coat color is bright orange and the tip of the tail is red. The substitution of the b or b^l allele for B in the above genotypes makes little difference to the phenotype. As a consequence, the red may have several different genotypes. This is reflected in the breeding behavior when mated to other varieties. The cream Abyssinian is the dilute form of the red. The genotypes for the color will be identical to those of the red except that the d allele replaces D. The color is a clear cream.

The tortoiseshell Abyssinian is a mixture of red and non-red areas, with the basic genotype A-OoT^aT^a. The non-red areas will be the color of the corresponding tortoiseshell variety-usual (ruddy), sorrel, chocolate etc., with the appropriate genotype to match. A problem with the tortoiseshell Abyssinian, unlike the other tabby pattern tortoiseshells, is that they are not always easy to identify, especially if the red areas are dispersed throughout the coat. This can be a challenging problem in some colored varieties.

Introducing the inhibitor gene I into the breed has created the silver series of varieties. Effectively, a white undercolor is produced, with the red or cream ground color disappearing completely. The colored tipping to the hairs will be one of the varieties described previously. All the colors described thus far may be bred as silver varieties. Their respective genotypes contain the I gene in addition to the usual complement. For instance, the genotype of the fawn silver tortoiseshell is AAb^lb^lddI-OoT^aT^a, to cite the variety with the maximum number of mutant alleles. In all, there can be 28 varieties of the Abyssinian. However, it must be mentioned that selective breeding for clear, white undercoat in the silver varieties is at odds with the improvement of depth of ground color in the non-silver varieties. Programs should specialize in either silver or non-silver varieties.

Somali

The Somali is a longhaired version of the Abyssinian. The name is fanciful, of course, as the breed was developed in the USA by the retention of longhaired kittens produced by the Abyssinian. The basic genotype is $AAllT^aT^a$. The Somali can be bred in all the color varieties found in the Abyssinian. Their genotypes are identical but with the addition of the longhaired allele l. The Somali variant is a shorthaired Somali with longhaired ancestry, such as may arise from a cross with the Abyssinian to maintain good conformation. These variants may be mated to Somalis but not to Abyssinians because of the probability of inadvertently introducing the long gene into the Abyssinian breed.

Siamese

The Siamese is an elegant animal and represents, in many people's eyes, the quintessence of cat breeding. The breed may be taken as archetypal of the foreign or oriental body type. The phenotype is a form of 'Himalayan albinism' that is found in many animals (e.g. rabbit and mouse) but displaying more pigmentation than is typical. For instance, the eyes are blue (instead of pink) and the body is slightly shaded (instead of stark white). Apart from this, the Siamese is typical in that the kitten is born devoid of pigment but begins to form pigment on the nose and ears within a few days. This behavior is characteristic of this class of mutations.

Production of pigment in the hair of the Siamese is temperature dependent. This phenomenon is responsible for the contrast between the color of the body and the points. Pigment forms on the points because the temperature of these areas is sufficiently low. However, the temperature of the body is too high for full pigment to be produced. As a result, the coat varies from pale to medium sepia, according to a number of factors. Individual Siamese will not all shade to the same degree even if kept at the same room temperature. Some cats respond to changes of temperature whereas others do not. In general, the cooler the surrounding temperature, the darker the color; the higher the temperature, the paler the color.

The albinism allele has other affects on the Siamese cat. The visual pathway is disrupted, preventing these cats from having full binocular vision. These cats neurologically compensate for this abnormality, however, and the cat's brain probably does not receive a distorted picture. A result of this disruption can be the crossed eyes that are historically a fault of this breed. Nystagmus, or tremors of the eyes, is a fault that can occur in pointed cats of any breed.

The seal Siamese is a non-agouti black with the addition of the Siamese allele c^s, i.e. $aaB-c^sc^sD-$. Note that the color of the points is not black but a dark seal brown. Such degrading of color intensity is characteristic of this albinism allele and fading of color applies to all varieties of Siamese. The color of the points differs slightly from the corresponding self color. The blue Siamese has the genotype $aaB-c^sc^sdd$, the chocolate $aabbc^sc^sD-$ and the lilac $aabbc^sc^sdd$ (frost point in some associations).

The seal tabby point or seal lynx Siamese (sometimes called Colorpoint Shorthair in the USA) has the genotype $A-B-c^sc^sD-$ and displays tabby markings on the head, feet and tail. The genotypes of the other three colors are: blue tabby point A-B-c^sc^sdd, chocolate tabby point A-bb-c^sc^sD- and lilac tabby point A-bbc^sc^sdd. Note that the type of tabby pattern is not included because so little of the tabby is expressed that this item is relatively unimportant. If it is desirable that no tabby markings are apparent on the body, the ticked tabby pattern will be preferred and selection should aim at minimizing and diffusing the expression of the striping.

The red and tortie point Siamese and their dilutes (also called Color-point Shorthairs in some USA registries) express the sex-linked orange gene. The formula for the red is c^sc^sO in the case of the male and c^sc^sOO for the female. The O gene is carried by the X chromosome and the inheritance of the gene is identical to that of an ordinary yellow (Table 4.1). Since O masks both A/a and B/b, the alleles at these two genes cannot be determined in the red point. Consequently, these are omitted from the genotype. The presence or absence of either of these genes can only be postulated from knowledge of the genotype of the parents or from breeding behavior. The cream point has the genotype c^sc^sddO (male) or c^sc^sd-dOO (female); the color being produced by the d gene acting upon the red pigment.

The tortie point Siamese can exist in a large number of different varieties. The seal point is aaB-c^sc^sD-Oo, with seal and reddish tortoise-shell markings. It should be clear that the various tortie points are simply the combination of Siamese and tortoiseshell, the expression of the latter being almost exclusively confined to the points. The blue tortie point is aaB-c^sc^sddOo, the chocolate $aabbc^sc^sD$-Oo and the lilac $aabbc^sc^sddOo$.

A similar series of four colors occurs for the tabby tortie points, with the substitution of the A gene for a. For instance, the seal tabby tortie is A-B-c^sc^sD-Oo and so on. All Siamese are c^sc^s and this must be added to the genotypes shown in Table 10.2. The Balinese/Javanese colors have identical genotypes to the above but with addition of c^sc^sll, that is, the breed is a longhaired Siamese. The red and red tabby have identical phenotypes, as do the cream and cream tabby.

Both a red point and a red tabby point Siamese are recognized. The former denotes the non-agouti red genotype, aac^sc^sOO, while the latter denotes the agouti red genotype, A-c^sc^sOO. The reason for the distinction

Table 10.2 Genotypes of Siamese colors

Color	Genotype	Color	Genotype
Seal	aa	Seal Tortie	$aaOo$
Chocolate	$aabb$	Chocolate tortie	$aabbOo$
Blue	$aadd$	Blue tortie	$aaddOo$
Lilac	$aabbdd$	Lilac tortie	$aabbddOo$
Seal tabby		Seal tabby tortie	A-Oo
Chocolate tabby	bb	Chocolate tabby tortie	A-$bbOo$
Blue tabby	dd	Blue tabby tortie	A-$ddOo$
Lilac tabby	$bbdd$	Lilac tabby tortie	A-$bbddOo$
Red	$aaO(O)$	Red tabby	A-$O(O)$
Cream	$aaddO(O)$	Cream tabby	A-$ddO(O)$

is to avoid the situation of mating a red point to a seal point and producing tabby point kittens instead of the desired seal points. This is possible because the two red Siamese cannot be distinguished visually. The breeding policy is to assume that all red Siamese are agouti until proven otherwise. This may be done by mating a red to one of the self colors (seat, blue, chocolate or lilac) or self tortie (same colors) and noting that all of the non-red progeny are self colored. Red points bred from proven red point Siamese parents would be acceptable. However, be on guard not to mate a proven red point to an unknown red Siamese. This would undo all previous careful breeding. The above comments apply with equal relevance to the differences between the cream point and the cream tabby point Siamese.

Foreign White/Oriental Shorthair/Havana

Non-pointed cats of similar conformation to the Siamese have been developed. Among the many varieties of Foreign or Oriental shorthaired cats, the Foreign White deserves special mention. Apart from the fact that it is a beautiful cat, the breed was created by the application of known genetic principles. The object was to produce a true-breeding blue-eyed white cat. This was accomplished by combining the Siamese allele c^s with the dominant white gene W. The coat is completely white due to the W gene and the eyes are always blue due to the $c^s c^s$ genotype. The eye color may vary in intensity and the correct shade must be maintained through selective breeding. The genotype of the breed is $c^s c^s W$-. The mating of two cats with the genotype $c^s c^s WW$ will consistently produce blue eyed offspring due to Siamese albinism and white due to W. It is unfortunate that deafness may still remain a recurring problem. Where there is epistatic white, there will always be the potential for deafness.

The other colors of foreign cats, known as Oriental Shorthairs in the USA, are shorthaired varieties produced by the usual combination of genes. Hundreds of potential colors can be produced through combinations of the inhibitor, dilute, chocolate/cinnamon, tabby pattern and piebald mutations. The chestnut brown Oriental has been isolated in the USA into a separate breed, the Havana Brown.

Balinese/Javanese

These cats are a longhaired relation of the Siamese. The names are as fanciful as that of Somali, as the breed was developed in the USA by selective breeding of longhaired offspring of Siamese. The basic genotype is $c^s c^s ll$. Other genes are added to create particular color varieties, for example $aac^s c^s ll$ for the seal point Balinese or $aac^s c^s ddll$ for the blue point Balinese. All of the colors recognized for the Siamese may be bred in the Balinese, with the tabby and red factored pointed colors being called Javanese by some US registries. The Balinese variant is a shorthaired Balinese with longhaired ancestry, such as may arise from a cross with the Siamese to improve conformation. These variants may be mated to Balinese but not to Siamese to avoid the probability of inadvertently introducing the long hair gene into the Siamese breed.

Angora/Turkish Angora/Oriental Longhair

Non-pointed cats of Oriental conformation have been developed as the Angora breed in the UK. They are not to be confused with the Turkish Angora cats of the USA, which are a longhaired breed of cat derived solely from cats imported from the Ankara Zoo, Turkey. Both breeds come in a variety of colors, with white being the majority color of the Turkish Angora. In the USA, longhaired non-pointed cats of Siamese heritage are known as Oriental Longhairs. They exist in the same numerous varieties as the Oriental Shorthair.

Burmese

The gene characteristic of the Burmese breed is a member of the albino series, a step up from Siamese in terms of the amount of pigment produced in the coat, but failing to attain the full production level of the normal colored cat. The result is that the black is changed to a dark sepia brown (seal) and the orange to a golden red. The points are darker than the body color, the difference being very obvious in kittens but becoming less perceptible in the adult. This effect confirms that the formation of pigment in these cats is also temperature sensitive, as in the Siamese. Another indication of temperature sensitivity is the fact that Burmese kittens are born much paler than their adult counterparts, as in the Siamese. Pigment expression in the Burmese is just below full strength. Thus, the four basic colors are recognizable, but are subtly paler in tone. The genotypes are listed in Table 10.3.

The exhibition Burmese bred at the moment are non-agouti. The brown or sable has the genotype $aaB\text{-}c^bc^bD\text{-}$, and is a dark seal brown. The blue is $aaB\text{-}c^bc^bdd$, and is a bluish gray, the chocolate is $aabbc^bc^bD\text{-}$. and is a medium chocolate brown. The lilac is $aabbc^bc^bdd$, a delectable dove gray. In the USA, the chocolate and lilac are known as 'champagne' and 'platinum', respectively. Generally, the fur color is lighter in the kitten but darker in the adult coat. Also, traces of tabby striping may be evident in the kitten but this fades upon adulthood. It is of interest that most, if not all, Burmese have the genotype for Abyssinian pattern, not the more usual mackerel or blotched pattern. This may be of significance as the Ta allele would minimize the expression of tabby pattern in the coat, resulting in more even body color.

The red Burmese has the genotype $c^bc^bD\text{-}O$ (male) and $c^bc^bD\text{-}OO$ (female) and is golden red in color. This color results from a reduction of

Table 10.3 Genotypes of Burmese cat colors

Color	Genotype	Color	Genotype
Brown	*aa*	Brown tortie	*aaOo*
Chocolate	*aabb*	Chocolate tortie	*aabbOo*
Blue	*aadd*	Blue tortie	*aaddOo*
Lilac	*aabbdd*	Lilac tortie	*aabbddOo*
Red	*aaO(O)*	Cream	*aaddO(O)*

Note: All Burmese colors are c^bc^b and this must be added to the genotypes intensity caused by c^b, on the one hand, and a policy of breeding for minimal tabby marking. The latter would result in a dissipation of the deeper pigment which is produced by the tabby pattern in red cats. The cream is a lighter-colored variation of the red and has the genotype $c^b c^b ddO$ and $c^b c^b ddOO$, depending on gender. The tortie and blue-cream varieties are simply Burmese analogues of the usual tortie and blue-cream, with genotypes aaB-$c^b c^b D$-Oo and aaB-$c^b c^b ddOo$, respectively. The chocolate tortie ($aabbc^b c^b D$-Oo), and lilac tortie ($aabbc^b c^b ddOo$) complete the series of varieties of Burmese. The red and cream varieties are non-agouti aa because of the method by which the Burmese are bred at this time.

Singapura

The popularity of the Burmese has lead to the development of cats with the conformation of Burmese, but in different colors. The Singapura is a sleek cat of striking coloration. The breed results from a combination of the Abyssinian ticked tabby pattern and agouti allele with the Burmese allele. The foundation cats were carefully test bred and culled in order to establish the homozygous genotype $AABBc^b c^b DDT^u T^u$. The Abyssinian pattern is clearly evident, while the color is a pleasing tone of dark sepia brown, shading over the body, upon a cream background.

Burmilla/Bombay/Asian

The Burmilla originated from a mating between a lilac Burmese and a Chinchilla. The first cross cats were so striking in appearance and type that these were developed by assiduous selection into a breed. The coat is short, with a white undercoat, profusely shaded with tipping of various colors. All of the colors found in the Burmese are permitted. The fundamental genotype is A-$c^b c^b I$-, with addition of the pertinent other genes to engender each of the colored varieties. The shaded Burmilla is agouti, and when non-agouti (aa) is added to the genotype the smoke Burmoire is produced. These have light or white undercolor but are more heavily shaded. The basic genotype is aaI- $c^b c^b$, together with the pertinent genes for the color varieties. All of the above have the dominant allele of the I gene to produce the white undercoat. Varieties which lack the I allele also occur within the breed. Continuing with the theme of the conformation of Burmese in non-traditional colors is the patent-leather jet black variety known as the Bombay (aaB-D-C-) and the agouti varieties known as Asians. Associations around the world are beginning to recognize the popular Burmese breed in a wider range of color possibilities and the definition and limitations of these breeds vary widely between countries and registries.

Tiffany/Tiffanie

Although the original cats bearing this name in the USA were chocolate brown cats, completely unrelated to the Burmese breed, the Tiffany/Tiffanie breed independently developed in the UK is a longhaired variety of the Burmese with the genotype $aac^b c^b ll$. The long coat produces a greater contrast between the sepia-brown tones over the body and the darker points.

Tonkinese

As the Burmese c^b allele is incompletely dominant to the Siamese c^s allele, it is possible to have a light phase Burmese. This has become known as the Tonkinese. The fundamental genotype is aac^bc^s. Other genes are added to produce the color varieties. The seal or natural mink variety has the genotype $aaB\text{-}c^bc^sD\text{-}$, while the chocolate is $aabbc^bc^sD\text{-}$, and so on for all of the recognized color varieties. The difference between the darker Burmese (also known as sepia) and the lighter mink phases is most obvious for kittens. The body color of the light phase is distinctly lighter and the contrast between the depth of pigment of the points and that of the body is emphasized. There is some variation, and the lightest may the appearance of dark Siamese while the darkest can approach the Burmese in color. As adults, the difference between the phases can be less noticeable.

Eye color is often a unique shade of aqua in this breed, an apparent midpoint between the deep blue eyes of the Siamese used in their development and the weak yellow to gold eye color of the Burmese. As exhibition Tonkinese (the 'mink' colors) are heterozygous, variant cats of Siamese and Burmese coloration are produced when these are mated together.

Albino

The complete albino with pink eyes and white coat is almost unknown in the cat. There have been two reports of albinism in the past, one from North America and one from France. In the most authenticated case, the pupil is described as blood red and the iris a translucent white. It is a little surprising that the true albino has not been established in cats because this mutation is extremely common among mammals and has been accepted by most fanciers as a respectable breed.

The 'Albino Siamese' bred in the USA is a Siamese-type cat with a completely white coat (no points) and eye color of a pale bluish-pink. It is inherited as a recessive to both normal color and Siamese. This form of albinism has also been observed in the Himalayan/Colorpoint.

More recently, an albino variety has been bred in Belgium under the name of 'European albino'. The coat is fully white while the eyes are ruby-red, with pale translucent blue irises. The body type is that of the European shorthair. The color is inherited as a recessive. Apart from body conformation, which is immaterial, the similar phenotype and heredity would imply that the two mutants are similar if not actually identical. Both forms are ascribed to a mutant allele c^a which is assumed to be just short of true albinism. However, the structure of the feline eye may be such that the pink iris color seen in other species may not be attainable. It may be the reflective/refractive qualities of the eye itself that produce the blue eye color seen in the reported albinos.

The blue-eyed albino is sometimes confused with the blue-eyed white produced by the dominant W allele. The two are similar, but only superficially, for close examination will reveal that the eye color differs between the two. Concern has been expressed that the albino may suffer from eye defects or deafness but this does not seem to be so. There is some photo-sensitivity, but this is also shown by the Siamese to some extent. Deafness is not a property of albinism. It must be emphasized that W and c^a are unrelated genetically.

Egyptian Mau

The Egyptian Mau is a spotted tabby of graceful foreign type. The inter-esting aspect of the breed is that it was the first to adopt the spotted tabby phenotype as its 'hallmark'. It is unknown if the spotted form is a distinct genetic entity or if it is a modified mackerel tabby of basic genotype A-M^c-. Because of the consistency with which the spotted pattern is produced, a separated spotted gene, provisionally indicated by Sp, seems likely, masking an underlying mackerel pattern. There is some variation in sharpness of definition, size and roundness of the spots but this can be overcome by selective breeding. Careful and diligent selection is essential to maintain the ideal spotted pattern.

The ordinary Egyptian Mau is a black tabby (A-B-D-) while the Bronze Mau is the chocolate tabby (A-bbD-). These are uniquely attractive cats, with rich chocolate spots against a yellowish background. The cinnamon Mau (A-b^lb^lD-) is also an attractive cat, differing from the Bronze in having lighter brown spots. Introducing the dilution gene produces the blue Mau (A-B-dd), the lilac Mau, and the fawn (A-b^lb^lD-). The fawn form is described as having a rosy-pink aura. One further variety which certainly merits comment is the silver Mau (A-B-D-I-), with its contrast-ing pattern of black spots on a white background. It has also been bred in the five other basic colors. A non-agouti cat with the inhibitor gene, the smoke, shows the extent to which 'ghost striping' can be accentuated by selective breeding and a white undercoat.

Chinese Harlequin

An attempt was made some years ago to popularize a nearly all-white oriental style cat under the name of 'Chinese Harlequin', based upon an alleged, probably mythical, ancient Chinese cat. The variety is mainly white except for small patches of black on the head, sometimes on the body, and a black tail. The genotype is aaB-SS. Only black were produced but presumably the blue (aaB-$ddSS$) would be an excellent alternative to the black. The phenotype is undoubtedly 'pretty', more perhaps to the casual cat keeper than to the serious breeder.

Longhairs/Persians

It has been said that the longhaired cat is one of nature's most beautiful creations. There is little doubt that the breed, known as Persian in the USA, has been brought to a high level of perfection. The coat is due mainly to homozygosity of the longhair gene (ll). In the exhibition animal, the coat is long, full bodied and exquisitely soft. In the mongrel longhaired cat, the coat is usually not so long, is often less dense and can be coarse to the touch. These differences are due to modifying polygenes which are inherited independently of the *l* gene. This fact also explains why the coat may differ in length or texture between shorthaired breeds. The coat, of course, is the most important feature of the Longhair and particular attention should be given to its quality in a breeding program.

Any of the colors found in shorthaired cats may be found in the Longhair. There can be subtle differences, however, due to the extra hair length. The tabby pattern, for example, is less well defined and less easily recognizable. The main factor to remember in longhaired cats is that the hairs overlap each other to a greater extent and not always regularly. A much greater length of the hair shaft is exposed and, as this is less intensely pigmented than the tip, it often produces an apparent reduction of color. Breeders have countered this effect to some extent by selection for sound color. This is most desirable for the black.

The black and the blue Longhair have the genotypes *aaB-D-ll* and *aaB-ddll*, respectively. Quality of coat, uniformity and depth of color, and richness of eye color are of prime importance in breeding programs. These traits are not necessarily of equal importance, and each line will have its particular strengths and weaknesses. The self chocolate has the genotype *aabbD-ll* and the self lilac, *aabbddll*. The whole color spectrum may be produced in this breed, with the exception of the cinnamon and fawn varieties which do not exist in the gene pool at this time.

The brown tabby has the genotype *A-B-D-mcmc*, or occasionally, *A-B-D-Mc-*. The red tabby (*D-Omcmc*, male; *D-OOmcmc*, female) should possess all of the qualities of the shorthaired breed, but in a long coat. Similarly, for the tortoiseshell (*aaD-Oossmcmc*) and the tortoiseshell and white (*aaD-OoS-mcmc*). The red self is of the same basic genotype as the red tabby except that the tabby pattern has been encouraged to spread into a large patch of deep red, covering the cat's body. Long hair tends to blur the pattern but, in developing the variety, reliance should not be placed upon this. Nor should one rely upon the chance occurrence of well colored individuals deriving from ordinary red tabbies. There should be deliberate selection for cats with this extended blotched pattern where the whorls and spirals have joined to form patches of intense pigmentation. These animals are distinct from the ordinary blotched tabby and probably would be regarded as too heavily patterned. However, these should be eagerly sought after for self red breeding. An alternate way to produce a seemingly self red cat is to selectively breed for a very faint mackerel tabby pattern, with a wide agouti band. This will result in a lighter body color, however, than the above approach.

The Maine Coon, Siberian and Norwegian Forest cats are longhaired breeds with firm coats, lacking the fullness associated with the British Longhairs/Persians. These cats have distinct conformation from the traditional longhair and can occur in all of the usual colors, although the tabby colors, with or without white spotting, seem to be the most common.

Colourpoint

A crossing of longhairs with pointed cats has resulted in the development of the Colourpoint or Himalayan Longhair. These lovely cats are not

Table 10.4 Genotypes of Colourpoint colors

Color	Genotype	Color	Genotype
Seal	*aa*	Seal tortie	*aaOo*
Chocolate	*aabb*	Chocolate tortie	*aabbCa*
Blue	*aadd*	Blue tortie	*aaddCo*
Lilac	*aabbdd*	Lilac tortie	*aabbddOs*
Seal tabby		Seal tabby tortie	*Oo*
Chocolate tabby	*bb*	Chocolate tabby tortie	*bbOo*
Blue tabby	*dd*	Blue tabby tortie	*ddCo*
Lilac tabby	*bbdd*	Lilac tabby tortie	*bbddCo*
Red	*aaO(O)*	Cream	*aaddO(O)*
Red tabby	*O(O)*	Cream tabby	*ddO(O)*

simply longhaired Siamese, for the conformation is completely different and identical to that of the traditional longhair. The Colourpoints tend to have clearer body color than the Siamese, due to temperature insulation from the dense coat, and this emphasizes the contrast between the body and the points.

Colourpoints may be bred in all of the colors known for Siamese. The genetic constitutions are the same, with the addition of the longhair gene: seal (*aaB-c^sc^sD-*), blue (*aaB-c^sc^sdd*), chocolate (*aabbc^sc^sD-*), lilac (*aabbc^sc^sdd*), red (*c^sc^sD-OO*), cream (*c^sc^sddOO*), tortoiseshell (*c^sc^sD-Oo*) and blue-cream (*c^sc^sddOo*). The addition of the *A* allele also results in a series of tabby or lynx points and smoke or silver points are also possible.

All Colourpoints are *c^sc^sll* and this should be added to the genotypes shown in Table 10.4. Red and red tabby (as well as cream and cream cabby) look alike but have different genotypes. The blue and lilac torties are also known as blue-cream and lilac-cream, respectively. The Birman and Ragdoll colors have identical genotypes to the above but with the addition of *c^sc^sS-ll*; that is, the breed is a Colourpoint with white spotting.

Birman

The Birman is an unusual, longhaired pointed cat. It is not, as one might think, simply a variation of the Colorpoint, although the Colorpoint has been bred to the Birman in the past. While the seal variety of each breed has the genotype *aac^sc^sll*, the Birman has white 'gloves' on the feet whereas the Colorpoint docs not. The white should not be too extensive so as to appear as a 'stocking'. The observations of K.J. Clark have lead to the hypothesis that a unique recessive gene for minor white spotting is involved, provisionally denoted by the symbol *g*. However, other crossings of Birmans with non-white spotted cats has proven that the white gloving is a dominant trait. This could be due to the white spotting allele depicted as *S*, another allele at that locus, or a different gene. The control of white spotting to limit it to the feet could be the result of polygenetic factors and not a major gene. All the colors of the Colorpoint may occur in the Birman.

Ragdoll

The Ragdoll is another longhaired breed that has elements of the Color-point in the background, together with piebald spotting. This results in a cat of very pleasing appearance. All Ragdolls are pointed and longhaired. It can occur in any of the colors listed above for the Colorpoint, although some associations limit the colors to seal, blue, chocolate and lilac. Each of the above can be combined with piebald S allele to produce one of two grades of white pattern: A limited amount of white on the face and feet is called the mitted pattern, while a more extensive white pattern, where white also occurs on the body, is called the bicolor pattern. The former appears to be the heterozygous Ss expression of piebald, while the latter often is the homozygous SS. Polygenetic factors influence the amount of white spotting and its pattern.

The name Ragdoll was given to these cats because of their exceptional relaxed, docile and affectionate behavior. These qualities were claimed to be enhanced by a car accident which befell the original queen, a textbook example of the fallacy of the inheritance of acquired traits.

Turkish

The Turkish (or Van) has extensive white spotting combined and long hair. The basic genotype is $llSS$. The colored areas are confined mostly to the head, elsewhere only on occasion, with a colored tail. In some registries these may only be orange (D-$llOOSS$), indicating the presence of O. An interesting variation is the cream Turkish of genotype $ddllOOSS$. Black and blue varieties, of genotype $aallSS$ and $aaddllSS$, respectively, are also bred.

Snowshoe

These are rather pretty short-coated cats of Siamese pattern with white 'gloves' to the feet. The gloves are produced by the heterozygous expression of the piebald gene S. The heterozygote Ss typically induces white toes but also small streaks of white on the face and stomach.

Rex

The two most established rex breeds are the Cornish and Devon rexes. These differ in body conformation and in the nature of the rex coat. The Cornish Rex lacks the primary guard hairs but, in general, has the denser and more complete coat. The Devon Rex coat possesses guard hairs but tends to have a thinner coat and is more prone to have bare areas, especially on the chest and stomach. The density of coat and the ability to retain the coat from one molt to the next are items that can be controlled through careful breeding. These aspects are under polygenic control.

Any of the colors known to occur in the normal furred cat may be found, or can be produced, in either of the rex breeds. It only requires patience and familiarity in manipulating the relevant genes. For example, the black or blue Cornish would have the genotypes *aaB-D-rr* and *aaB-ddrr*, respectively. The seal Devon Si-rex (Siamese rex) would have the constitution *aaB-c^{s}c^{s}D-rere* and the white Devon Rex, *rereW-*. These examples could be almost endlessly extended. The Devon color range includes the spectrum of burmese colors from outcrosses to that breed.

It has been decreed by the rex breed societies that the two rexes be kept separated and never be crossed. Crosses between Devon and Cornish rexes produces cats heterozygous at both loci (*RrRere*) and therefore straight coated. During the early days of the rex, a presumptive double rex (*rrrere*) was bred, combining features of both rexes and having a soft, thin coat.

Also during the initial development of the Cornish Rex, the longhaired rex (*llrr*) was produced. The coat was longer than normal, but not as long as the Persian, and very fine in texture. The whiskers were bent and curled, a sure sign of the presence of a rex gene. The phenotype was not particularly attractive and was not pursued.

Selkirk Rex

The Selkirk Rex is another curly coated breed, this one developed from a mutation occurring in the USA. It is characterized by the dominant gene *Se*. Curliness of the coat is apparent from birth. These cats have been developed into a different conformation than either the Devon or Cornish Rex. The cat is heavy boned with a rounded head and short muzzle. They have been developed in both shorthaired and longhaired varieties, although the coat length is not as long as Persian in the latter. This breed also occurs in a wide spectrum of colors, self, pointed, tabby, piebald, smoke and silver as well as the full range of Burmese colors. Homozygous cats (*SeSe*) have a different type of coat, one that is finer, curlier and sparser than that of the heterozygote. Exhibition Selkirks are heterozygous cats.

American Wirehair

Another coat mutation that first appeared in the USA is the dominant wirehair mutation (*Wh*). This trait has been developed into a breed with the general conformation of the American Shorthair. The coat is bristly and develops slowly as the cat matures. The fur can be brittle and prone to breakage. Breeders select for cats that are densely coated. This gene has incomplete penetrance where cats with the dominant allele may have normal coat appearance but are capable of producing wire coated offspring.

Sphynx

The Sphynx is described as a hairless cat, but this is not strictly true. The Sphynx kitten has a soft covering of hair which is lost as the kitten develops. The adult animal may have a transitional covering of fine hair but this is lost as the cat matures until the skin is permanently hairless except for a few thin hairs on various parts of the body. The trait is recessive and symbolized by *hr*. The whiskers are short and bent, similar to those of the rex. In fact, the similarity of Sphynx to the Devon Rex induced breeders to cross the two breeds, a practice which led to the finding that the Sphynx hairlessness is dominant to the rex coat.

American Curl

The American Curl breed was developed from a dominant mutation *Cu* which causes the external ear (pinna) to curve gently backwards. The effect is caused by a change in cartilage formation. The pinnae are of normal appearance for the first 12 to 16 weeks of kittenhood but then begin to develop the curve, which is permanent. This gives the cat a rather alert appearance. There is variation in the degree of curvature and selection must be practiced to arrive at the desired curve. The American Curl can be bred in any color, together with long- or shorthair. Large numbers of homozygous curl *CuCu* cats have been produced, with no reported anomalies.

Scottish Fold

The Scottish Fold takes its name from the country in which it was found and from the fact that the apex of the ear pinna is bent forward because of a defect in cartilage development. The ear fold is not present for the first four weeks or so of life but then the peak tilts forwards to become a permanent feature at about 12 weeks. The fold is produced by a dominant allele *Fd* with incomplete penetrance. Unfortunately for the popularity of the breed, the cartilage defect is echoed throughout the skeletal system, but appears to cause no other symptoms for the majority of heterozygotes. However, the homozygote may have a crippling overgrowth of the cartilage of the bones known as osteodystrophy. The bones of the tail become palpably thickened and stiffened, and the bones of the legs become thickened and arthritic, especially around the feet. Normal bone growth is disturbed because of abnormalities of the epiphyseal plates. Ossification is also deficient and irregular. Eventually in these cats, they lose the ability to walk properly and suffer considerable discomfort.

To avoid the breeding of the homozygote, the Scottish Fold cat should only be mated to other breeds (British Shorthairs have been used for this purpose) or normal-eared cats which have been bred from Scottish Folds. The problem with the latter approach is that because this is a dominant gene with incomplete penetrance, some Folds with the mutant allele have normal appearing ears. It is disturbing that even in the most careful breeding program, a small proportion of the cats produced develop the crippling form of this abnormality. Very rarely heterozygote cats also suffer from the abnormality. A myth surrounding this breed is that they are prone to deafness and more susceptible to ear infections. Neither is true. The Fold may be found in any color, pattern or coat type.

Manx

The Manx cat, associated with the Isle of Man, is one of the most well-known breeds, even by people who do not keep cats. Similar mutations have occurred in many parts of the world. It is bred in a number of colors and in both coat lengths. Any of the known colors could be combined with the Manx gene *M*, although some associations limit the color spectrum. The trait is dominant, with a wide variety of expression from a slightly foreshortened tail to complete lack of coccygeal vertebrae ('rumpy').

The homozygote *MM* has been declared a prenatal lethal, although this presumption has been recently questioned by Manx breeders. Initial studies noted that 25 per cent of kittens from Manx to Manx breeding were reabsorbed in utero. However, fetal death seems to be fairly common in all cats. The Manx is associated with various anomalies of the lower vertebrae and anal region. A stilted or stiff-legged gait can be the symptom of pelvic defects. Constipation, megacolon and both urinary and bowel incontinence can be symptoms of abnormal anal and perineal denervation. The colon and bladder can be enlarged. Spina bifida is also seen in this breed. Selective breeding for severely shortened bodies can precipitate these defects.

These various anomalies arise from the action of the *M* allele in causing the taillessness and are inescapable in Manx breeding. This allele disrupts the normal development of the caudal neural tube during embryological growth. The spinal cord may terminate abruptly because of a missing sacral cord segment, the part of the spinal cord that provides innervation to the colon, bladder, perineum region and hind leg muscles. It is urged that only the most robust and healthy cats should be allowed to breed.

The longhaired Manx (*llMm*) has been produced in the USA under the name of 'Cymric'. Despite the appellation, the variety has no connection with Wales. Several different colors are known.

Japanese Bobtail

The Japanese Bobtail is a form of short tail common in Far Eastern cats which is different from that seen in the Manx. It is the result of a mutation. The tail is shorter, rather than absent, and there are no overt signs of any other skeletal abnormality. The breed has been popularized in the USA. The tail length is variable but usually less than 4 inches (10 cm) long. It is often curved and rigid, not always flexible. The fur on the tail is often bushier than that of covering a normal tail, creating a pom-pom type appearance that is unique to the breed. Cats with high-grade white spotting (*aaSS*) are popular varieties, with the tricolor (*aaOoSS*), or 'Mike' being exceptionally prized. These are individuals, mostly white, with patches of orange and black, either occurring as separate islands of color or composed of patches of color with minimal brindling.

Technical Appendices

A: Color likelihood from matings involving chocolate and dilute alleles

Table 10.5 Statistical distribution of offspring from matings involving the chocolate and dilute alleles. These numbers give guidance on the likelihood of a particular colored offspring being produced in a litter, but each individual litter may not exhibit the precise distributions described here, due to the small sample size represented by a single litter

Parental types (either parent)	Statistical odds (%) of color of offspring								
	Black				Chocolate		Blue		Lilac
	BBDD	BBDd	BbDD	BbDd	bbDD	bbDd	BBdd	Bbdd	bbdd
BBDD (black) × BBDD	100								
× BBDd	50	50							
× BbDD	50		50						
× BbDd	25	25	25	25					
× bbDD			100						
× bbDd			50	50					
× BBdd		100							
× Bbdd		50		50					
× bbdd				100					
BBDd (black carrying dilute) × BBDd	25	50					25		
× BbDD	25	25	25	25					
× BbDd	12.5	25	12.5	25			12.5	12.5	
× bbDD			50	50					
× bbDd			25	50				25	
× BBdd		50					50		
× Bbdd		25		25			25	25	
× bbdd				50				50	
BbDD (black chocolate) × BbDD	25		50		25				
× BbDd	12.5	12.5	25	25	12.5	12.5			
× bbDD			50		50				
× bbDd			25	25	25	25			
× BBdd		50		50					
× Bbdd		25		50		25			
× bbdd				50		50			
BbDd (black carrying both) × BbDd	6.25	12.5	12.5	25	6.25	12.5	6.25	12.5	6.25
× bbDD			25	25	25	25			
× bbDd			12.5	25	12.5	25		12.5	12.5
× BBdd		25		25			25	25	
× Bbdd		12.5		25		12.5	12.5	25	12.5
× bbdd				25		25		25	25
bbDD (chocolate) × bbDD					100				
× bbDd					50	50			
× BBdd				100					
× Bbdd				50		50			
× bbdd						100			
bbDd (chocolate carrying dilute) × bbDd					25	50			25
× BBdd				50				50	
× Bbdd				25		25		25	25
× bbdd						50			50
BBdd (blue) × BBdd							100		
× Bbdd							50	50	
× bbdd								100	
Bbdd (blue carrying chocolate) × Bbdd							25	50	25
× bbdd								50	50
bbdd (lilac) × bbdd									100

B: List of color and coat mutant genes and symbols

Table 10.6 Color and coat mutant genes and symbols

Symbol	Name	Symbol	Name
a	Non-agouti	mc	Blotched tabby
b	Chocolate	O	Orange
b^l	Cinnamon	r	Cornish Rex
c^b	Burmese	re	Devon Rex
c^s	Siamese	ro	Oregon Rex
c^a	Blue-eye albino	Se	Selkirk Rex
c	Pink-eyed albino	S	White spotting
d	Dilution	T^a	Abyssinian
hr	Sphynx	T^a	Abyssinian
I	Melanin inhibitor	W	Dominant white
l	Long hair	Wh	Wire hair
Mc	Mackerel tabby		

Note: The following mutant genes are probable but can only be listed as provisional at present: Dm dilute modifier; Sp spotted tabby modifier. See text for details of each gene.

C: Blood types

During the 1990s, research published by the University of Pennsylvania has indicated that domestic cats possess several different blood types. Those identified so far are A, B and AB. It is important to note that these do not bear the same relationship to each other as do the similarly-named blood types in humans.

Survey work in the USA indicates that the frequency of type B varies widely among specific breeds. In addition, the interplay between blood types has been identified as a primary cause of what breeders know as 'fading kitten syndrome', or neonatal isoerythrolysis. Specifically, neonatal isoerythrolysis seems to occur when a B queen is nursing A kittens. Blood type testing is available for adults and can be used at the delivery of kittens. This means that breeders can avoid noenatal isoerythrolysis in many cases by withdrawing kittens at risk from nursing on the queen for about 18 hours.

However, the fact that the samples have been largely limited to the USA precludes the development of any list which can state with certainty the frequency with which B occurs in each breed. Time will undoubtedly change that.

D: Breeds and outcrosses

Every cat registry has its own rules relating to the ability of registered pedigreed cats to be crossed with other breeds of cats. It is important for both the breeder and the veterinarian to understand that it is possible for one breed to have one, two or even three allowable outcrosses in its pedigree. Table 10.7 describes the current status of such allowable outcrosses for recognized and provisional breeds in two of the world's major registries, CFA and FiFE. This list does not include outcrosses which have been permitted in the past.

Table 10.7 Permitted outcrosses for recognized and provisional breeds – 1998

Breed	Allowable outcrosses	
	CFA	FiFe
Abyssinian	None	Somali
American Curl	Domestic short/longhair	N/R
American Shorthair	None	N/R
American Wirehair	American Shorthair	N/R
Balinese	Siamese	Javanese, Oriental, Siamese
Birman	None	N/R
Bombay	American Shorthair, Burmese	N/R
Burmilla	N/R	Burmese
British [Shorthair]	None	None
Burmese	None	None
Chartreux	None	None
Colorpoint Shorthair	Siamese	N/R
Cornish Rex	None	None
Devon Rex	American Shorthair, British Shorthair	None
European	N/R	None
European Burmese	None	N/R
Egyptian Mau	None	None
Exotic	Persian	Persian
German Rex	N/R	None
Havana Brown	None	N/R
Japanese Bobtail	None	None
Javanese	Balinese, Colorpoint Shorthair, Siamese	Balinese, Oriental, Siamese
Korat	None	None
Maine Coon	None	None
Manx	None	British, European
Norwegian Forest Cat	None	None
Ocicat	Abyssinian	None
Oriental	Siamese, Colorpoint Shorthair, Balinese, Javanese	Balinese, Javanese, Siamese
Persian	None	Exotic
Ragdoll	None	None
Russian Blue	None	None
Sacred Birman	N/R	None
Scottish Fold	British Shorthair, American Shorthair	N/R
Selkirk Rex	British Shorthair, Persian, Exotic	N/R
Siamese	None	Balinese, Javanese, Oriental
Siberian	N/R	None
Singapura	None	N/R
Sokoke	N/R	None
Somali	Abyssinian	Abyssinian
Tonkinese	None	N/R
Turkish Angora	None	None
Turkish Van	None	None

Notes: N/R Not recognized (under this name). In some cases, the differences in breeds is only one of nomenclature; in others it is more significant.

For some breeds, the allowable outcrosses have other significant restrictions, such as date after which they are no longer allowed, or a limitation of which color or hair length is permitted for outcrossing.

Chapter 11

Genetic anomalies

> - Classification
> - Specific anomalies
> - Technical appendix:
>   List of genetic anomalies and symbols
> - Historical appendix:
>   The elimination of craniofacial defects in the Burmese cat – a
>   case study of responsible breeding

Classification

A wide variety of genetic anomalies have been found in cats. In an attempt
to classify these the following system has been developed which encompasses three major divisions and eight subdivisions:

- **Lethal**
  Classical lethal – lethal in utero, no kittens survive.
  Tetralogical lethal – lethal at birth (stillborn) or shortly following
  birth.
  Deferred lethal – lethal in full manifestation, e.g. autosomal
  dominant polycystic kidney disease (PKD).
- **Impairing**
  Non-cosmetic, non-lethal but currently difficult or impossible to
  control with medical or surgical therapy.
  Non-cosmetic, non-lethal, but currently requiring surgical therapy
  for the cat to survive or to live a relatively painless life.
  Non-cosmetic, non-lethal, but currently requiring prolonged or life-
  time medical management.
- **Cosmetic**
  Cosmetic, but having medical or physical repercussions.
  Cosmetic, but not requiring surgical or medical intervention to
  permit the cat to live a healthy life indoors.

These classifications are based on veterinary medicine as it is practiced
today. Thus, an anomaly which is now considered as deferred lethal may,
over time, more properly be reclassified as impairing (non-cosmetic, non-
lethal, but currently requiring surgical therapy for the cat to survive or to
live a relatively painless life). In addition, some anomalies can be classified
under more than one of these divisions or subdivisions, depending on how
they are expressed. For example, while polycystic kidney disease in its full
expression is fatal, experimental kidney transplant surgery appears to have
been effective in preventing complete kidney failure in some cases. Thus
polycystic kidney disease may currently be classified as deferred lethal,

with the possibility of it also being impairing (requiring surgical therapy for the cat to survive) in a few cases.

[Hypertrophic cardiomyopathy], unlike defects such as a kinked tail, affects a cat's quality of life and quantity of life. Any disease that causes pain and suffering (and heartbreak to owners) and yet can be silent, must be dealt with proactively, ethically, and openly.
Jody A. Chinitz, Marcia J. Munro (Maine Coon breeders)
and Mark D. Kittleson, DVM, PhD (Veterinary researcher) (1996)

Specific anomalies

The anomalies covered here appear to have genetic components and are currently present in the population of pedigreed cats. For each, the broad classification into which most of the cases currently appear to fall has been noted in the heading in the square brackets. Until molecular genetic research (see Chapter 3) can be used to state, with certainty, that a particular anomaly is, or is not, genetically-based, anomalies which almost certainly have genetic components, as well as some which may have such components are covered. As research proceeds, the uncertainty will decrease.

Achondroplastic dwarfism [cosmetic]

A short-legged condition was regarded by Schwangart and Grau in 1931 as being inherited. No details were given at that time for the mode of inheritance. Following this report, various short-legged cats were found over time in various parts of the world. These cats lived in the wild and apparently functioned as well as long-legged cats.

Cats with achondroplastic dwarfism are now being bred under the name 'Munchkin'. While this breed is still relatively new, the anomaly appears to be cosmetic only. Dr David Biller, in his study of these cats, concluded that this form of chondrodysplasia affects the long bones with less apparent changes in the forelimbs. The skull, spine and pelvis were not affected in the cats he studied.

Two congenital bone problems were found to occur in this breed but they are also in the general cat population. The two problems are lordosis which is a downward dip in the spine starting just behind the shoulder blades and pectus which is an inward displacement of the caudal sternum and costal cartilages.

The gene causing dwarfism appears to be an autosomal dominant gene. Due to the decrease in the size of litters when short-legged cats are bred to short-legged cats, the gene also appears to be a homozygous lethal gene.

Amyloidosis [lethal]

Amyloidosis is a disease in which an amlyoid substance is deposited in many organs of the body, including the kidneys, where it is especially detrimental. The symptoms are listlessness, bedraggled coat, loss of weight detrimental. The symptoms are listlessness, bedraggled coat, loss of weight and appetite, accompanied by excessive thirst and urination.

The overall incidence of the ailment is rare, but was relatively high with respect to the kidneys in a strain of Abyssinians. A 1980s paper reported evidence of a familial propensity in the breed, but was not able to determine the mode of inheritance.

Studies in the 1990s suggest that there was another feline amlyoid, this one in Siamese and related breeds (e.g. Oriental Shorthair), impacting the liver. Again, only a familial propensity was found.

It appears that the transmission of amyloidosis may be genetic, but no precise mode (or modes) of inheritance has yet been determined. In addition, it has been suggested that different breeds may have different genes for the precursor proteins (O'Brien, 1998).

Bent and short tails [cosmetic]

Many cases of nodulated, kinked, bent or loss of the terminal portion of the tail are known to occur. In the majority, the defect is traceable to injury, possibly at parturition or at a later stage. Occasionally, however, the defect may occur in individuals of one particular strain or in blood lines. When this occurs, the likelihood of a genetic influence should be considered.

A form of partial tail loss is not uncommon in certain strains of Siamese. It has been thought for some time that the condition could be inherited although exactly how is unknown. However, one geneticist claims to have found that a shortened tail, observed in a strain of Siamese, is inherited as a simple recessive. There was variation in length for the affected animals but the tail was regularly shorter than normal. The gene is symbolized by *br* from brachyury ('short tail'). In other strains, there may be little or no shortening of the tail. Instead, there are kinks or swellings such as would arise from a fusion of adjacent vertebrae. It is debatable whether these are an aspect of the same genetic situation which underlies the tail shortening or due to something entirely different. In the absence of critical experiments designed to probe this question, it is almost impossible to offer a worthwhile answer. The simpler explanation is that these are variable manifestations of the same genetic entity, the difference in expression being caused by the background of the individual strain.

In most, and very probably in all, strains of Siamese bred to conform to the standard for the breed in the cat fancy, there has been selection against deformed tails. The effect of this selection has been to reduce the frequency of occurrence and to alleviate the severity. Shortening of the tail is now rare but there are instances where the tail may be slightly kinked. When the manifestation of the deformity is slight it is conceivable that some impenetrance may occur. This could imply that the descent of the deformity could be irregular and make accurate determination of the defect difficult, if not impossible. It also may hamper elimination of the defect by means of simple culling of all affected animals.

The Japanese Bobtail is a breed where the tail-shortening gene distinguishes the breed and is one of its major characteristics. The short tail may be viewed as a deformity, but it is only a cosmetic one, as the general health is not affected. Because this mutation can cause tail abnormalities in heterozygotes, it should be considered a dominant mutation with incomplete penetrance. However, as the complete folding of the tail that is characteristic of this breed requires homozygosity for the mutation, it is commonly considered a recessive character by breeders.

Regardless of its nature, in Japanese Bobtail breeding programs, only Japanese Bobtail cats are used with no outcrossing to other breeds permitted, so breeding experience with the Japanese Bobtails will not resolve this question. When the Japanese Bobtail breeding program is followed, different examples of the twisted tail appear in kittens with some tails being longer than others and some more twisted than others.

Cataract [impairing]

An inherited cataract, or opacity of the lens of the eye, in the Himalayan (Colorpoint Persian) breed has been observed. The cataract occurred in both eyes and was extensive as early as 12 weeks of age. The breeding data was scanty but suggestive of recessive monogenic heredity.

Cardiac stenosis [lethal]

Cardiac stenosis is the constriction of any of the orifices leading to or from the heart or between chambers of the heart. There is generally an achalasia of the cardia involved with this condition. This means that the lower segment of the esophagus fails to relax which causes a difficulty in passage of food to the stomach. Affected kittens have difficulty in retaining food after weaning. There is intermittent vomiting and unproductive retching. Before development of the cardiac stenosis, the esophagus is usually dilated. The growth of the kitten is severally retarded and there is some emaciation. Death may occur from a variety of causes.

A recessive mode of inheritance is suggested by the breeding data but it is insufficient for this to be definitely established at this time.

Chediak-Higashi syndrome [impairing]

The most obvious feature of Chediak-Higashi syndrome is a lightening of the coat to produce a bluish color. The iris tends to be yellow-green while the 'eye-shine' is reddish instead of bright yellowish green. This is due to a marked reduction or absence of pigmentation of the tapetum. The tapetum is a layer of fibers leading from the corpus callosum which form a roof and the lateral walls of the inferior and posterior horns of the lateral ventricles of the brain. These fibers pass to the temporal and occipital lobes of the brain. Because of this lack of pigmentation, photophobia, or an unusual sensitivity to light, is common in some individuals. The bleeding time of the cat is prolonged, even following minor surgery, and small hematomas may form in tissues. There is misrouting of optic ganglian in a similar manner to that described for Siamese and albino animals. The syndrome is inherited in a recessive manner and symbolized by *ch*.

Corneal mummification [impairing]

A specific corneal mummification which recurred in adult Colorpoint cats could be inherited. The affected eye showed signs of a dark area in the cornea which was accompanied by chronic inflammation and ulceration. No breeding data was available but a study of the pedigrees showed extensive inbreeding with common ancestors in both the maternal and paternal lines. These observations would certainly be indicative of a genetic predisposition but without necessarily revealing the mode of inheritance. Vawer (1981) proposed that the condition is caused by a recessive gene.

Corneal edema [impairing]

An apparently inherited corneal edema has been reported. Fluid accumulates in the layers of the cornea to produce a haziness or cloudiness in the eyes of kittens at about four months of age. The condition is progressive and leads to breakdown of corneal tissue, followed by bacterial infection. The condition is familial, possibly monogenic, but the exact mode of heredity could not be determined.

Cryptorchidism [cosmetic]

A few people have surmised that the failure of either both testes to descend properly (bilateral cryptorchidism) or merely one (unilateral cryptorchidism) could be genetically determined. Unfortunately, there is no evidence of this. Bilateral cryptorchidism usually results in infertitlity. Unilateral cryptorchids are usually fertile but there should be great hesitation in placing these at stud until the genetic mode of transmission of this anomaly has been determined.

The likelihood that cryptorchidism could have a genetic basis becomes a fascinating question as the defect is the outcome or failure of the testes to pass through the inguinal canal into the scrotum. From a genetics point of view, the problem may actually be a malformation of the inguinal canal making it too small to allow the passage of the testes. There may even be a maladjustment of development, so that the testes are not ready to descend at the appropriate time. These are the factors which would be genetically determined, rather than the phenomenon of cryptorchidism itself. The fact that the cryptorchidism can be unilateral could be an indication that the real problem is with the inguinal canal.

Breeders consider cryptorchidism to be undesirable as the cat is not perfect and can not be exhibited in many cat associations. Geneticists find this anomaly interesting because it is an example of sex-limited inheritance. Only the male can have undescended testes. Whether, or not, the female may show a comparable primary defect to that presumed to occur in the male is unknown. Externally, the female is normal although she may carry the propensity for cryptorchidism and be fully capable of transmitting the condition to her sons. In this respect, the carrier female is as big a problem as the unilateral cryptorchid. In a breeding program where cryptorchidism is found, selective culling is necessary. The breeder should also be just as careful of the apparently normal siblings of affected individuals as they are of the cat who manifests cryptorchidism. Other factors being equal, the sensible course would be to eliminate these siblings from the breeding program as well as the affected cat.

One study found that during a 10 year period, 1.7 per cent of 1345 cats admitted for neutering were cryptorchid. Two of these cats (0.1 per cent) were monorchid. This study also found more cryptorchidism in Persians. Of the 17 Persians in the study, five (29 per cent) were cryptorchid. In contrast, only 1.4 per cent of non-Persian cats were cryptorchid. Of the 64 Siamese in the study, only one was cryptorchid; and of the 58 cats of other breeds in the study, none was cryptorchid. They only found one cat who had another congenital defect in this group of cryptorchids; the cat had a kinked tail.

Published recommendations are that the testicles should be descended into the scrotum by 16 weeks of age at the very latest. Some authorities will declare cryptorchidism by eight weeks of age. Usually, they are palpable by four to six weeks of age (although very small); they are actually supposed to be in the scrotum at birth.

Susan Little, DVM

Curled ears [cosmetic]

A feature of the American Curl Cat is the remarkable backward curve of the ear pinnae. This genetic anomaly is an excellent example of a purely cosmetic anomaly as it does not have any effect on the health of the cat. The condition is caused by a dominant gene Cu. A large number of heterozygotes have been bred which have shown no signs of other anomaly. Only the homozygote $CuCu$ may possibly turn out to possess undesirable defects but, since this breed has been in existence, this has never been found to be true.

Cutaneous asthenia [impairing]

The skin is excessively loose in cutaneous asthenia. This enables folds of skin to be held away from the body. The skin is also very fragile which results in lacerations and wounds from minor accidents and play. Even simple scratching of its skin by the cat can produce multiple lacerations. The condition is caused by defects in the collagen packing of both fibrils and fibers in the reticular layer of the dermis which determines the tensile strength of the skin. Breeding experiments have indicated that the anomaly is inherited as a dominant gene. The causative gene may be symbolized by Cut.

Deafness [cosmetic]

It is well known that white cats may be deaf but the association is not complete. Among a group of 240 white cats in which blue eye color and deafness was recorded, 39 per cent had blue eyes and were deaf, 29 per cent were blue eyed with normal hearing, seven per cent were gold eyed and deaf, while 25 were gold eyed with normal hearing. The association is clearly evident. 'Odd eyed' cats, those with one blue eye and a gold or green one, are a different story. An independent study found that those odd eyed cats which were deaf, were deaf on their 'blue-eyed side'. This deafness in odd eyed cats is, however, rare.

The genetic explanation for the association is that the W gene has several effects, of which only the white coat is constant. The gene also produces blue iris color and deafness in 60 to 70 per cent and in 40 to 50 per cent of cats, respectively. The eyes of white cats with orange or yellow irises are normally pigmented but those with blue irises had deficiencies. The tapetum may be absent in these cats on a regular basis (see Chediak-Higashi syndrome).

Numerous studies have been carried out on the cause of the deafness. These have revealed that the onset of deafness is gradual and is due to degeneration of the canal of Corti. This canal is an elongated spiral structure which runs the entire length of the cochlear duct and rests on the basilar membrane. It is the end organ of hearing which contain hair cells, supporting cells and neuroepithelial receptors which are stimulated by sound waves. However, there is wide variation of time of onset and the extent to which the hearing structures are affected.

Diabetes mellitus [impairing]

Diabetes mellitus is a disorder of carbohydrate metabolism. It appears to result from inadequate production of insulin but why this happens is still unknown. A cat exhibiting symptoms such as increased thirst, increased urine production and increased food intake should be checked for an increase in blood sugar and sugar in the urine. In an Australian study of over 4000 cats, researchers found that Burmese cats were significantly over represented among cats with diabetes mellitus. Irrespective of breed, however, the risk of diabetes in the study population increased with age.

Epibular dermoids [impairing]

Fifteen cases of a similar epibular dermoid or skin-like growth have been described in an inbred group of Birman kittens. The dermoids were hairy, pigmented and attached to the conjunctiva at the corner of the eye. In each case, the dermoid was unilateral and developed in the lateral corner of either the left or right eye. The dermoid hairs tended to be an irritant and gave rise to an early inflammation of the cornea (keratitis).

Removal of the dermoid gave complete relief. From the similarity between cases and because the affected cats were related, some closely, a genetic predisposition may be assumed. The mode of inheritance could not be determined but it was speculated that the condition could be due to threshold heredity.

Episodic weakness [impairing]

Episodic weakness is an abnormal behavior pattern which manifests itself between the ages of four and 10 months of age, with the average age being 7.4 months. Both sexes may be affected. The cat may appear normal until the attack is precipitated by various factors, such as excitement or mildly stressful situations. The head is held characteristically close to the chest when walking or at rest. When walking, the head position nods up and down, the fore legs are stiff, straight and high stepping, and the hind legs flex normally but are held more widespread. Afflicted cats can only walk for short distances and, if forced to jump, cannot land properly. Dilation of the pupils and extension of the claws were also noted during episodes. The condition was observed in the Burmese breed and was shown to be inherited recessively. The gene may be provisionally symbolized by *em* until a precise cause of the condition has been ascertained.

Flat-chested kitten syndrome [lethal]

In this syndrome, the chest of afflicted young kittens appears compressed, or 'flat chested' instead of being nicely rounded. Depending on the degree of compression, the kitten may show signs of breathing difficulties, distress and poor growth. Autopsy findings have revealed more or less severe dislocation of internal organs which can cause early death. On the other hand, kittens which are mildly affected can recover and appear to have normal chests. In the Burmese breed, there is good evidence that the condition is inherited in a recessive manner and the gene may be provisionally symbolized by *fck*.

Folded ears [cosmetic]

The ears of the normal cat are carried in a 'pricked' position. The ears of the folded-eared cat, however, are bent forward in a characteristic manner. At birth, and until about four weeks of age, the ears appear to be normal. From approximately four weeks of age, the tip of the ear tends to turn inwards and the fold is fully formed by approximately three months. When fully developed, the apexes of both ears are folded forward. The condition is inherited as an incomplete dominant (symbol *Fd*). The folded ear is a characteristic of the heterozygote *Fdfd*. While the majority of these animals are healthy, a few suffer from the same anomaly which besets the homozygote. The homozygote *FdFd* has the folded ear, but it also may be afflicted with a crippling epiphyseal dysplasia which results in a short, thickened tail, swollen feet and a marked decrease in activity. This condition was once prevalent in Scottish Fold cats but now appears to have been significantly reduced in incidence by selective breeding.

Four-ears [impairing]

A curious head anomaly produces a small extra pair of 'ears' in affected animals, hence it is known as 'four-ears'. The eyes are reduced in size and the jaw is slightly undershot. The head appears to be a peculiar shape. While growth and size do not appear to be abnormal, the affected cat seems to be relatively inactive and lethargic. This could imply that the functioning of the brain is affected. The condition is inherited as a recessive and the responsible gene is symbolized by *dp*.

Gangliosidosis GM1 [lethal]

Gangliosidosis GM1 is a degenerative disease of the brain and spinal cord. The clinical signs are a fine tremor of the head and hind limbs which begin at about two to three months of age. This tremor increases in severity until the cat cannot stand up. This usually happens at about seven to eight months of age. By one year of age the affected cats have seizures and may suffer some loss of vision. The disease is due to an enzyme deficiency. Although this problem behaves as a recessive, the enzyme deficiency can be detected in heterozygotes.

Gangliosidosis GM2 [lethal]

Gangliosidosis GM2 is another degenerative disease affecting the nervous system. A fine tremor of the head may be noticed at about six to 10 weeks of age. This progresses to muscular incoordination (ataxia) and falling. The head has an unusual rounded appearance while the cornea of the eye is slightly opaque. The disease is inherited recessively and is produced by an enzyme deficiency which may be detected in heterozygotes when the need arises for carriers to be identified. It is detected most frequently in Korat cats. For this reason Korat cats are being used as an animal model to develop a gene therapy.

Both gangliosidosis GM1 and GM2 are lysomal storage diseases which result from a mutation in the genetic code for one of 40 enzymes. These diseases are inherited as autosomal recessive traits.

If breeders understand that they would be able to select for non-carrier cats to perpetuate the breed, and perhaps sell the others for pets after neutering, the pain might not be severe enough to continue tolerating the presence of the mutation in their stock and the breed.

Professor Henry J. Baker, Auburn University

Globoid leukodystrophy [lethal]

Kittens with globoid leukodystrophy show a tremor, weakness and lack of coordination of the back legs at about five to six weeks of age. Later, the condition becomes worse, the clumsy behavior spreading to the front legs. Degenerative changes in the brain produce these symptoms. The malady was shown to be familial, but the data were too meager to do more than hint at recessive heredity.

Hemophilia A [impairing]

Hemophilia is the most well known of the 'bleeding diseases'. The disease manifests itself with protracted bleeding following injury and surgery. Hematomas are common at the joints or under the skin. The gene (*Hma*) is carried on the X chromosome and healthy queens transmit it to their sons, regardless of the male to which they may be mated. Hemophiliac males have heightened mortality but they can survive if the bleeding is of a mild character and if they are kept in a sheltered environment.

Hemophilia B [impairing]

Hemophilia B is a bleeding disease very similar to that described in hemophilia A. The gene (*Hmb*) is borne on the X chromosome and is transmitted to sons by carrier queens. The bleeding is prolonged but is somewhat milder than usually found for hemophilia A.

Both hemophilia A and B are X-linked recessive traits and are usually found in the progeny of asymptomatic carriers. One study noted its presence in British Shorthair cats. However, this was probably due to inbreeding rather than being a breed specific anomaly.

Hageman factor deficiency [impairing]

A deficiency of one of the factors involved in blood clotting can result in a bleeding disease called Hageman factor deficiency. It is, however, unusual for the malady to result in prolonged bleeding. The deficiency is inherited as an incompletely dominant trait, with the symbol *Hag* for the mutant gene.

Hairlessness [cosmetic]

The 'hairless cat' is not truly hairless. Various parts of the body may be nude while the remainder (e.g. muzzle, feet) is covered by fine down or fuzzy hair. Quite often the condition progresses with age, the fine covering of the young adult giving way to bare wrinkled skin and complete hairlessness over much of the body. This progressive loss usually distinguishes the true hairless animal from a temporary loss which may be due to a variety of factors. No improvement of feeding or nursing can produce a normal coat on the truly hairless cat. Hairless individuals may turn up spontaneously in any litter but it is rare.

Three of the hairless conditions have been investigated, those occurring in France, Canada and England. In each case, it was evident that this abnormal deficiency of hair, or hypotrichosis, was due to a recessive gene (symbolized by *h*, *hr* and *hd*, respectively). The Canadian hairless is currently being bred under the name of 'Sphynx'. It is difficult to ascertain if the same or different mutant alleles are producing the various hairless conditions, mainly because the alleles are being expressed against different genetic backgrounds. However, Hendy-Ibbs believes that the various hairless conditions can be explained in terms of two distinct alleles, on the basis of absence or presence of short and curled vibrissae. There are breeding data to suggest that the *hr* gene is either closely linked to, or is an allele of, the Devon Rex gene *re*.

Sphynx kittens are only released to homes where there is a guarantee by the new owners that they will not be permitted out of doors. This is the general way responsible breeders assure that the kittens they sell as pets are safe from the outdoor hazards which are generally unknown to pedigree cats.

It is a disputable point whether hairless cats found in a litter that is other than a litter of Sphynx cats, should be kept. The lack of hair could mean that they will suffer from debilitating heat loss during cold weather. It would seem humane to have them destroyed at an early age. However, if this seems unnecessarily heartless, they should certainly be kept in a warm environment and be provided with a knitted woollen 'over-coat' in very cold spells.

Veterinarians need to be aware of the fact that the Sphynx build up a lot of wax in their ears, due to the lack of fur in the ears. This is always mistaken for ear mites, but it is not in most cases. The internal body temperature of the Sphynx is the same as other cats, but they feel warm to the touch due to the lack of an insulating coat. Also, too many veterinarians tell their clients to get a Sphynx if they are allergic to cats. This is not the case.

Lisa Bressler, Sphynx breeder

Rex cats have a tendency to lose their fur, sometimes in the form of a premature molt or sometimes more permanently in old individuals. This may be represented as a hairless condition, although it is not a true independent loss of hair. The condition is part of the rex syndrome, for the rex coat itself is anomalous. The guard hairs are abortive and the down hairs are thin. In some animals, the anomaly is possibly intensified to cause a deficiency of the down hairs or to produce a baldness where the thin hairs either break off or are pulled from a weakly gripping hair follicle by the habitual incessant grooming of the cat. The Devon Rex is the more prone of the two English rexes to baldness. Its hair fibers are particularly fragile. The loss of hair in the rex is termed baldness to distinguish it from the hairless condition due to the *h* gene.

Hare-lip and cleft-palate [lethal to impairing]

The two often associated anomalies of hare-lip and cleft palate, are thought to be inherited. The basis for this statement stems from the case of a female cat with a slight hare-lip which produced kittens with a similar defect. One kitten was undersized and possessed a cleft-palate. The animal's ability to suckle was impaired and it eventually died. This information is interesting but scarcely sufficient in itself to more than hint at a genetic basis. As an isolated observation, little more can be expected but if a number of such familial associations are reported, perhaps a more positive conclusion can be reached.

Hip Dysplasia [impairing]

Hip dysplasia is an abnormal development of tissue in the hip, generally a replacement of bone tissue with fibrous tissue. This can lead to debilitating arthritis in affected cats. Hip dysplasia can be completely eradicated if breeders would have their cat's hips X-rayed and certified by the Orthopedic Foundation for Animals (OFA) and by a private veterinarian using the OFA guidelines. Only cats who are considered 'clean' for hip dysplasia by the OFA guidelines should be used in a breeding program. While no breed is immune to hip dysplasia, there are indications that it is more common in larger breeds, such as the Maine Coon and Persian. Cats with hip dysplasia can have this defect corrected surgically.

Hydrocephalus [lethal]

Hydrocephalus is a morbid condition associated with a swelled edematous head region, often with other defects. Such animals occur at odd intervals, usually as a result of development mishaps. However, such conditions can be inherited and a case has been reported for the cat. The breeding evidence indicates that a single recessive gene is involved. The mutant gene has been symbolized by *hy*.

The abnormality is readily identifiable at birth. The affected kitten is always very large and bloated in appearance around the head and limbs. It may also have various degrees of hare-lip, cleft-palate or talipes (foot deformities). However, it is uncertain if these abnormalities are strictly a part of the hydrocephalus condition.

Hyperoxaluria [lethal]

Cats with hyperoxaluria succumb to acute renal failure at between five and nine months of age. They become anorexic, dehydrated and exceedingly weak, death occurring within a few days. Palpation of the stomach reveals painful kidneys. Kidney failure is caused by the disposition of oxalate crystals in the tubules. The condition was shown to be inherited in a recessive manner. The gene is symbolized by *ho*.

Hyperchylomicronemia [lethal]

Although growth is more or less normal, kittens with hyperchylomicronemia show a persistent lipemia (an excess of fatty substances in the blood). At approximately eight to nine months of age, affected kittens are unable to move their eyelids and chew food properly. They cannot extend the toes and the patella, or knee reflex, is lost. Clinically, the occurrence of multiple hematomas appears to compress the peripheral nerves, resulting in loss of sensation. The malady is inherited recessively and is symbolized by *hce*.

Hypertrophic cardiomyopathy [lethal]

Hypertrophic cardiomyopathy is characterized by a marked papillary muscle hypertrophy, progressive left atrial enlargement when the disease is severe and systolic anterior motion of the mitral valve. This anomaly appears to be an autosomal dominant trait with 100 per cent penetrance in which the stillborn kittens represent lethal homozygotes.

Hypothyroidism [impairing]

A 1991 study diagnosed congenital hypothyroidism in related Abyssinian cats. The article argued that the disease appeared to be inherited as an autosomal recessive trait with affected homozygotes showing signs of reduced growth rate, shorter stature with kitten-like features, constipation and goiter. However, it did not indicate that this is breed specific.

'Kangaroo' cat [cosmetic to impairing, depending upon defects]

A number of extraordinary animals were described by Dr H. Williams-Jones in the 1940s. These cats possessed unusually short front legs but otherwise appeared to be normal. The gait of these creatures tended to resemble that of a ferret in their smooth but hunched-up movements. When induced to sit back, the posture was that, if anything, of a miniature kangaroo. The peculiarity is said to be inherited because the affected animals were observed in at least four litters. Unfortunately, precise details which might have established the mode of inheritance are lacking. This curiosity has occurred at least twice in widely separated localities. It may have turned up once again in the late 1990s. Unfortunately, in this instance, these cats were being affirmatively bred and were called the 'twisty cats', due to twisted limbs and paws caused by this anomaly in conjunction with polydacylism.

Mannosidosis [lethal]

The majority of kittens with mannosidosis are either stillborn or die at birth. For those which survive, the initial signs develop during the first few days or weeks as a general apathy with diarrhea, followed by tremor and ataxic behavior. The individual appears unable to stand properly. The voice becomes weaker and the stomach appears swollen because of an enlarged liver. The anomaly is induced by an enzyme deficiency which adversely affects the central nervous system. The anomaly manifests through recessive inheritance (symbol *man*).

Manx taillessness [classical lethal]

It has been known for some time that Manx taillessness is inherited as a dominant trait, with the symbol *M*. This has been confirmed and, what is more important, the accumulation of breeding data has shown that individuals homozygous for the Manx gene die before birth. The evidence for this is: an apparent absence of pure-breeding strains of Manx and a decrease of the average number of young per litter for matings of Manx to Manx. The reduction is from an average of about four to three living offspring per litter.

Thus, the Manx gene for taillessness seems to be lethal when homozygous. One aspect of this is a preponderance of females among the viable Manx offspring, as if the males are less likely to survive. Also, examination of Manx stillborn kittens, and those which died before the age of 12 months, revealed a greater number of both skeletal and organ anomalies than was shown by those Manx cats which lived beyond the 12 months.

The absence of a tail is readily apparent although careful examination has shown that the loss can be relative. In all, four types of Manx taillessness have been distinguished. The true Manx is known as a 'rumpy'. In rumpies, no tail vertebrae can be observed. Indeed, there is often a small dimple where the vertebrae would normally issue. A second type is 'rumpy-riser', in which an extremely small number of tail vertebrae can either be seen or felt as an upright projection, usually immovable. The third type is 'stumpy'. Here, the tail is longer and usually moveable although often deformed, nobbly and kinked. The fourth type is the 'longie' and possibly is the rarer of the four. The tail is longer than many of the above, though shorter than normal, and is of a more normal appearance. One series of experiments are suggestive that the various expressions of the Manx taillessness are controlled in part by modifying polygenes.

The influence of the Manx genes may be observed for the whole length of the vertebral column. In the fore-part of the column, this seems to be little more than a slight decrease in the length of the individual vertebrae but, in the hind-part, there is also a decrease in number and, particularly, a fusion of vertebrae. The sacral and pelvic bones are also drawn into the general fusion and maldevelopment. In a number of cases, variable degrees of spina bifida has been found upon autopsy. Spina bifida is a congenital defect where the walls of the spinal canal are affected by a lack of union between the laminae of the vertebrae. Spina bifida is characterized by the membranes of the cord being pushed through the opening forming a tumor known as spina bifida. Occasional a recurrent bowel stoppage may occur because of a narrowing of the anal opening. This may be observed when the kitten is weaned. The spinal cord frequently terminates prematurely. This could lead to a failure of innervation of certain organs and their proper functioning, such as the loss of control of the hind legs.

It is well known that the homozygous Manx is a prenatal lethal condition, but it is only comparatively recently that the moribund fetuses have been identified. These have been detected at as early as five weeks gestation as abnormally small and globoid fetuses with gross malformation of the central nervous system. The responsible Manx breeder must be prepared at all times to have young kittens euthanazed if they begin to manifest problems which affect the quality of life.

Meningoencephalocele [lethal]

Meningoencephalocele is a congenital defect of the cranium which allows fatal herniation of meninges and brain tissues in the newborn kitten. Externally, the anomaly manifests as soft swellings on the forehead and face of the newborn. A study of the incidence in a strain of Burmese revealed that the condition is inherited as a recessive trait, with the mutant gene being symbolized by *mc*. It was thought that the selection for a short nose and rounded skull for the American Burmese may have been conducive for the presence of the gene in the breed but this does not seem to be so. Defective kittens have been bred from Burmese cats with relatively long skulls.

Mucopolysaccharidosis 1 [lethal]

The profile of cats with mucopolysaccharidosis 1 is subtly altered; the nose is short and broad, with a depressed nasal bridge, prominent forehead, small ears and opacity of the cornea. The afflicted cat sits in a crouching position, with spread forelegs. The cervical vertebrae are wider than normal, asymmetrical and frequently fused, while the sternum is unusually concave. The stomach may be swollen because of enlarged liver and spleen. The neurons of the brain and spinal cord are grossly abnormal. Phenotypically, the anomaly behaves as a recessive trait (symbol *mps-1*) but the malady arises from an enzyme deficiency which can be detected in heterozygotes as well as homozygotes.

Mucopolysaccharidosis 6 [impairing]

Cats with mucopolysaccharidosis 6 tend to resemble those described for mucopolysaccharidosis 1. The nose is short and broad and the nasal bridge is depressed, giving the face a flattened appearance. The eyelids appear to be narrow, with the upper lid swollen and drooping. The cornea of the eye is slightly opaque. The vertebral column is deformed, especially the cervical, thoracic and lumbar regions. Clinically, the anomaly is inherited as a recessive trait (symbol *mps-6*). However, the affliction has been traced to an enzyme deficiency which may be detected in both heterozygotes and homozygotes. Interestingly, two different mutant *mps-6* alleles have been discovered. These produced very similar or identical diseases but were found to be biochemically distinct. The progress of the malady can be corrected by bone marrow transplantation.

Neuroaxonal dystrophy [lethal]

Neuroaxonal dystrophy is a behavioral disorder associated with a pale coat color. The color is described as similar to 'lilac' on a non-agouti background. Affected kittens display a progressive ataxia: by five weeks of age, nodding of the head is apparent, by six weeks, the head is definitely shaking and by eight weeks, the gait shows signs of incoordination. These symptoms steadily worsen. There is probably an impairment of vision and some deafness. Body size is reduced. The cause of the disease is a degeneration of the main neurons of the brain stem and is caused by a recessive gene *no*.

Onion hair [impairing]

This anomaly is characterized by 'onion-like' swellings to the hairs. The swelling usually occurs at the tip of the hair but may arise at sites along the hair shaft. The swelling is just visible to the naked eye. The coat appears lustreless and feels rough when stroked. The whiskers and guard hairs normally taper to a fine point. In one cat, however, the anomaly was confined to the whiskers. The swelling is caused by an enlargement of the inner core of medulla cells. Examination of the skin revealed that the hair follicles and appendages were apparently normal.

Onion hair was observed in the Abyssinian breed. Although no breeding data are reported, cats with the abnormal coat were produced by normal-coated parents. The implication is that the anomaly could be inherited as a monogenic recessive trait.

Patella luxation [impairing]

Patella luxation is displacement of the patella from its normal position in the trochlear groove, either by force or spontaneously. The condition may recur if the groove is unusually shallow or incorrectly formed. A survey of breeds for the anomaly revealed that the Devon Rex showed a notably high incidence. The condition may rectify itself with but temporary discomfort to the individual. However, in a minority of cases, the condition can lead to lameness. The breed incidence implies a genetic predisposition but without indicating the mode of inheritance nor the precipitating factors. It is possible that the condition is inherited in a polygenic manner, perhaps as a threshold character, affecting the form of growth of the trochlear groove. It appears that cats with patella luxation are also three times more likely to have hip dysplasia than those without. Cats with patella luxation may be able to have this condition corrected with surgery.

Pelger-Huet anomaly [impairing]

The Pelger-Huet anomaly is a defect causing an abnormal segmentation of the nuclei of granulocytes, one of the several forms of leukocyte (white blood cell). The trait is inherited in a dominant way (symbol *Ph*) but, as far as can be ascertained, the defect does not have any adverse effects on the health of the cat.

Polycystic kidney disease [lethal]

In one form of polycystic kidney disease, kittens are born with greatly enlarged abdomens and death ensues at about six to seven weeks of age. Affected kittens were shown to have enlarged kidneys, composed of dilated cystic channels, and cystic bile ducts of the liver. In the most common form of polycystic kidney disease, renal function deteriorates leading to renal disease by three to 10 years of age.

> *According to our experts, by far the most of the cases are easy to call, especially in cats over eight to 10 months old. If the cat has no kidney cysts by that time, the cat does not have PKD. If a cat has multiple cysts in both kidneys (always bi-lateral, remember), then the cat almost assuredly has PKD. The gray area for diagnostic purposes comes in cats that are of middle to later years, that have a few cysts in both kidneys. There are cases of acquired multicystic disease – these are not PKD and not hereditary. In these gray area cases, Dr Biller says that knowing the family history can be the only determinant on which is which. Otherwise, the simple fact that the cat is a Persian will be enough for most veterinarians to pronounce that the cat has PKD.*
>
> Anna Sadler, Persian breeder

Polycystic kidney disease is seen as an autosomal dominant gene. While potentially present in all breeds, experience indicates that it occurs significantly more frequently in Persian cats and those breeds which have used Persian cats in their pedigrees, such as Exotic Shorthairs and Himalayans.

Fortunately, cats can be scanned with the use of ultrasound equipment at the age of nine to 10 months to determine whether or not the kidneys are cystic. If the kidneys do prove to be cystic, the cat can be withheld from the breeding program. False negatives are rare, but known to occur with ultrasound screening. Rescreening particularly influential cata may be prudent.

> *You don't have to euthanize a cat with PKD, unless it's seriously ill. Healthy cats should be neutered and kept as pets. If every responsible breeder would scan their cats, we could be rid of the problem within a generation.*
>
> Monique Malm, Persian breeder

Polydactyly [impairing]

If the number of separate reports is anything to judge by, the presence of extra toes on the foot, polydactyly, is something that attracts attention. This anomaly has been noted as early as 1868, if not earlier, and on many occasions since that date. There is considerable variation from animal to animal in the number of extra toes and how perfectly formed they may be. This may range from an enlargement of the inside digit to resemble a thumb to the formation of three apparently well formed extra toes making a total of seven toes on one foot. This variation in expression may occur between different feet on the same cat. In fact, the hind feet are never, or rarely, affected unless the front are abnormal.

Reviewing the various reports of polydactyly, it is remarkable how many give either direct or indirect evidence of a dominant mode of heredity. This aspect is remarkable as not all of the separate cases need be caused the same mutant gene. It is possible that the same gene may have arisen by mutation in different localities, and at different times. This could account for the similar heredity. However, it would be wise to remember that other cases of polydactyly might behave somewhat differently. At the moment, only one polydactyly gene is recognized which is symbolized by *Pd*.

Porphyria [impairing]

Porphyrins are precursor substances for the production of haem, a major component of hemoglobin. These substances arise in the bone marrow and, when they are produced in excessive amounts, are deposited in the body tissues such as the skin, bones and teeth. They are also eliminated in the urine. When this occurs, the teeth appear to be unusually discolored and the urine turns bloody. These symptoms are usually expressed from an early age. The diagnosis of the porphyric cat may be easily accomplished by examination of the teeth or bones under ultraviolet light. The impregnated teeth and bones exhibit a bright pinkish-red fluorescence. The condition is inherited as a dominant trait which is symbolized by *Po*.

A second form of porphyria has been reported. The symptoms were similar to those described above but were accompanied by noticeable lethargy and anemia. The data were consistent with monogenic transmission of the malady but the precise mode of heredity could not be determined.

Progressive retinal atrophy [impairing]

A number of accounts may be found in the literature on the occurrence of this degenerative disease of the retina. The age of onset may vary and the degeneration may take various forms, but the outcome is invariably loss of vision. The typical signs are a dilation of the iris, increased tapetal reflectability, cautious behavior, especially in leaping from heights, and clumsy behaviour such as blundering into obstacles which a cat with normal vision would easily avoid.

Two early studies were indicative that the anomaly is inherited. That of West-Hyde and Buyukmihci showed that the condition was transmitted to the offspring in a possible dominant manner but the breeding data were too few to establish this with certainty. Somewhat better data were reported by Rubin and Lipton but here the inheritance was recessive. The anomaly could be detected at between 12 to 15 weeks of age by pupil dilation and hesitant behavior.

Two cases which coincidentally occurred in the Abyssinian breed have been investigated in detail. The first was found in Swedish Abyssinian cats and was determined to be inherited in a recessive way (symbol *rdg*). Early stages of the defect could be diagnosed in many affected individuals by 18 to 24 months of age, but the advanced stages of retinal degeneration were not reached until three to four years.

The second case was found in English Abyssinian cats and was inherited as a dominant trait (symbol *Rdy*). In these cats the onset could be seen as early as four to five weeks and the advanced stages were reached by 12 weeks of age. The differing ages of onset and progression of the disease, as well as modes of heredity, would seem to indicate two independent mutant genes, despite their occurrence in the same breed of cats.

Pyloric stenosis [impairing]

Pyloric stenosis or pylorospasm is a malfunction of the lower opening of the stomach. The condition can be diagnosed by X-ray analysis following barium feeding. The symptoms are persistent, and sometimes violent, vomiting after weaning. The vomiting occurs usually after a meal but not necessarily. The inability to retain food leads to a slow-down of growth. The observations of Pearson and others imply that the defect could be inherited, although it was not possible to decide on the manner of the inheritance.

Sparse-fur [impairing]

Sparse-fur is a marked alopecia which results in a thin straggly coat that is rough to the hand. All guard hairs are short and deformed, with few down hairs. The whiskers are bent and curled. A reddish-brown exudate leading to encrustation forms along the rim of the eyelids, about the nostrils and mouth, frequently affecting the hairs of the chest and stomach. The eyelids become thickened and inflamed, and the bulbus shows signs of sepsis if left untreated. The condition is inherited as a recessive trait (symbol *sp*).

Spasticity [impairing]

Spasticity is a name given to a muscular disorder which has been found in the Devon Rex. The symptoms usually develop between four and seven weeks of age but may be delayed until 12 to 14 weeks. The kitten is active but displays an unusual posture, with the shoulder blades held high and the neck arched downwards. At rest, the body lies flat with the head held to one side. Eating is a problem for the kitten as the arched neck inter-feres with the normal feeding action of extending the neck. When drink-ing, the nose may be plunged below the surface of the liquid. These symptoms are usually interspersed with short periods, measured in days, of apparent normality. As the kitten matures, the condition becomes worse. The cat remains active but rests more often, either by lying flat with the head to one side or by leaning against an upright object. An analysis of the frequency of normal and spastic kittens born to normal parents indicated that the condition is inherited as a recessive trait, symbolized as *spt*.

Spheroid lysosomal disease [lethal]

The initial symptoms of spheroid lysosomal disease arise at about eight to 12 weeks of age as a tremor. This progresses to nodding of the head and swaying of the body. Movement is slow, with ataxia and much falling. The cat's sense of direction is impaired and seizures may occur when the cat is handled. Appetite is not disturbed but feeding is a messy affair. The cause was traced to anomalous inclusions in the tissues of the brain and spinal cord. The anomaly occurred in the Abyssinian and is caused by a recessive gene *SI*.

Sphingomyelinosis [lethal]

Kittens with sphingomyelinosis display a loss of interest in their surround-ings and develop a tremor, followed by ataxic behavior. Appetite is impaired or lost. This nervous disease is caused by an enzyme deficiency which is inherited as a recessive trait (symbol *spi*) as regards clinical manifestation. The heterozygotes can be detected by biochemical analy-sis.

Split-foot [impairing]

The typical manifestation of split–foot is that of a central cleft of either one or both front feet. Other disturbances may be present, however, such as an absence of toes or fusion to produce double claws and abnormal foot-pads. Considerable disorder of the bones, particularly the metacarpals and carpals, is shown on X-rays. The defect does not appear to interfere with normal activities, except that of climbing. The hind feet were unaffected in those animals studied.

The split-foot condition is inherited as a dominant trait and the responsible gene is symbolized by *Sh*. As the number of defective animals observed is less than expected, it is suggested that a proportion of the genetically split-foot individuals may appear normal footed. This could easily occur as a result of the variability of expression of the gene.

Squint [cosmetic]

The Siamese breed is sometimes regarded as possessing a convergent squint as a breed characteristic (Pedersen, 1991). This squint is possibly caused by a disrupted visual pathway in some strains of Siamese. However, it does not seem to have been proven correct as a general statement. Whatever may have happened in the past, there are many strains in existence at the present time which do not show this affliction. It will be appreciated, of course, that a squint may occur in any individual or breed in addition to that of Siamese.

The situation is complicated by the fact that a kitten may display a mild squint while young which is slowly corrected as it becomes older. This means that genetically 'squinted' animals may appear as normal if the early life of the cat is unknown. Only one report on the condition in Siamese has made any attempt to interpret the mode of inheritance. However, the results of a number of crosses have not yielded clear cut results. The condition seems to be inherited but seemingly as the outcome of the interaction of two or more genes. It seems possible that the squint is inherited as a polygenically controlled threshold character; alternatively, of course, it could be determined monogenetically but with impenetrance.

Testicular feminization [impairing]

Although only one case of testicular feminization has been reported in the cat, the anomaly so resembles comparable inherited conditions in other mammals that an account is warranted. The adult cat was an apparently normal female but with no signs of estrus behavior. Upon examination, it was found that the sex chromosomes were male and that the sex organs had been incompletely developed as female. In general, the condition is due to a mutant gene (adopted symbol *tfm*) on the X chromosome which disrupts development of normal male secondary sex structures. The feminized male is identified because of the accompanying sterility. Female sterility may arise from numerous causes and testicular feminization must now be added to the list.

Tremor [impairing]

Tremor is characterized by a continuous, whole body, tremble which begins at about two to four weeks of age. The kitten rolls and bobs in an undulating fashion while the tail weaves in circles. The trembling only ceases when the animal is completely at rest or is held firmly. Even when held by the nape of the neck, the tremble is still obvious. A single recessive gene *tr* is postulated for the anomalous behavior. There is no sign of underdeveloped cerebellum which typifies the virus-induced ataxia.

Umbilical hernia [cosmetic to impairing]

Two research veterinarians, Henricson and Bornstein, have observed a particularly high incidence of umbilical hernia among the Abyssinian breed in Sweden. The precise mode of inheritance could not be determined but the influence of heredity is unmistakable in their data. For example, the chances of the offspring being herniated is about 75 per cent when one parent is known to have an hernia, against 3 per cent for the offspring of parents which are known to be normal or are unknown. These figures are cited merely as a guide and must not be taken too literally.

The fact of the high incidence among the progeny, when one parent is known to be herniated, prompted the suggestion that the predisposition towards the occurrence of an hernia might be inherited as a dominant. This may be the case, and the data is certainly suggestive in this respect, but it may be wise to be cautious. When the breeding data are closely examined, too many individuals are marked as 'unknown' for positive conclusions to be drawn.

Umbilical hernia is usually caused by an inherent defect in the umbilical ring. A weakness can result in a part of the abdominal contents being extruded as a soft bulge. However, even if the musculature is defective, a hernia need not always develop or the development may be so slight as to escape notice. This means that if attention is focused entirely upon the presence or absence of hernia the fundamental or primary defect will not be detected in some cases. The hernia condition is a 'secondary' manifestation of a probable anomaly of the umbilical region. The descent of the hernia from one generation to the next could appear to be irregular, in spite of the probability that the primary defect is inherited along regular lines. However, it must be admitted that the problem is complex. The simplest hypothesis is that the incidence of hernia is a threshold character.

Urolithiasis [impairing]

There is a case of urolithiasis, or formation of urinary calculi, which reveals a familial tendency. A male cat showed the disease and so did three kittens out of four from matings with his sister. Full details of the urolithiasis are not given except the statement that the disease failed to respond to any treatment, including surgery. The affected animals are otherwise healthy and there was no evidence of environmental factors at play. It is possible that a hereditary influence may be involved.

Though intriguing, these observations would carry little weight, standing alone, but they are the sort that could contribute towards something tangible should a number of similar reports come in over the years. For this reason, if no other, this condition deserves to be cited. It is quite likely that a predisposition towards the formation of urinary calculi could be determined to some extent by heredity. A genetic propensity towards urolithiasis is suspected in the dog.

Visual pathways misrouting [impairing]

True albino animals are completely without pigment, hence the coat is white and the pupil of the eye is pink or red, surrounded by a translucent iris. In the cat, the Siamese allele is a form of partial albinism with a limited amount of pigment to create a blue iris.

A curious feature of albinotic animals is a misrouting of the visual ganglion axons from the retina to the brain. An unusual number pass to the wrong side of the brain. However, this may not seriously impair vision as the cat's brain is apparently able to compensate. Both albino and Siamese cats are affected, the latter to a lesser extent than the former. It is of interest that, while white coat color is recessive to fully colored, the heterozygotes *Ccs* and *Cc* have misrouted pathways although to a lesser degree than the homozygotes *cscs* or *cc*.

Cats with the Chediak-Higashi syndrome also show misrouting of the pathways but to a lesser extent than the albino. Incidentally, neither the Burmese of the albino series of alleles nor dominant white exhibit signs of visual misrouting. There are many reports on the anomaly.

Weeping eye [impairing]

A perpetually weeping or running eye could be due to several causes: injury to the eyelid, entropion or inward turning of the eyelid, so that hairs irritate the eyeball, or to blockage of either the nasolacrimal canal or the lacrimal duct which are responsible for draining excess tears. The blockage could result from a foreign body in the canal or duct. It is advisable to consult a veterinary surgeon if the condition persists.

However, the condition can arise as a consequence of selective breeding for an excessively short nose in some breeds. This may lead to distortion, narrowing or even blockage of the nasolacrinal canal or lacrinal duct. The eyes overflow with tears which trickle down the side of the nose. In this case, the condition may be held to be genetic, probably polygenically, as a result of changes in skull shape. If affected animals recur in related litters or over several generations, the breeding policy should be reviewed. The responsible breeder will not breed from afflicted cats even if they are surgically corrected. It would also be wise to retire from breeding any animal which produces such offspring.

Technical appendix

List of genetic anomalies and symbols

Table 11.1 Genetic anomalies and their symbols

Symbol	Name	Symbol	Name
br	Brachyury	hy	Hydrocephalus
ch	Chediak-Higashi syndrome	M	Manx tailnessness
Cu	American Curl	man	Mannosidosis
Cut	Cutaneous asthenia	mc	Meningoencephalocele
dp	Duplicate pinnae	no	Neuroaxonal dystrophy
ew	Episodic weakness	Pd	Polydactyly
fck	Flat-chest kitten syndrome	Ph	Pleger-Huct anomaly
Fd	Folded ears	Po	Porphyria
ga-1	Gangliosidosis GM1	rdg	Progressive retinal atrophy
ga-2	Gangliosidosis GM2	Rdy	Progressive retinal atrophy
h	French hairless	rt	Retinal degeneration
Hag	Hageman factor	Sh	Split-foot
hce	Hyperchylomicronemia	sl	Spheroid lysosomal disease
hd	Redcar hairless	sp	Sparse fur
Hma	Hemophilia A	spl	Sphingomyelinosis
Hmb	Hemophilia B	spt	Spasticity
ho	Hyperoxaluria	tr	Tremor
hr	Canadian hairless		

Historical appendix

The elimination of craniofacial defects in the Burmese cat – a case study of responsible breeding

The Burmese cat has a standard that calls for 'roundness' everywhere. This look is especially apparent in the head. The face of the Burmese presents a rounded head with round cheeks, round chin and rounded ear tips. In order to meet this standard, Burmese breeders began to breed for a very rounded look in the head. This look became known as the 'contemporary' (or 'eastern' or 'extreme' or 'new') look. However, in striving to perpetuate this look, the breeders of Burmese cats began to see significant deformities in their litters. The deformity is known as incomplete cojoined twinning. The defect basically is a duplication of the upper maxillary. Kittens are born alive but are not able to survive.

As soon as the Burmese breeders became aware of the fact that this defect was occurring in Burmese litters across the country and was not an isolated incident or an environmental problem, they began to send affected kittens to Cornell University School of Veterinary Medicine for study. In the 1980s, they also asked the Winn Foundation to fund a study and initiated the Burmese Cooperative Research Group to study this defect.

The studies found that the 'Contemporary phenotype is the expression of the incomplete penetrance of the dominant and its presence insures that the cat is a carrier for the lethal gene or genes'. To date it appears that the contemporary phenotype is always linked to the head defect.

At the present time, responsible breeders of Burmese cats are working to eliminate the head defect in their cats. They are to be given credit for finding the defect, working with research veterinarians to study this defect and for using the results to better their breed and produce healthy, viable Burmese kittens.

Glossary

This glossary covers terms found in this edition as well as additional ones which may be encountered in genetic texts.

A

Abyssinian tabby See Ticked tabby.

Adult For purposes of cat shows, a cat which is at least eight months old. Its age is measured at the time of the show.

Agouti The natural coloring of most species of mammals. The wild type color phenotype in coat color genetics. Includes classic (blotched), mackerel, spotted and ticked tabby. The hairs are banded with yellow, especially at the base. The coat of the Abyssinian is a good example. The hairs are banded with yellow. The wider the band, the lighter the coat.

Albino The pink or red-eyed white mutant which is completely devoid of pigment is a true albino. The red-eye is caused by the blood in the translucent eye structures. Blue or dark- eyed white individuals are not albinos. Siamese coloration is a form of incomplete albinism.

Allele Mutant form(s) of the normal gene. There may be more than one at a locus. Often employed as an alternative term for any gene, although this usage is strictly incorrect. Gene is the more general term.

Allelic series A series of mutant alleles which have arisen from a normal gene by mutation. A number of alleles at the same locus.

Allelomorph Obsolete term for allele.

Alter A class where spayed and neutered cats are judged (see Premier). Also, a cat who has been surgically corrected to prevent breeding. See Neuter and Spay.

Alternative heredity Mendelian inheritance involving the genetic assortment of major genes, as opposed to blending heredity.

Anestrus Interval between successive estruses.

Anomaly Anything which is contrary to the general rule. An organ or structure which is abnormal with reference to form, structure, position; a malformation.

Anorexia Loss of appetite.

Antenatal Before birth.

Antibodies Proteins, produced by the immune system, which are generated in response to the presence of a foreign substance such as bacteria.

Artificial fertilization The union of ovum and sperm by various artificial techniques. It also involves artificial insemination.

Artificial selection The action by man to ensure that certain individuals are preserved in preference to others. Different breeds of the single species of domestic cat are created in this manner. Such action can counter natural selection.

Assortative mating The mating of individuals with similar characteristics. Like-to-like matings.

Assortment of genes The random combination of genes from each parent to create a unique individual.

Atavism Appearance of an ancestral form among litters of kittens. Now an obsolete term.

Autosomal gene A gene present on the autosomes, as opposed to those on the sex chromosomes. See Sex-linked genes.

Autosomes The ordinary chromosomes of the complement, as opposed to the sex chromosomes X and Y.

B

Backcross Mating of the F_1 to one of the parents, usually to the parent with the recessive genotype of interest. See Testcross.

BC Symbol to denote a backcross mating.

Bicolor Having a patched coat of one color and white.

Bigenic A character which is determined by alleles at two independent loci.

Blastodermic The embryonic disk of an embryo. A disk of cells which lies between the yolk sac and the amniotic cavity from which the embryo develops.

Blaze Having white on the face in the form of a inverted V.

Blending heredity Where ancestral traits 'blend' to produce intermediate expression in matings, as opposed to alternative (Mendelian) inheritance.

Bloodline Breeder's rather than genetic term. Roughly equivalent to a strain but used to denote descent from a famous but remote ancestor.

Blotched tabby See Classic tabby.

Bottleneck Point where a population decreases to few individuals from any cause and from which it increases in size. In cats, this could occur where a once popular breed loses popularity rather sharply before regaining usual numbers.

Breed An interbreeding group of individuals with uniform and distinctive characteristics.

Breed Club A group of cat owners and exhibitors where membership is limited to owners of the breed in question. It may be independent or affiliated with one of the cat registries.

Breed standards The written list of characteristics formulated by a cat federation for use in judging a particular breed. The standards describe the ideal specimen of that breed. They are sometimes called 'standards of perfection' or 'points of excellence'.

Breeder quality A pedigree cat that is basically sound in appearance, and of good health and overall quality (when measured against the standards of the breed), and thus would prove an asset to a breeding program. However, while it shows no disqualifying characteristics, it would not win in competition. A breeder's term.

Brindling Coat of a mixture of black and orange (or blue and cream) colored hairs. Opposite of patching. Also brindle.

C

Calling Female cat's vocalization during estrus.

Carrier An individual which is heterozygous for a particular recessive gene; commonly used with reference to a lethal or other undesirable gene. Breeder's term rather than genetic.

Castration Removal of testes from the male.

Cat Fancy A term often used to describe a cat federation. It is also used in the broader sense of the entire universe of those breeding purebred cats and showing both purebred and household pet cats at cat shows. There it is usually just called 'the Fancy'.

Cat Federation An association of persons and clubs involved in breeding, showing and judging cats. Among its activities are sanctioning shows and registering cats. See also Registry.

Cat For cat shows, a feline, of either sex, over eight months of age. Usually, but not always, denotes an unaltered (whole) cat.

Cattery A name registered by a cat breeder to identify the breeder's line of breeding. A registered cattery name always appears as a prefix to the name of a cat bred by that cattery/breeder. Also used to describe the facility where the breeding or boarding of cats takes place.

Cell The fundamental unit of tissues and organs of the body.

Cervix Region where the two uteri join to form the vagina.

Character A feature considered as an entity in heredity. The expression of major genes. Also see Trait.

Checkerboard A diagram to facilitate the derivation of phenotypes and genetic ratios produced by two or more assorting independently genes.

Chiasma The physical expression of exchange of segments of chromosomes during the first stage of meiosis. Important for recombination of genes.

Chiasmata Plural of chiasma.

Chimera One individual formed from the fusion of two fertilized eggs. May be of unique appearance but sometimes grotesque. Some tortoiseshell males are chimeras.

Chromatid Primitive chromosome formed during the early stages of meiosis, before separation into two fully fledged chromosomes.

Chromosome Strands of DNA which are bearers of genes. These can be seen as small bodies in the nucleus of cells. One of the fundamental units of heredity.

Chromosome complement The number of chromosomes for a species. In the cat, the number is 38, or 19 pairs.

Classic tabby Maximum expression of pattern, with the fine vertical stripes of the mackerel being replaced by bars and whorls. Also called blotched tabby.

Classical lethal Lethal gene which causes death of the individual before birth. Responsible for much prenatal or uterine mortality.

Closed stud A system of breeding whereby individuals are selected from within the breeder's own stock or strain. Outcrosses to another strain are only undertaken for a special purpose.

Cobby A compact body type.

Codominance When the phenotypes of two genes are shown in the heterozygote. Do not confuse with incomplete dominance. Uncommon.

Coefficient of inbreeding A numerical measure of the amount of inbreeding in ancestry of a cat. An important quantitative determination in the art of breeding.

Coital crouch Characteristic squatting posture by the female to receive the male at coitus (for copulation).

Coitus Act of mating.

Colostrum A queen's 'milk' which is produced during the first 48 hours after the birth of kittens. This very special substance is very high in protein and antibodies.

Comparative genetics The study of comparing the location and function of genes between species.

Compensatory mating A method of breeding whereby good and bad characters are balanced against each other in arranging matings between individuals. The object is to achieve an overall improvement in the population.

Conception Product of a successful mating. Initiation of pregnancy.

Conformation The 'look' or physical type of a cat, usually when measured against its written breed standard.

Congenital Character present at or from birth.

Copulation Act of mating.

Copulatory ovulator A species in which copulation results in hormonal changes resulting in the release of ova.

Corpus lutea Yellowish scar tissue of a burst Graafian follicle on the surface of the ovary.

Cosmetic genes Those genes which produce cosmetic changes in a cat, but which are neither lethal nor impairing. They are of two types: those having medical or physical repercussions and those which do not require any surgical or medical intervention to permit the cat to live a healthy life.

Crossbred Individual from a purposeful mating between two distinct breeds. Do not confuse with the general term mongrel.

Crossover When genes pass from one partner of a pair of chromosomes to the other as a result of exchange of DNA during meioses. Also called crossing over.

Cryptorchidism Disruption of the descent of testes into the scrotum. Bilateral when both testes fail to descend, unilateral when one testis fails to descend. Monocryptorchidism is an incorrect term for the latter.

Culling The rejection or removal of inferior individuals from breeding. Act of selective breeding. As used in the practice of breeding pedigree cats, this refers to the practice of spaying or neutering a kitten or cat that does not measure up to the show standard (or other standard being applied) for that breed. In no way does culling, as used by responsible breeders, signify the killing of healthy kittens or cats if they fail to meet the applicable standard.

Cytogenetics Combination of the study of chromosomes and genetic analysis of characters.

Cytology Scientific study of cells and tissues.
Cytoplasm Contents of a cell other than the nucleus.

D

Dam Female parent. Also queen.
Deferred lethal A gene which is lethal in full manifestation, that is it is not lethal in utero, at birth, or shortly following birth.
Deoxyribonucleic acid Major biochemical constituent of the chromosome. Abbreviation DNA.
Dermatitis An inflammation of the skin.
Differentiation Biological process where precursory cells divide to form more specialized cells to make tissues and organs.
Digitigrade Walking on the tips of the toes, like a cat.
Diploid number The usual complement of two of each chromosome in the body cells of the individual. Twice the basic, haploid, number.
Disassortative mating Mating of individuals with dissimilar characteristics. Mating of unlike to unlike. See Compensatory mating. Cf. Assortative mating.
DNA Abbreviation for deoxyribonucleic acid.
Doctoring Vernacular term for spaying or neutering.
Domestication The adaptation of a wild species to life in captivity, as wild *Felis libyca* developed into the tame domestic cat.
Dominance When the expression of a gene completely over-rides the expression of another at the same locus. Not to be confused with epistasis.
Dominant gene The allele whose expression completely over-rides that of another at the same locus. The allele which manifests in the F_1. See Recessive gene.
Double recessive Individual homozygous for two recessive genes.
Drift See Genetic drift
Dysplasia Development that is not normal. Hip dysplasia is a concern in some breeds of cats.

E

Ectopic pregnancy Development of an ovum other than in the uterus.
Effective population The number of individuals which actually contribute offspring to the next generation, as opposed to the general population or a population before culling.
Egg The ovum after fertilization by a sperm.
Ejaculate The seminal fluid. Semen.
Ejaculation Expression of seminal fluid.
Embryo Stage of development of a fertilized egg before becoming a fetus.
Endocrine glands Those ductless glands which secrete hormones. These are important for many biological functions, including sex development and behavior.
Entire Said of an individual which has not been neutered. See Whole.
Environment All non-genetic influences affecting the growth, maturity and well-being of the individual.
Epididymus The duct in which the sperms produced by the testes are stored before ejaculation.

Estrus Period when the female will accept a mating.

Estrus period The duration of estrus.

Epistasis When the expression of an allele masks the effects of one or more alleles at different loci. Not to be confused with dominance. Cf. Hypostasis.

Eumelanin One of the basic pigments, usually called brown or black.

Expression The variation of the phenotype of a gene.

Expressivity The measurement of the variable expression of a gene by a convenient scale.

F

F_1 Symbol for the first filial generation. The first cross offspring.

F_2 Symbol for the second filial generation. The offspring from mating the F_1 inter se.

Factor Obsolete term for a gene.

Fallopian tube Thin tube leading from the ovary to the uterus. Also called oviduct.

False pregnancy Pseudopregnancy.

Familial selection Selection which is based not exclusively on the excellence of the individual but also, or alternately, on the excellence of closely related individuals as a group, usually siblings.

Fancy Short for 'the Cat Fancy'.

Fecund Highly fertile.

Fecundity The ability to produce numerous offspring.

Feral Domestic individual which has returned to living in the wild.

Feral Non-domesticated cat. This can refer to cats who are 'wild' such as bobcats, tigers, etc. The term is also used to denote a colony of cats who live outside in a community but are not cared for by humans.

Feral blood Referring to the presence of a 'wild' cat, such as a bobcat, that is bred into the lines of a pedigree cat.

Fertilization Fusion of ovum and sperm. Cf. Conception.

Fertility The ability to produce offspring.

Fixation The stage where genes become homozygous or 'fixed' as a consequence of either drift, selection or inbreeding, usually the latter.

Fix Vernacular term for spaying or neutering.

Fixing To 'fix' a characteristic in the individual either by selection or by inbreeding. Breeder's term rather than genetic.

Fetal atrophy Loss of fetuses before birth. Death and resorption of a fetus within the uterus. Common in species with multiple birth.

Fetus Stage of development when the embryo has become a recognizable kitten.

Foster To transfer offspring from the dam to another female for nursing.

Foster mother Female who nurses another female's offspring.

Founder principle Population with unique features due to their derivation from a few individuals, the 'founders'. Many cat breeds were 'founded' in this manner.

G

Gametes Genetic term for the reproductive cells. Sperms and ova of the male and female, respectively. Opposite to somatic cells.

Gene The basic unit of heredity, as carried by the chromosomes like 'beads on a string'.

Gene frequency Proportion or percentage of individuals in a population expressing a particular gene, usually the mutant allele.

Gene mapping The process of determining the location of a particular gene on a chromosome.

Gene pair Two alternative genes assorting at a locus, usually the normal gene and a mutant allele, but these could be two mutant alleles.

Gene pool The collective number of genes and hence potential somatic diversity in an interbreeding population; usually shown as 2n, where n is the number of individuals in the population, as the genes occur in pairs in the individual. Also a breeder's term describing the genetic constitution of a group of individual cats.

Gene symbols Genes are denoted by letters of the Latin alphabet, usually as a convenient shorthand for writing genotypes and to work with checkerboards. By convention, capital letters denote dominant genes and lower case letters denote recessive genes or alleles.

Genealogy The study of pedigrees, bloodlines and ancestry. Important for the art of breeding.

Genetic Pertaining to the genes.

Genetic constitution The genetic endowment of the individual. The genotype as opposed to phenotype.

Genetic drift Random fixation of genes, usually due to a limited breeding group within a strain, breed or species. Can occur if selection is relaxed.

Genetic fingerprinting Pattern of fragmented and stained DNA which is unique to the individual. Shared patterns only exist in cases of identical twins or very closely related, highly inbred individuals.

Genetic marker A piece of genetic material highly associated with a particular disease or gene and used to determine its presence.

Genetic ratio Ratios of phenotypes produced by assorting genes

Genetics The study of heredity and phenotype variation in a population.

Genitals External sex organs.

Genic Pertaining to the genes. See Genetic.

Genome The totality of the genetic endowment of the individual. Employed in a more general sense than genotype, as it includes genes not yet completely characterized.

Genotype Genetic constitution of the individual expressed in terms of gene symbols. A more limited definition than genome, as it only includes genes which have been characterized. Cf. Phenotype.

Genetic anomaly An inherited abnormality. Not all congenital abnormalities are genetic in nature. In cats, they are of three major types: lethal, impairing and cosmetic.

Germ cell Reproductive cell or gamete.

Germ cell lineage Concept of an immortal lineage of cells bridging generations. The lineage consists of an alternation of the germinal cells (gonads) of the individual and the germ cells (ova and sperm) which these produce.

Germinal cells Pertaining to the germ cells (ova and sperm) of an individual.

Germinal mutation Mutation within the germ cell lineage giving rise to inherited or genetic variation. Mutation in the body cells may be expressed in the phenotype but are not inherited. See Somatic mutation.

Gestation Pregnancy.

Gestation period Duration of a pregnancy; period of carrying offspring from conception to parturition.

Ghost pattern Tabby pattern to be seen in the coats of solid colored kittens, revealing the tabby pattern masked by the non-agouti gene. Often disappears with successive molts.

Gonads Organs of the body which produce the germ cells or gametes. More specifically when the organs have not differentiated into testes (male) and ovaries (female).

Graafian follicle Sac or pimple on the surface of the ovary containing the ova. In cats, the act of copulation results in the elevation of a hormone which causes these to rupture, releasing ova. After release of ova, a yellowish scar is formed. See Corpus lutea.

Grading Assessment of the quality of characters either by measurement (weight or size) or by grading on a scale of points for excellence. Cf. Scoring.

Grading up Improvement by repeated matings of inferior animals to those from a superior strain. Rapid method of improving inferior stock.

Gravid Pregnant.

Gynander See Gynandromorph.

Gynandromorph Individual with a mixture of male and female sex organs. It is possible for an individual to be male on one side of the body and female on the other. Cf. Hermaphrodite; Intersex.

H

Haploid number The number of chromosomes in the gamete, being half that normally found in the body or somatic cells. Cf. Diploid.

Heat The period when a female will accept a mating. See Estrus period.

Hemolysis Destruction of red blood cells, with the liberation of hemoglobin, which diffuses into the fluid surrounding the cells. When this occurs, the body is unable to retain the hemoglobin, which is lost through the kidneys and imparts a red color to the urine.

Herd management Practices necessary to the health and well-being of a group of animals, usually a herd of farm animals but also applied to a breeding cattery.

Heredity The transmission of inherited variation from parent to offspring.

Heritability The variation between individuals may be partitioned into that caused by environment and that due to heredity. Heritability is the latter expressed as a proportion of the total variation.

Hermaphrodite Individual with both male and female reproductive organs (ovaries and testes) which are more or less functional. Cf. Gynandromorph; Intersex.

Heterogametic sex Producing two types of germ cells or gametes. In particular, the gender which produces both gametes containing X chromosomes and gametes containing Y chromosomes. In cats and other mammals, this is the male. Cf. Homogametic sex.

Heterochromia Where the iris of one eye is normal but the other is partially or wholly blue. Cats exhibiting this phenomenon are commonly called 'odd-eyed'.

Heterosis The exceptional vigor which may be observed in the offspring from crosses between inbred strains. Also known as hybrid vigor.

Heterotic effect When the heterozygote displays exceptional expression compared with the parents. Heterosis or hybrid vigor may be cited as a special case.

Heterozygosis Genetic transmission of a particular quality or trait from parent to offspring.

Heterozygosity Proportion of heterozygous loci in an individual. Proportion of heterozygous individuals in a population. Cf. Homozygosity.

Heterozygote Individual with two dissimilar alleles (*Aa*) at a locus as opposed to two similar alleles (*AA* or *aa*). See Homozygote.

Heterozygous advantage When the heterozygote (*Aa*) is superior to either homozygote (*AA* or *aa*). The accepted basis for heterosis.

HHP Abbreviation for household pet (cat or kitten) in a cat show.

Homogametic sex Producing only one sort of gamete. In particular when all of the gametes carry the X chromosome. In cats and other mammals, this is the female. Cf. Heterogametic sex.

Homologous Genes with similar function and phenotype between genes species. Many coat color genes are homologous between species. Dogs, cats and rodents have many genes in common.

Homozygosity Proportion of homozygous loci in the individual (*AA* or *aa*). Proportion of homozygous individuals in a population. Cf. Heterozygosity.

Homozygote Individual with two similar alleles (*AA* or *aa*) at a locus, as opposed to an individual with dissimilar alleles (Aa). See Heterozygote.

Homozygous Possessing a pair of identical alleles at a given locus, that is *AA* or *aa*.

Hormones Chemicals produced within the body which control many biological functions, including sexual development and reproductive processes in general. Cf. Androgen; Estrogen.

Household pet A non-pedigree cat or kitten or a pedigree cat or kitten being exhibited in a class with non-pedigree cats or kittens. Some cat federations have a separate procedure for registering household pets. Some federations also permit household pets to earn titles equivalent to those won by pedigree cats. Household pets are usually required to be altered by a certain age and may or may not be permitted to be declawed.

Hybrid Offspring of a cross between two species. To use the term for offspring between two breeds is strictly incorrect.

Hybrid vigor Common term for heterosis.

Hypostasis When the expression of one or more alleles are masked by the expression of another allele at a different locus. Not to be confused with dominance/recessiveness. Cf. Epistasis.

I

Idiogram Diagramic representation of chromosomes of a karyotype.

Impairing genes Genes which produce conditions which are not lethal, but which impair the ability of the cat to function. They are of three types:

those which are difficult or impossible to control with medical or surgical therapy; those which require surgical therapy for the cat to survive or to live a relatively painless life; and those which require prolonged or life-time medical management.

Impenetrance When the expression of a gene fails to manifest, as may occur for the poor expression of a gene. See Incomplete penetrance.

Implantation Attachment of the developing egg to the wall of the uterus.

Impregnation Insemination.

Inbred strain A group of animals which have been closely inbred for many generations. Such strains can be remarkably uniform.

Inbreeding Mating of closely related individuals. The two most common are brother–sister or parent–offspring.

Inbreeding depression Decline of vigor and vitality as a consequence of inbreeding because of the fixation of impairing genes with small cumulative effects.

Inbreeding index A ratio describing the intensity of inbreeding.

Incomplete dominance When the heterozygote (Aa) has a phenotype which is intermediate in expression to those of the two homozygotes (AA and aa). Do not confuse with codominance.

Incomplete penetrance See Impenetrance

Independent culling levels A method of selection whereby the individual is culled if it fails to surpass a given level of excellence for any one of a number of characters.

Individual merit Straightforward selection based on the excellence of the individual.

Induced ovulation Ovulation which is induced by the stimulus of coitus, as opposed to spontaneous ovulation. Cats are induced ovulators. Cf. Spontaneous ovulation.

Infertile Inability to produce viable offspring; sterile.

Inherited That which is transmitted from parent to offspring.

Insemination Introduction of semen into the vagina, either from coitus or artificially.

Intermediate heredity Blending inheritance.

Intersex Individual with imperfectly formed sex organs, neither fully functional as male or female and often mixed. Cf. Gynandromorph; Hermaphrodite.

Intromission Insertion. In breeding, vaginal penetration.

Isolate Population bred in isolation from the general population. Individual breeds of cats are examples of isolates.

K

Karyogram Schematic representation of a karyotype; idiogram.

Karyology Study of the nucleus of cells, especially the number and form of the chromosomes.

Karyotype An account of the number and physical description of the chromosomes of an individual, breed or species.

Keratin Biochemical substance which forms the hair and nails.

Keyhole breeding A breeder's term, identifying breeding practices that focus on the use of one select stud cat or particular line, usually representing successful competitors. The term may come from the idea that one is looking for breeding partners, but can see only one when looking through a keyhole. While this tends to fix the look or type of a breed, it also reduces genetic diversity very quickly.

Kitten A feline, of either sex, under the age of eight months. For purposes of cat shows, a cat that is at least four months old, but less than eight months old. Its age is measured at the time of the show.

L

Lactation Production of milk in the queen and the suckling of offspring.

Lethal gene A gene which causes death of the recipient. Of three types: classical lethal, tetratological and deferred.

Libido Sex drive or urge.

Like-to-like mating Assortative mating.

Line Group of interbreeding individuals with acknowledged distinctive characteristics. Sometimes referred to as a strain. See Strain

Line breeding A form of inbreeding intended to concentrate the genes of a certain individual, usually by repeated backcrosses. A term frequently but wrongly used by breeders to denote less intense forms of inbreeding.

Linkage Presence of two or more genes on the same chromosome. These genes do not always sort at random, but tend to stay together if derived from the same parent, or do not recombine if derived from different parents.

Linkage map Linear representation of order of genes on a chromosome.

Litter Numerous kittens produced at a single parturition.

Litter registration The recording by a cat federation of the birth of a litter, giving the date of birth, number of kittens, as well as the sire and dam. Litter applications are submitted by the breeder of the litter.

Litter siblings Offspring belonging to the same litter regardless of sex.

Littering Giving birth. Also queening.

Livestock Domestic animals kept for breeding.

Loci Plural of locus.

Locus The precise location of a gene on the chromosome. Normally the gene occupies the same position on the same chromosome in all individuals.

Long day Encouragement of breeding by provision of artificial illumination during the shorter daylight hours of the autumn, winter and early spring.

Lordosis A severe condition affecting the spine of a cat just behind the shoulder blades.

M

Mackerel tabby The wild-type tabby pattern of gently curving vertical stripes.

Major genes Genes with large effects on the phenotype, as opposed to genes which have small effects or traits that are polygenetic in nature. Cf. Minor genes.

Mammae Mammary glands.

Mammary glands Milk secreting glands of the female.

Manifestation Expression of a gene.

Masking When a genotype is concealed by the actions of a gene at another loci, such as the effect of dominant white over other color genes. See Epistasis.

Maternal impressions Discredited belief that impressions received by a pregnant female influence the character of her offspring.

Mating Placing two animals together for coitus. Copulation.

Matrilineal Descent through the female line or ancestry. Cf. Patrilineal.

Meiosis Specialized cell divisions which result in the halving of the diploid number of chromosomes present in the individual, before the formation of the gametes with the haploid number. Cf. Reduction division.

Melanin Coloring pigment of the hair, iris of the eye and skin. See Eumelanin and Phaeomelanin.

Melanism Black or very dark phenotypes in a population; as with black cats in a feral population.

Mendelian character A trait produced by a single major gene and which is inherited according to Mendelian principles of independent sorting.

Mendelian factor Obsolete term for a gene.

Mendelian When the inheritance of a character conforms to simple principles of the independent sorting and expression of dominant and recessive alleles.

Mendelism Obsolete term for elementary genetics. After Gregor Mendel who discovered the basic laws of heredity.

Microsatellites Highly polymorphic pieces of genetic material, randomly distributed throughout the genome, with no known function. Used as markers for other genes or to determine identity, paternity, etc.

Minor gene Gene with minor effects on the phenotype. As opposed to major genes. See Polygenes.

Minority breed A breed which is small in terms of the total number of kittens born each year, thus tending to produce fewer numbers of whole adults.

Misalliance Said of a litter from an accidental mating.

Mismating Said of a litter from an accidental mating.

Missed mating When a mating failed to produce a litter.

Mitosis Cell division which produces tissues and organs of the body.

Modifiers Genes which modify the expression of other genes. Commonly applied to those polygenes which mold the expression of major genes. Important in shaping the finer points of breeds or phenotypes.

Modifying gene A gene which modifies the expression of another gene. May be either a major or minor gene, usually the latter.

Molecular genetics The study of genes and their effects at the molecular level. Also molecular biology.

Mongrel Individual from indeterminate breeding, as opposed to purebred or even crossbred. Slang, Moggie.

Monogenic A character which is determined by a single major gene.

Morph Variant form in a polymorphic population.

Morula Solid mass of cells, resembling a mulberry, resulting from segmentation of an ovum.

Mosaic Individual composed of tissues with differing genetic make-up. Some tortoiseshell males are mosaics.

Molt Replacement of hairs in the coat to maintain its quality. Molting in the cat is diffuse, replacing a few at a time.

Multiple alleles Series of mutant alleles which have arisen from the same wild-type gene.

Multiple factors Polygenes.

Mutagenic Factors which are capable of inducing mutation of the genes, including atomic radiation and certain chemical substances. These mutations be either germinal or somatic.

Mutant An individual displaying the effects of a mutated gene.

Mutant allele A variant of a gene which has arisen by mutation from a wild-type gene.

Mutation The process of producing a mutant allele; an obvious deviation from the normal which is genetically caused.

N

Natural selection The survival of certain individuals at the expense of others, mediated by natural events.

Necropsy Autopsy of a non-human animal.

Neonatal Pertaining to newborn offspring.

Neonatal erythrolysis Hemolysis in the newborn kitten. A disease condition caused when the kitten's red blood cells are destroyed by the actions of the maternal antibodies ingested in the queen's colostrum. This can occur in the blood type A kittens delivered by a blood type B queen.

Neuter Desexing of either gender. For breeders, a male cat who has been castrated to prevent breeding.

Neutering Castrating a male cat. See Neuter.

Neoteny Persistence of juvenile characteristics into adulthood. Important concept for the process of domestication.

Normal gene The gene which produces the normal phenotype, as opposed to that produced by a mutant allele. The original gene for a locus. See Wild type.

Normal phenotype The typical phenotype for the species. The phenotype against which the effects of mutant alleles are compared. Also known as the 'wild type'. In the cat, this is the mackerel striped *Felix libyca*.

Nucleus The body within the cell which contains the chromosomes, among other important constituents.

O

Obligate carrier The offspring of a cat that is homozygous for a given allele.

Odd-eyes Having eyes with different colored irises. Usually yellow and blue. See Heterochromia.

Offspring The progeny from a mating. Kittens from a particular mating.

Ontogeny Stages of development of the individual.

Oogenesis Cell divisions which produce the female germ cells of gametes (ova).

Outbred stock An interbreeding population in which inbreeding is carefully avoided.

Outbreeding Method of breeding in which inbreeding is deliberately avoided.

Outcross Breeder's term meaning the breeding one cat to another unrelated cat.

Ovariohysterectomy Removal of ovaries and uterus.

Ovary Female organ for the production of germ cells or gametes (ova).

Overdominance When the heterozygote *Aa* is more extreme in expression than the homozygote *AA*.

Overlaps When the phenotype of one gene has the phenotype of another gene. Typically when the phenotype of a mutant allele mimics that of the normal gene. Particularly when an impairing gene appears normal in action or appearance.

Oviduct Tube which conveys the ova from the ovary to the uterus.

Ovulation Release of ova from the Graafian follicles. The cat is one of the few species which requires the stimulus of mating to induce ovulation.

Ovum Singular of ova.

P

Panmixis Random mating within an interbreeding population. Random mating where inbreeding is not deliberately avoided.

Papers One way to refer to a cat's certificate of registration and pedigree form.

Parental generation Initial generation which produces the F_1.

Parthenogenesis Development of ovum without fertilization by a sperm. Also known as 'virgin birth'. Almost impossible in mammals.

Parturition Moment of birth.

Partial dominance Incomplete dominance.

Pathogenic Inducing a disease condition. Said of a lethal or impairing gene.

Patrilineal Descent through the male line or ancestry. Genes on the Y chromosome will display patrilineal inheritance, but these are rare.

Pedigree Formalized presentation of the ancestry or ancestors of an individual; a document showing a cat's background for three, four or five generations. A three-generation pedigree includes the cat, plus three generations back. A pedigree gives names, colors and registration numbers for each cat in the pedigree. Show titles are usually also given.

Pedigree cat This usually refers to a cat whose heritage is known, documented and registered. See Pedigree.

Penetrance The proportion of individuals that express a particular gene. See Impenetrance.

Penis Male organ for depositing the semen in the female vagina.

Perinatal At the moment of parturition.

Pet quality A pedigree cat that the breeder believes that it is not suitable for show competition against other pedigree cats for one or more reasons. These reasons include matters such as color and color placement, relative size or perfection of physical features, such as ears, tail etc. and other subjective, cosmetic features, measured against the standards of perfection. Pet quality does not mean that the kitten is unhealthy. A breeder's term.

Phaeomelanin Yellow coloring pigment of the hairs. Often called red or orange as well.

Phenocopy Variation which mimics a known mutant phenotype but is not genetic. When experimentally induced, it is important in the study of development and genetic diseases.

Phenotype The expression of a gene in the individual. Also phenotypical.

Pheromone Scent given off by individual which influences the behavior of another individual. Specially sex pheromones to advertise estrus.

Phylogeny Evolutionary history of a species. Such as the study of extinct felid-like creatures which gave rise to the modern cats species and ultimately to the domestic cat.

Piebald Individual with patches of white fur.

Pigment granules Minute melanin-containing bodies which color the hairs.

PKD Autosomal dominant polycystic kidney disease.

Placenta Organ by which the fetus is attached to the uterus, through which it receives nourishment.

Pleiotropy The quality of a gene to manifest itself in more than one way, that is to produce more than one phenotypic expression.

Pleiotropism When a gene has several apparently unrelated effects on the phenotype. However, usually these can be traced to a common genetic cause.

Pointed A cat on which the mask (face), ears, legs, feet and tail are clearly a darker shade.

Points Extremities of the body the nose, ears, feet and tail.

Polycystic kidney disease A defect of the kidneys which is sometimes inherited. Fatal when both kidneys involved.

Polydactyly The presence of more than the normal number of toes.

Polygenes Genes with small but cumulative effects on the expression of a character These minor genes are as important as major genes, if not more so.

Polygenic Character determined by several genes, usually with reference to minor genes or polygenes.

Polymorphism Presence of one or more variant forms in a population, such as coat colors in mongrel cat populations.

Polymerase chain reaction (PCR) A technique used to amplify small amounts of genetic material.

Population Group of interbreeding individuals, such as a strain, breed or species. Very flexible but important term in breeding practice.

Population genetics Branch of genetics concerned with the composition and genetics of groups of individuals or populations. Of considerable relevance for animal breeding as it embraces the consequences of both selection and inbreeding.

Postnatal After parturition.

Postpartum After parturition.

Pregnant Condition of carrying viable offspring.

Premier In some cat associations, a class where altered cats are judged.

Prenatal Before parturition.

Primary sex ratio Number of males per 100 females at fertilization.

Primiparous Producing offspring for the first time.

Progeny Offspring.

Progeny selection Assessment of the breeding worth of an individual by examination of the quality of the offspring.

Progeny testing Testing of the individual for the possibility of it being heterozygous for a lethal or impairing recessive gene.

Protoplasm Total contents of a cell. Nucleus and cytoplasm.

Pseudopregnancy Condition of not carrying offspring in spite of appearing pregnant.

Puberty Sexual maturity.

Purebred Individual of a recognized breed, as opposed to crossbred or mongrel.

Pyometria An infection in the uterus.

Q

Qualitative variation Abruptly changing variation caused by the assortment of major genes.

Quantitative variation Variation which moves continuously through a range from one extreme of expression to another. Usually indicative of determination by polygenes.

Queen Female cat, especially one used for breeding.

R

Random bred A way in which breeders of pedigree cats often refer to cats that are not pedigree.

Random breeding The probability of any male cat being bred with any female cat is a directly related function of the number of females in the population. Which cat breeds with which cat is a matter of chance. See also Random mating.

Random mating Mating in which neither inbreeding or outbreeding is encouraged nor avoided. Usually applied to populations where the mating is uncontrolled.

Recessive gene Allele whose expression is over-ridden by another at the same locus. The allele whose expression vanishes in the F_1 but reappears in the F_2.

Reciprocal mating Where a character is involved in two matings, in the first via one sex and in the second via the other sex. Usually performed to ascertain the possible influence of sex on the character.

Recombinant Individual which has received a new combination of alleles, especially in the F_2 generation.

Reduction division Special division during meiosis which halves the number of chromosomes.

Registered cat A cat (whether purebred or household pet) which has completed the requirements for registration with one of the cat federations.

Registration The initial recording of a cat's individual cat name/owner record in a cat federation. This also refers to the registration certificate issued by a cat federation to the registered owner of the cat.

Registration rules The rules and guidelines set up by a cat federation for the registration of cats, litters, catteries etc.

Registry One term used to describe a cat federation, taken from one of its primary roles, registering the birth and pedigree of cats.

Reproductive cells Germ cells or gametes.

Reproductive tract The passage in the female comprising the oviduct, uterus, cervix, vagina and vulva.

Repulsion When two alleles at different loci enter a mating from different parents.

Reticulation Formation of a network mass.

Reversion Appearance of wild-type phenotype, typical expectation of a mating between individuals homozygous for different recessive, mutant alleles at the same locus.

Rufinism The degree of expression of orange/yellow pigment.

S

Scaling Assessment of the quality of characters by scoring on a scale of points for excellence. The points scale is usually from 1 to 10.

Scoring Assessment of the quality of characters by either measurement (weight or size) or by grading on a scale of points for excellence.

Scrotum Sac containing the testes.

Season Estrus.

Secondary sex ratio Number of males per 100 females at parturition.

Segregation Assortment of major genes.

Selection Choice of certain individuals for breeding in preference to others. The basis of genetic improvement in animal breeding.

Selection index The total score of the individual divided by the maximum total score. The quotient is usually expressed as a percentage.

Selective breeding Choice of certain individuals in preference to others so as to favor desirable characters. The basis of the art of breeding.

Self A cat whose parents are of the same (solid) color.

Semen Fluid ejaculate containing sperms.

Semi-dominance Incomplete dominance.

Seminal fluid Semen.

Sex Male or female of the species.

Sex chromosomes Two special chromosomes (X and Y) which determine gender. In mammals, the heterozygote XY is male, the homozygote XX is female.

Sex linkage Genes which display association with sex because they are located on one of the sex chromosomes, usually the X.

Sex organs Reproductive organs, testes in the male, ovaries in the female.

Sex ratio Number of males per 100 females.

Sex-limited genes Genes which can only find expression in one sex. Do not confuse with sex-linked genes.

Sex-linked gene Genes on one of the sex chromosomes, usually the X because the Y is small and has few gene loci.

Show A series of rings of judging sponsored by a cat club.

Show quality A cat that, when measured against the written standards of the breed, would be expected to achieve a title in competition relatively easily. Breeder's term. Some breeders use the term 'top show' to designate a cat that is expected to do extraordinarily well.

Show rules Rules formulated by a cat federation governing all of the aspects of how shows sanctioned and licensed by that federation are to be managed. This includes how the cats are judged and how titles are awarded.

Siamese pattern Coloration where the points are dark and the body is light sepia or almost white. Also known as the Himalayan or colorpoint pattern.

Sib Shortened form of sibling.

Sib mating Mating of brother to sister.

Sib selection Selection based on the quality of all individuals from the same parents or of a litter.

Siblings Brothers and sisters. The term is not necessarily limited to litter siblings, although this is the usual implication.

Sire Male parent.

Soma Body cells of the individual as opposed to the germinal cells.

Somatic mutation Mutation in the body (soma) cells, as opposed to mutation in the germinal cells. Such mutation gives rise to mosaics and are not inherited unless the germinal cells are involved.

Spay A female cat who has had a ovariohysterectomy to prevent breeding and heat cycles.

Spaying Removal of ovaries in the female; altering a female cat. See Spay.

Spermatogenesis Cell divisions which produce the male germs cells or gametes (sperms).

Spermatozoa Sperms.

Sperms Male germ cells or gametes.

Spotted tabby Color pattern in which the large or small dark spots appear against a lighter background.

Spraying A male cat's habit of urinating anywhere, usually associated with establishing territory. Sometimes a female cat will also spray.

Standards of perfection Another name for breed standards. Often just referred to as 'standards'.

Sterile Inability to produce offspring.

Stock Group of interbreeding individuals of insufficient distinction to be called a strain.

Striped tabby Mackerel tabby.

Strain Group of interbreeding individuals with acknowledged distinctive characteristics. Sometimes referred to as a line. See Line.

Stud Male individual kept for breeding; also called a 'Working Male'. Older way of referring to a cattery, probably due to the fact that smaller catteries may have only one stud male.

Subvital gene Gene which lowers the vitality of the individual without producing a visible anomaly. Responsible for the effects of inbreeding depression.

Superfecundation Offspring sired by different males in the same litter.

Superfetation Production of offspring of different ages at same or spaced parturitions. Usually caused when ova are released at different estrus cycles and develop in different horns of the uterus.

Superovulation Production of unusually large numbers of ova. Usually hormone induced, rather than a natural event.

Syndactyly The absence of normal number of toes. See Polydactyly.

Syndrome Association of several characteristics induced by a common root cause.

T

Tandem selection Method of selection whereby each character is improved in turn before moving to another.

Tabby pattern Overlay of pattern on the agouti ground color. Vestigial in the Abyssinian, but strongly apparent in the classic, spotted and mackerel.

Tapetum lucidum A layer of pigment cells behind the retina which enables the cat to see more clearly in dim illumination.

Telegony Discredited belief that the sire of a previous mating can influence the characteristics of the offspring of the succeeding sire.

Tertiary sex ratio Number of males per 100 females at puberty.

Testcross Backcross of the F_1 to the parent with the recessive gene(s). See Backcross.

Testes Male organs for the production of male germ cells or gametes (sperms).

Testicles Testes.

Testis Singular of testes.

Tetratological lethal A lethal gene which is lethal at birth (stillborn) or shortly following birth.

Threshold character Character which simulates alternate heredity but in reality is determined by polygenes.

Throw back Reversion to the phenotype of ancestors. Breeder's term rather than genetic.

Ticked tabby Tabby pattern with the minimum of markings, confined to the face, feet and tail. Also called Abyssinian tabby. Each hair of the coat is tipped with darker color.

Tom Common name for a male cat.

Tortie A short-hand way of describing a tortoiseshell cat.

Tortoiseshell A cat with intermingled patches of black and orange color.

Total score Method of selection whereby characters are scored for excellence and totaled to assess the quality of the individual. See Breeding index.

Toxic Poisonous.

Trait A character. Typically when inherited.

Transgenic Incorporation of genic material of one species into the genome of another.

U

Unit character A character determined by a single gene. Obsolete term.

Unigenic A character which is determined by a single major gene.

Unlike mating Disassortative mating.

Urethra Passage in the penis for transmitting semen. Females have one as well.

Uterus Organ for carrying and nourishing offspring during pregnancy.

Uteri Plural of uterus.

V

Vagina Passage for receiving semen deposited by the male.

Variant A form which deviates from the wild type; usually but not necessarily genetic.

Variable expressivity A defect with variable expressivity is one where the same abnormality may be expressed differently in different animals.

Variety Distinctive form within a breed, such as color or coat type of many breeds of cat.

Vas deferens Duct for conveying the sperms from the testes to the urethra.
Virgin birth Parthenogenesis.
Vitality The normal health, growth and reproductive ability of the individual.
Vulva The external opening of the female vagina.

W

Whole (intact) male A male cat who has not been castrated and is still able to breed.
Whole (intact) female A female cat who has not surgically altered to prevent pregnancies.
Wild type The normal phenotype of the species. Employed as a standard to which the effects of mutant alleles are compared.
Womb Uterus.

X

X chromosome The 'female' chromosome, so called because females have two X chromosomes, whereas the male has only one.

Y

Y chromosome The 'male' chromosome, so called because it is present only in males. The main function of the Y is to induce development of the fertilized egg to be a male.

Z

Zygote The individual which results from the fusion of the male and female gametes.

Bibliography

General (including genetics, breeds, registries and health)

Angell, K. (1996). Purrsonality Profile: Niels C. Pedersen DVM, PhD. *Cats*, November 10.

Angell, K. (1996). Genetic disorders produced in breeding. *Cats (Exhibitor Edition)*, September 3.

Angell, K. (1997). Mei Toi Cats. *Cats*, July 20.

Anon. (1993). Castle-Hardy-Weinberg equilibrium – a study of gene frequencies in a population of domestic cats. Purpose – to calculate the frequencies of the several genes that act to determine the coat color and patterning in the random-bred cat. *American Biology Teacher*, **55**, 175–177.

Anon. (1997). The biotechnology century. *Business Week*, 10 March, 78–92.

Associated Press. (1997). Researchers link domestic dogs to wolves. *Reading Eagle/Reading Times*, 13 June, A9.

Ballard, D. (1981). The siamese cat reviewed: Coat pattern and color. *The Cat Fanciers Association, Inc. Yearbook*, **12**, 545–549.

Bearden, H.J. and Fuquay, J.W. (1996). *Applied Animal Reproduction*, 4th edn. Prentice Hall.

Bernstein, J. (1980). Those terrific Tonkinese. *The Cat Fanciers Association, Inc. Yearbook*, **11**, 434–445.

Bourdon, R.M. (1996). *Understanding Animal Breeding*. Prentice Hall.

Burns, M. (1966). *Genetics of the Dog. The Basis of Successful Breeding*. Oliver and Boyd.

Cat Fanciers Association, Inc. (1993). *The Cat Fanciers Association Cat Encyclopedia*. Simon & Schuster.

Cat Fanciers Association, Inc. (1998). An important note on feline structure. *The Cat Fanciers Association, Inc., 1998 Show Standards*.

Childs, B. (1963). A brief summary of general genetics. In *Birth Defects*, ed. Fishbein, M., JB Lippincott.

Chinitz, J.A., Munro, M.J. and Kittleson, M.D. (1996). Responsible breeding and hypertrophic cardiomyopathy. *Maine Coon International*, Summer, 6.

Cho, K.W. et al. (1997). A proposed nomenclature of the domestic cat karyotype. *Cytogenetics and Cell Genetics*, **79**, 72–78.

Clark, R. (ed). (1992). *Medical Genetic and Behavioral Aspects of Purebred Cats*. Cortlandt Group.

Crick, F. et al. (1961). General nature of the genetic code for proteins. *Nature*, **192**, 1227.

Deal, V.Z. (1983). A Burmese cat tale. *The Cat Fanciers Association, Inc. Yearbook*, **14**, 626–639.

Doernberg, D. (1984). What is a breed? *Cat Fanciers' Association Almanac*, June.

Givney, A. (1986). Why there are two: the story of the Cornish Rex and the Devon Rex. *The Cat Fanciers Association, Inc. Yearbook*, **17**, 624–31.

Gorin, M.B. et al. (1993). The cat RDS transcript – candidate gene analysis and phylogenetic sequence analysis. *Mammalian Genome*, **4**, 544–548.

Graf-Webster, E. (1982). In priase of the 'east coast' Burmese. *UBCF Newsletter*, **24(1)**, 11–14.

Hanvey, K. (1997). Gene wise. *ACFA Bulletin*, **43(2)**, 13–25.

Haukenberry, B. and Federico, M. (1982). Early longhairs: facts and speculations. *The Cat Fanciers Association, Inc. Yearbook*, **13**, 302–303.

Helmrich, H. and Libott, S. (1991/92). Abyssinians in America – the era of expansion 1980–1990. *The Cat Fanciers Association, Inc. Yearbook*, **22**, 131–143.

Hirota, J. et al. (1995). The phenotypes and gene frequencies of genetic markers in the blood of Japanese crossbred cats. *Journal of Veterinary Medicine and Science*, **57**, 381–3.

Hoger, H. (1994). Mutant allele frequencies in domestic cat populations in Austria. *Journal of Heredity*, **85**, 139–142.

Horowitz, N.H. (1956). The gene. *Scientific American*, **195(4)**, 78.

Howard, J. (1981). Gold fever: the Golden Persian – a beginning. *The Cat Fanciers Association, Inc. Yearbook*, **12**, 217–23.

Jeffreys, A.J. et al. (1987). DNA fingerprints of dogs and cats. *Animal Genetics*, **18**, 1–15.

Jolly, R.D. et al. (1986). Screening for carriers of genetic diseases by biochemical means. *Veterinary Record*, **119**, 264–7.

Kajon, A., Garcia, D.C. and Ruizgarcia, M. (1992). Gene frequencies in the cat population of Buenos Aires, Argentina, and the possible origin of this population. *Journal of Heredity*, **83**, 148–152.

Kidwell, J.F. (1951). The number of progeny required to test a male for heterozygosity for a recessive gene. *Journal of Heredity*, **42**, 215–216.

Kiester, N.R. (1994). American Curls in focus: the early years. *The Cat Fanciers Association, Inc. Yearbook*, **24**, 168–171.

Klein, K. et al. (1986). Mutant allele frequencies in cats of Minneapolis-St Paul. *Journal of Heredity*, **77**, 132–134.

Koerner, B. (1997). Silence of the genes. *US News & World Report*, December 8, 69–70.

Leveque, N.W. (1998). Feline genetic disease conference initiated. *Journal of the American Veterinary Medical Association*, **213**, 465.

Liddell, M. (1995). D.M. Siamese. *The Cat Fanciers Association, Inc. Yearbook*, **25**, 201–203.

Lorimer, H.E. (1996/97). Genetic myths: Part 1 – What are the odds. *Cat Fanciers' Journal*, Winter, 4–5.

Lorimer, H.E. (1997). Genetic myths: Part 3 – News and old mutations. *Cat Fanciers' Journal*, Summer/Fall, 7.

Lyons, L.A. (1996/97). The feline genome project; eradicating genetic disease in cats. *Cat Fanciers' Journal*, Winter, 44–46.

Lyons, L.A. (1998). The feline genome project and the cat fancy. *Cat Fanciers' Journal*, **17(4)**, 3–7.

Lyons, L.A. (1996). The feline genome project and its relevance to cat fanciers. *Cat Fanciers' Almanac*, **14(4)**, December, 88–90.

Lyons, L. (1997). Feline gene mapping. *Winn Feline Foundation Presentation*, June.

Masuda, R. and Yoshida, M.C. (1995). Two Japanese wildcats, the Tsushima cat and the Iriomote cat, show the same mitochondrial DNA lineage as the leopard cat *Felis bengalensis*. *Zoological Science*, **12**, 655–659.

Mazia, D. (1961). How cells divide. *Scientific American*, **205**, 100.

Menotti, R.M. et al. (1997). Genetic individualization of domestic cats using feline STR lock for forensic applications. *Journal of Forensic Science*, **42**, 1039–1051.

Meyers-Wallen, V.N. (1993). Genetics of sexual differentiation and anomalies in dogs and cats. *Journal of Reproduction and Fertility Supplement*, **47**, 441–452.

Miller, J. (1998). 'Strategies to avoid detrimental breed characteristics' in University of Pennsylvania, School of Veterinary Medicine. (1998). First International Feline Genetic Disease Conference – Workbook.

Miller, J. (1996). The domestic cat: perspective on the nature and diversity of cats. *Cat Fanciers' Almanac*, **14(2)**, 103–105.

Obrien, S.J. et al. (1997). Comparative gene mapping in the domestic cat (*Felis catus*). *Journal of Heredity*, **88**, 408–414.

Obrien, S.J., Wienberg, J. and Lyons, L.A. (1994). Comparative genomics – lessons from cats [Review]. *Trends in Genetics*, **13**, 393–399.

Patterson, D.F. (1993). Understanding and controlling inherited diseases in dogs and cats. *Tijdschrift Voor Diergeneeskunde*, **118**, S23–S27.

Pedersen, N.C. (1991). *Feline Husbandry: Diseases and Management in the Multiple-Cat Environment*. American Veterinary Publications, Inc.

Peltz, R.S. (1978). The seventies find Burmese entering a new era. *The Cat Fanciers Association, Inc. Yearbook*, **9**, 306–28.

Peltz, R.S. (1992/93). Genetics – practical aspects of breeding cats. *The Cat Fanciers Association, Inc. Yearbook*, **23**, 290–1, 294–5, 708–12.

Piacchi, N. and Bittaker, A. (1982). The Havana Brown – the felicitous feline. *The Cat Fanciers Association, Inc. Yearbook*, **13**, 289–296.

Powell, G. (1998). DNA testing in cats (part 1). *TICA Trend*, **19(1)**, April/May, 15–17.

Rankin, G.R. (1998). Abyssinians in America. *The Cat Fanciers Association, Inc. Yearbook*, **28**, 150–158.

Rettenberger, G. et al. (1995). ZOO-FISH analysis – cat and human karyotypes closely resemble the putative ancestral mammalian karyotype. *Chromosome Research*, **3**, 479–486.

Ritter, D. and Ritter, L. (1990/91). Somalis; the first decade and beyond. *The Cat Fanciers Association, Inc. Yearbook*, **21**, 133–140.

Ruizgarcia, M. (1993). Analysis of the evolution and genetic diversity within and between Balearic and Iberian cat populations. *Journal of Heredity*, **84**, 173–180.

Ruizgarcia, M. (1994). Genetic profiles from coat genes of natural Balearic cat populations – an eastern Mediterranean and North-African origin. *Genetics Selection Evolution*, **26**, 39–64.

Ruizgarcia, M. (1994). Genetic structure of the Marseilles cat population – is there really a strong founder effect? *Genetics Selection Evolution*, **26**, 317–331.

Sager, R. (1961). *Cell Heredity*. Wiley.

Scollard, D.L. (1998). Munchkin research. *Cat Fanciers' Journal*, **17(4)**, 66–67.

Schuler, L. and Borodin, P.M. (1992). Influence of sampling methods on estimated gene frequency in domestic cat populations of East Germany. *Archiv Fur Tierzucht (Archives of Animal Breeding)*, **35**, 629–634.

Siegal, Mordecai (ed) (1997). *The Cornell Book of Cats: A Comprehensive and Authoritative Medical Reference for Every Cat and Kitten*. Villard.

Smith, F.O. (1984). Is It Inherited? *UBCF Newsletter*, **26(1)**, Spring, 15.

Thompson, J.C. and Cobb, V.C. (1973). Genetics of the Burmese cat. In *The Burmese Cat* (R. Pocok, D. Silkstone Richards, M. Swift and V. Watson, eds), pp. 145–149.

Torio, T. and Torio, V. (1983). The Ankara cat (original Turkish Angora) fact sheet – July 1968. *The Cat Fanciers Association, Inc. Yearbook*, **14**, 641–649.

University of Pennsylvania, School of Veterinary Medicine. (1998). *First International Feline Genetic Disease Conference – Workbook*.

Vella, C. and McGonagle, J. (1997). *Breeding Pedigreed Cats*. Howell Book House.

Vella, C.M. and McGonagle, J.J. Jr. (1990). *In The Spotlight: a Guide to Showing Pedigreed and Household Pet Cats*. Howell Book House.

Wastihuber, J. (1990). Gene pool expansion as a solution to breed health problems. *Cat Fanciers' Almanac*, October, 57–58.

Willis, M. (1989). *Genetics of the Dog*. Howell Book House.

Winn Feline Foundation (1995). Burmese Genetic Study Project – Progress Report. February.

Wright, S. (1922). Coefficients in inbreeding and relationship. *American Nature*, **56**, 330–338.

Anomalies and inherited traits

Albert R.A. and Thomas, K. (1982). Congenital anomalies of the head in Burmese cats. *UBCF Newsletter*, **24(3)**, Fall, 6–7.

Anderson, R.E. et al. (1991). Plasma lipid abnormalities in the Abyssinian cat with a hereditary rod-cone degeneration [letter]. *Experimental Eye Research*, **53**, 415–417.

Angell, K. (1986). 'Ears to 25 years: the Scottish Fold. *The Cat Fanciers Association, Inc. Yearbook*, **17**, 145–158.

Anon. (1997). APBC highlights common problems in dogs and cats. *Veterinary Record*, **140**, 414.

Anon. (1984). Report from the Burmese Breed Council breakfast. *UBCF Newsletter*, **26(2)**, Summer, 13–24.

Ault, S.J. et al. (1995). Abnormal ipsilateral visual field representation in areas 17 and 18 of hypopigmented cats. *Journal of Comparative Neurology* **354**, 181–192.

Berg, T. et al. (1997). Purification of feline lysosomal alpha-mannosidase, determination of its cDNA sequence and identification of a mutation causing alpha-mannosidosis in Persian cats. *Biochemical Journal*, **328**, 863–870.

Biller, D.S., Chew, D.J. and DiBartola, S.P. (1995). Polycystic kidney disease in a family of Persian cats. *Journal of the American Veterinary Medical Association*, **196**, 1288–1290.

Biller, D.S. et al. (1996). Inheritance of polycystic kidney disease in Persian cats. *Journal of Heredity*, **87**, 1–5.

Biller, D.S., DiBartola, S. and Lagerwerf, W. (1998). Autosomal dominant polycystic kidney disease in Persian cats. *Cat Fanciers' Almanac*, **15(9)**, 92–93.

Black, L. (1972). Progressive retinal atrophy. A review of the genetics and an appraisal of the eradication scheme. *Journal of Small Animal Practice*, **13**, 295–314.

Burmese Cooperative Research. (1984). N.T. *UBCF Newsletter* **26(1)**, Spring, 7–14.

Carr, A.P. and Johnson, G.S. (1994). A review of hemostatic abnormalities in dogs and cats. *Journal of the American Animal Hospital Association*, **30**, 475–482.

Casal, M.L. et al. (1994). Congenital hypotrichosis with thymic aplasia in nine Birman kittens. *Journal of the American Animal Hospital Association*, **30**, 600–602.

Chinitz, J.A., Munro, M.J. and Kittleson, M.D. (1998). Hypertrophic cardiomyopathy: an update and primer. *The Scratch Sheet*, Spring/March, 13–17.

Coates, J.R. et al. (1996). A case presentation and discussion of type IV glycogen storage disease in a Norwegian Forest cat. *Progress in Veterinary Neurology*, **7**, 5–11.

Dohrmann, H. (1998). Case history: hip dysplasia. *Cat Fanciers' Journal*, Spring, 71–72.

Dohrmann, H. (1998). Hip dysplasia: OFA report. *Cat Fanciers' Journal*, Spring, 73, 75.

Dohrmann, H. (1998). 'OFAing' your cats' hips. *Cat Fanciers' Journal*, Spring, 74–75.

Eaton, K.A. et al. (1997). Autosomal dominant polycystic kidney disease in Persian and Persian-cross cats. *Vet Pathology*, **34**, 117–126.

Ehinger, B. et al. (1991). Photoreceptor degeneration and loss of immunoreactive GABA in the Abyssinian cat regina. *Experimental Eye Research*, **52**, 17–25.

Foley, C.W. et al. (1979). *Abnormalities of Companion Animals: Analysis of Heritability*. Iowa State University Press.

Fyfe, J.C. et al. (1992). Glycogen storage disease type-IV – inherited deficiency of branching enzyme activity in cats. *Pediatric Research*, **32**, 719–725.

Giger, U. (1990). Genetics of feline blood groups in the United States – the frequency of feline A and B blood types and neonatal isoerythrolysis varies markedly between breeds. *Cat Fanciers' Almanac*, **7(7)**, 77 et seq.

Giger, U. and Akol, K.G. (1990). Acute hemolytic transfusion reaction in an Abyssinian cat with blood type B. *Journal of Veterinary Internal Medicine*, **4**, 315–316.

Giger, U., Bucheler, J. and Patterson, D.F. (1991). Frequency and inheritance of A and B blood types in feline breeds of the United States. *Journal of Heredity*, **82**, 15–20.

Gorin, M.B., To, A.C. and Narfstrom, K. (1995). Sequence analysis and exclusion of phosducin as the gene for the recessive retinal degeneration of the Abyssinian cat. *Biochemica Biophysica Acta*, **1260**, 323–327.

Griot Wenk, M.E. et al. (1996). Blood type AB in the feline AB blood group system. *American Journal of Veterinary Research* **57**, 1438–1442.

Haskins, M. and Giger, U. (1997). Lysosomal Storage Diseases. In *Clinical Biochemistry of Domestic Animals*, 5th edn, Kanko, J.J., Harvey, J.W. and Bruss, M.L. (eds). Academic Press, pp. 741–761.

Haskins, M.E. et al. (1992). Hepatic storage of glycosaminoglycans in feline and canine models of mucopolysaccharidoses I, VI, and VII. *Veterinary Pathology*, **29**, 112–119.

Inada, S. et al. (1996). A study of hereditary cerebellar degeneration in cats. *American Journal of Veterinary Research*, **57**, 296–301.

Jensen, A.L., Olesen, A.B. and Arnbjerg, J. (1994). Distribution of feline blood types detected in the Copenhagen area of Denmark. *Acta Veterinaria Scandinavia*, **35**, 121–124.

Jones, B.R. et al. (1992). Preliminary studies on congenital hypothyroidism in a family of Abyssinian cats. *Veterinary Research*, **131**, 145–148.

Kahraman, M.M. and Prieur, D.J. (1991). Animal models – prenatal diagnosis of Chediak-Higashi syndrome in the cat by evaluation of cultured chorionic cells. *American Journal of Medical Genetics*, **40**, 311–315.

Keller, R.S. (1996). Feline hip dysplasia. *Cat Fanciers' Journal*, Spring, 69–70.

Kruger, J.M. et al. (1996). Inherited and congenital diseases of the feline lower urinary tract. *Veterinary Clinics of North America – Small Animal Practice*, **26**, 265–279.

Lawler, D.F., Templeton, A.J. and Monti, K.L. (1993). Evidence for genetic involvement in feline dilated cardiomyopathy. *Journal of Veterinary Internal Medicine*, **7**, 383–387.

Libott, A. (1993). Feline blood type frequencies and their importance. *Cat Fanciers' Almanac*, **10(4)**, 83 et seq.

Lees, G.E. (1996). Congenital renal diseases. *Veterinary Clinics of North America – Small Animal Practice*, **26**, 1379.

Ling, G.V. et al. (1998). Renal calculi in dogs and cats: prevalence, mineral type, breed, age and gender interrelationships (1981–1993). *Journal of Veterinary Internal Medicine*, **12**, 11–21.

Littlewood, J.D., Shaw, S.C. and Coombes, L.M. (1995). Vitamin K-dependent coagulopathy in a British Devon Rex cat. *Journal of Small Animal Practice*, **36**, 115–118.

Maddison, J.E. et al. (1990). Vitamin-K-Dependent multifactor coagulopathy in Devon Rex cats. *Journal of the American Veterinary Medical Association*, **197**, 1495–1497.

Maggio-Price, L. and Dodds, W.J. (1993). Factor IX deficiency (hemophilia B) in a family of British Shorthair cats. *Journal of the American Veterinary Medical Association*, **203**, 1702–1704.

Malik, R., Mepstead, K., Yang, F. and Harper, C. (1993). Hereditary myopathy of Devon Rex cats. *Journal of Small Animal Practice*, **34**, 539–546.

Mason, K. (1988). A hereditary disease in Burmese cats manifested as an episodic weakness with head nodding and neck ventroflexion. *Journal of the American Animal Hospital Association*, **24**, 147–151.

Mathews, K.G.A.U. et al. (1995). Resolution of lameness associated with Scottish Fold osteodystrophy following bilateral ostectomies and pantarsal arthrodeses: a case report. *Journal of the American Animal Hospital Association*, **31**, 280–288.

Millis, D.L., Hauptman, J.G. and Johnson, C.A. (1992). Cryptorchidism and monorchism in cats: 25 cases (1980–1989). *Journal of the American Veterinary Medical Association*, **200**, 1128–1130.

Moreau, P.M. et al. (1991). Peripheral and central distal axonopathy of suspected inherited origin in Birman cats. *Acta Neuropathologica*, **82**, 143–146.

Muldoon, L.L. et al. (1994). Characterization of the molecular defect in a feline model for type II GM2-gangliosidosis (Sandhoff disease). *American Journal of Pathology*, **144**, 1109–1118.

Muns, M. (1996). Case study: Hip dysplasia. *Cat Fanciers' Journal*, Summer/Fall, 64–65.

Noden, D.M. and Evans, H.E. (1986). Inherited homeotic midfacial malformations in Burmese cats. *Journal of Craniofacial Genetics and Developmental Biology* Supplement 2, 249–266.

O'Brien, A. (1998). Amylodosis in pedigreed cats: A review of selected papers. *Cat Fanciers' Journal*, **17(4)**, 35–38.

Partington, B.P. et al. (1996). What is your diagnosis? Scottish Fold osteodystrophy. *Journal of the American Veterinary Medical Association*, **209**, 1235–1236.

Perry, J. (1998). A Matter of the Heart. *Cat Fancy*, March, 45–48.

Plummer, S.B. et al. (1993). Tethered spinal cord and an intradural lipoma associated with a meningocele in a Manx-type cat. *Journal of the American Veterinary Medical Association*, **203**, 1159–1161.

Piirsalu, K. et al. (1994). Role of I-123 serum amyloid protein in the detection of familial amyloidosis in Oriental cats. *Journal of Small Animal Practice*, **35**, 581–586.

Rand, J.S. et al. (1997). Over representation of Burmese cats with diabetes mellitus. *Australian Veterinary Journal*, **75**, 402–405.

Richardson, E.F. and Mullen, H. (1993). Cryptorchidism in cats. *Compendium on Continuing Education for the Practicing Veterinarian*, **15**, 1342–1345.

Robinson, R. (1993). Expressivity of the Manx gene in cats. *Journal of Heredity*, **84**, 170–172.

Robinson, R. (1992). Spasticity in the Devon Rex cat. *Veterinary Record*, **130**, 302.

Rozengurt, N. (1994). Endocardial fibroelastosis in common domestic cats in the UK. *Journal of Comparative Pathology*, **110**, 295–301.

Soute, B.A.M. et al. (1992). Congenital deficiency of all vitamin-K-dependent blood coagulation factors due to a defective vitamin-K-dependent carboxylase in Devon Rex cats. *Thrombosis and Haemostasis*, **68**, 521–525.

Stur, I., Roth, A. and Muller, S. (1991). Investigation into a familiar accumulated occurrence of congenital cardiac anomalies in Siamese-shorthaired-cats and Oriental-shorthaired-cats. *Kleintierpraxis*, **36**, 85–86.

Tanase, H. et al. (1991). Inherited primary hypothyroidism with thyrotrophin resistance in Japanese cats. *Journal of Endocrinology*, **129**, 245.

van der Linde Sipman, J.S. et al. (1997). Generalized AA-amyloidosis in Siamese and Oriental cats. *Veterinary Immunology and Immunopathology*, **56(1–2)**, 1–10.

Vitale, C.B. et al. (1996). Feline urticaria pigmentosa in three related sphinx cats. *Veterinary Dermatology*, **7**, 227–233.

Wiggert, B. et al. (1994). An early decrease in interphotoreceptor retinoid-binding protein gene expression in Abyssinian cats homozygous for hereditary rod-cone degeneration. *Cell Tissue Research*, **278**, 291–298.

Zuber, R.M. (1993). Systemic amyloidosis in Oriental and Siamese cats. *Australian Veterinary Practice*, **23**, 66–70.

Color and coat

Angell, K. (1997). Blue Eyes. *Cats*, September, 25–26.

Bradbury, M.W. et al. (1988). Changes in melanin granules in the fox due to coat color mutations. *Journal of Heredity*, **79**, 133–136.

Bultmen, S.J. et al. (1992). Molecular characterization of the mouse agouti locus. *Cell*, **71(7)**, 1195–1204.

Bultman, S.J. et al. (1994). Molecular analysis of reverse mutations from non-agouti (*a*) to black-and-tan (*at*) and white bellied agouti (*Aw*) reveals alternative forms of agouti transcripts. *Genes and Development*, **8(4)**, 481–490.

Cornelius, L. (1994). Altering the fate of the yellow cat. *Veterinary Medicine*, **89**, 843.

Doolittle, D.P. et al. (1975). The Goodale white-spotted mice: a historical report. *Journal of Heredity*, **66**, 376–380.

Everett, D. (1994/95). The Rex gene. *Maine Coon International*, Winter.

French, B. (1997). Color Me Purrfect. *Cats*, September, 28–33.

Hearing, V.J. et al. (1992). Functional properties of cloned melanogenic proteins. *Pigment Cell Research*, **5(5 pt 2)**, 264–270.

Heid, S., Hartmann, R. and Klinke, R. (1998). A model for prelingual deafness, the congenitally deaf white cat – population statistics and degenerative changes. *Hearing Research*, **115**, 101–112.

Hirobe, T. (1984). Effects of genic substitution at the brown locus on the differentiation of epidermal melanocytes in newborn mouse skin. *Anatomical Record*, **209**, 425–432.

Johnson, N. (1996). The Asian, a cat of many colors. *Cat World™ International*, April.

Kwon, B.S. (1993). Pigmentation genes: the tyrosinase family and the pmel 17 gene family. *Journal of Investigative Dermatology*, **100** (Supplement 2), 134S–140S.

Logan, A. et al. (1978). Pelage color cycles and hair follicle tyrosinase activity in the Siberian hamster. *Journal of Investigative Dermatology*, **71**, 295–298.

Lorimer, H.E. (1997/98). Genetic myths – part 4: Dilute or not dilute? *Cat Fanciers Journal*, Winter/Spring, 4–6.

Lorimer, H.E. (1995). Variations on the theme or how to paint a cat. *The Cat Fanciers Association, Inc. Yearbook*, **25**, 193–200.

Mayer, T.C. (1979). Interactions between normal and pigment cell populations mutant at the dominant spotting (*W*) and steel (*Sl*) loci in the mouse. *Journal of Experimental Zoology*, **210**, 81–88.

Miller, W.J. et al. (1986). The sex-linked black cat fallacy: a textbook case. *Journal of Heredity*, **77**, 463–464.

Movaghar, M. et al. (1987). Tyrosinase activity and the expression of the agouti gene in the mouse. *Journal of Experimental Zoology*, **243**, 473–480.

Murray, J.D. (1981). On pattern formation mechanisms for lepidopteran wing patterns and mammalian coat markings. *Philosophical Transactions of the Royal Society of London – Series B: Biological Sciences*, **295**, 473–496.

Ortonne, J.P. et al. (1993). Hair melanins and hair color: Ultrastructural and biochemical aspects (Review). *Journal of Investigative Dermatology*, **101** (Supplement 1), 82S–89S.

Osgood, M.P. (1994). X-chromosome inactivation: the case of the calico cat. *American Journal of Pharmaceutical Education*, **58**, 204–205.

Osier, C. (1997). What color is your cat? *Cat Fancy*, July, 32–35.

Ozeki, H. et al. (1995). Chemical characterization of hair melanins in various coat-color mutants of mice. *Journal of Investigative Dermatology*, **105**, 361–366.

Perry, W.L. et al. (1994). The molecular basis for dominant yellow agouti coat color mutations (Review). *Bioessays*, **16**, 705–707.

Pontier, D., Rioux, N. and Heizmann, A. (1995). Evidence of selection on the orange allele in the domestic cat felis catus – the role of social structure. *Oikos*, **73**, 299–308.

Prota, G. et al. (1995). Comparative analysis of melanins and melanosomes produced by various coat color mutants. *Pigment Cell Research*, **8**, 153–163.

Ragni, B. and Possenti, M. (1996). Variability of coat-colour and markings system in *Felis silvestris*. *Italian Journal of Zoology*, **63**, 285–292.

Richardson, D. (1998). The white spotting factor gene in the Ragdoll, www.users.bigpond.con/drdavid/white.htm, February 25.

Ryugo, D.K. et al. (1997). Ultrastructural analysis of primary endings in deaf white cats – morphologic alterations in endbulbs. *Journal of Comparative Neurology*, **385**, 230–244.

Searle, A.G. (1990). Comparative genetics of albinism. *Ophthalmic Paediatrics and Genetics*, **11**, 159–164.

Shelton, L.M. (1995). The Pigment Parade. *Persian News*, Winter (October), n.p.

Shibasaki, Y. et al. (1987). The R-banded karyotype of *Felis catus*. *Cytobios*, **51**, 35–47.

Siracusa, L.D. (1991). Genomic organization and molecular genetics of the agouti locus in the mouse. *Annals of the New York Academy of Sciences*, **642**, 419–430.

Thody, A.J. et al. (1992). Tyrosinase and regulation of coat color changes in C3H-heavy mice (review). *Pigment Cell Research*, **5(5 pt 2)**, 335–339.

Urabe, K. et al. (1993). From gene to protein: Determination of melanin synthesis (review). *Pigment Cell Research*, **6(4 pt 1)**, 186–192.

Vinogradov, A.E. (1997). Fine structure of gene frequency landscapes in domestic cat: the Old and New Worlds compared. *Hereditas*, **126**, 95–102.

Vinogradov, A.E. (1994). Locally associated alleles of cat coat genes. *Journal of Heredity*, **85(2)**, 86–91.

Wagner, A. et al. (1987). Pelage mutant allele frequencies in domestic cat populations of Poland. *Journal of Heredity*, **78**, 197–200.

Wagner, A. (1996). Coat color alleles in the domestic cat populations at the Adriatic coast. *Journal of Heredity*, **87**, 473–475.

Williams, J.A. (1990). Races of shorthaired and longhaired cats. *Tijdschrift Voor Diergeneeskunde*, **115**, 959.

Wilson, N. (1997). Ticking and the silvering gene in British Blues. *Cat World™ International*, **25–2**, Summer/Fall, 12.

Woolf, C.M. (1990). Multifactoral inheritance of common white markings in the Arabian horse. *Journal of Heredity*, **81**, 250–256.

Yaremchuk, J. (1984). Breeding tabby Persians: The genetics of stripes. *The Cat Fanciers Association, Inc. Yearbook*, **15**, 667.

Other physical aspects

Angus, K. et al. (1966). A note on the genetics of umbilical hernia. *Veterinary Record*, **90**, 245–247.

Anon. (1992). Diagnosis and medical therapy of congenital disorders. *Urologic Surgery of the Dog and Cat*, (Stone, E.A. and Barsanti, J.A., eds). Lea & Febiger, 201–204.

Anon. (1992). Postoperative management and surgical complications of congenital disorders. *Urologic Surgery of the Dog and Cat*, (Stone, E.A. and Barsanti, J.A., eds). Lea & Febiger, 210–211.

Anon. (1992). Surgical therapy for congenital disorders. *Urologic Surgery of the Dog and Cat*, (Stone, E.A. and Barsanti, J.A., eds). Lea & Febiger, 205–209.

Axner, E. et al. (1996). Reproductive disorders in 10 domestic male cats. *Journal of Small Animal Practice*, **37**, 394–401.

Beenirchke, K. et al. (1974). Trisomy in a feline fetus. *American Journal of Veterinary Research*, **35**, 257–259.

Blok, H. (1997). PRA in cats. *TICA Trend*, April/May, 8.

Bridle, K.H. and Littlewood, J.D. (1998). Tail tip necrosis in two litters of Birman kittens. *Journal of Small Animal Practice*, **39**, 88–89.

Christmas, R. (1992). Surgical correction of congenital ocular and nasal dermoids and third eyelid gland prolapse in related Burmese kittens. *Canadian Veterinary Journal – Revue Veterinaire Canadienne*, **33**, 265–266.

Cotard, J.P. (1993). Hepatic disorders in the dog and cat. *Recueil de Medecine Veterinaire*, **169**, 999–1006.

Court, E.A., Watson, A.D. and Peaston, A.E. (1997). Retrospective study of 60 cases of feline lymphosarcoma. *Australian Veterinary Journal*, **75**, 424–427.

Day, M.J. (1997). Review of thymic pathology in 30 cats and 36 dogs. *Journal of Small Animal Practice*, **38**, 393–403.

Deal, V. (1986). Research Committee. *UBCF Newsletter*, **28(1)**, Winter, 13–14.

Dohrmann, H. (1998). Case history: hip dysplasia. *Cat Fanciers' Journal*, Spring, 71–72.

Eason, P. (1998). Unusual ocular condition in Burmese cats [letter]. *Veterinary Record*, **142(19)**, 524.

Girelli, M. et al. (1995). Abnormal spatial but normal temporal resolution in the Siamese cat: a behavioral correlate of a genetic disorder of the parallel visual pathways. *Canadian Journal of Physiology and Pharmacology*, **73** 1348–1351.

Gunn Moore, D.A., Crispin, S.M. (1998). Unusual ocular condition in Burmese cats [letter]. *Veterinary Record*, **142**, 376.

Jacobberger, P. (1998). Surgical option for the treatment of prolapsed gland of the nictitans lacrimal gland (cherry eye) in Burmese cats. *NAAB Newsletter*.

Jonsson, N.N., Pullen, C. and Watson, A.D. (1990). Neonatal isoerythrolysis in Himalayan kittens. *Australian Veterinary Journal*, **67**, 416–417.

Kruger, J.M. et al. (1996). Inherited and congenital diseases of the feline lower urinary tract. *Veterinary Clinics of North America – Small Animal Practice*, **26(2)**, 265–279.

Lantinga, E., Kooistra, H.S. and Vannes, J.J. (1998). Periodic muscle weakness and cervical ventroflexion caused by hypokalemia in a Burmese cat [Dutch]. *Tijdschrift voor Diergeneeskunde*, **123**, 435–437.

Lisciandro, S.C., Hohenhaus, A. and Brooks, M. (1998). Coagulation abnormalities in 22 cats with naturally occurring liver disease. *Journal of Veterinary Internal Medicine*, **12**, 71–75.

Noden, D.M. (1985). Normal development and congenital birth defects in the cat. *The Cat Fanciers Association, Inc. Yearbook*, **16**, 426–431.

Saada, A.A., Niparko, J.K. and Ryugo, D.K. (1996). Morphological changes in the cochlear nucleus of congenitally deaf white cats. *Brain Research*, **736**, 315–328.

Sturgess, C.P. et al. (1997). Investigation of the association between whole blood and tissue taurine levels and the development of thoracic deformatiers in neonatal Burmese kittens. *Veterinary Record*, **141**, 566–570.

Internet sites

Health – http://ourworld.compuserve.com/homepages/GCCF_CATS/health/htm

Hip Dysplasia Awareness – http://www.netropolis.net/kazikat/FelineHD1.htm

Immunity – http://www.inch.com/~harbur/usf/articles/immungen.html.

PKD Statistics – http://www.indyweb.net/~lucky/Stats.html

Winn Feline Foundation, The – http://www.winnfelinehealth.org/

References from Roy Robinson, Genetics for Cat Breeders (third edition)

Baker, H.J., Lindsey, J.R., Mckhann, G.M. and Farrell, D.F. (1971). Neuronal GM1 gangliosidosis in a Siamese cat. *Science*, **174**, 838–839.

Bamber, R.C. and Herdman, E.C. (1993). Two new colour types in cats. *Nature*, **127**, 558.

Barnett, K.C. and Curtis, R. (1985). Autosomal dominant progressive retinal atrophy in Abyssinian cats. *Journal of Heredity*, **76**, 168–170.

Basrur, P.K. and Deforest, M.E. (1979). Embryological impact of the Manx gene. *Carnivor. Genet. Newsletter*, **31**, 378–384.

Berg, P.B.F., Baker, M.K. and Lance, A.D. (1977). A suspected lysosomal storage disease in Abyssinian cats. *Journal of the South African Veterinary Association*, **48**, 195–199.

Bergsma, D.R. and Brown, K.S. (1971). White fur, blue eyes and deafness in the domestic cat. *Journal of Heredity*, **62**, 171–185.

Bistner, S.I., Aguirre, G. and Shively, J.N. (1976). Hereditary corneal dystrophy in the Manx cat. *Investigation Ophthalmology*, **15**, 15–26.

Bogart, R. (1959). *Improvement of Livestock*. MacMillan.

Bosher, S.K. and Hallpike, C.S. (1965). Observation on the histological features, development and pathogenesis of the inner ear degeneration of the deaf white cat. *Proceedings of the Royal Society of Biology*, **162**, 147–162.

Centerwall, W.R. and Benirschke, K. (1973). Male tortoiseshell and calico cats. *Journal of Heredity*, **62**, 272–278.

Chapman, V.A. and Zeiner, F.N. (1996). The anatomy of polydactylism in cats with observations on genetic control. *Anat. Ret.*, **141**, 105–127.

Clifford, D., Soifor, F.K., Wilson, C.F., Waddell, E.D. and Guilland, G.L. (1971). Congenital achasia of the esophagus in four cats of common ancestry. *Journal of the American Veterinary Medical Association*, **158**, 1554–1560.

Collier, L.I., Bryan, G.M. and Prier, D.J. (1979). Ocular manifestation of the Chediak-Higashi syndrome in four species of animals. *Journal of the American Veterinary Medical Association*, **175**, 587–590.

Cooper, M.I. and Blasdel, G.G. (1980). Regional variation in the representation of the visual field in the visual cortex of the Siamese cat. *Comparative Neurology*, **193**, 237–253.

Cork, L.C., Munnell, J.F. and Lorenz, M.D. (1978). The pathology of feline GM2 gangliosidosis. *American Journal of Pathology*, **90**, 723–730.

Cork, L.C., Munnell, J.F., Lorenz, M.D., Murthy, J.V. and Baker, H.J. (1977). Gm2 ganglioside lysosomal storage disease in cats. *Science*, **196**, 1014–1017.

Cotter, S.M., Brenner, R.M. and Dodds, W.J. (1978). Haemophilia A in three unrelated cats. *Journal of the American Veterinary Medical Association*, **172**, 166–168.

Creel, D., Collier, L.L., Leventhal, A.G., Conlee, J.L. and Prier, D.J. (1982). Abnormal retinal projections in cats with the Chediak-Higashi syndrome. *Investigations in Ophthalmology and Visual Science*, **23**, 798–801.

Creel, D., Hendrickson, A.E. and Leventhal, A. (1982). Retinal projections in tyrosinase negative albino cats. *Journal of Neuroscience*, **2**, 907–911.

Crowell, W.A., Hubbell, J.J. and Riley, J.C. (1979). Polycystic renal disease in related cats. *Journal of the American Veterinary Medical Association*, **175**, 286–288.

Curtis, R., Barnett, K.C. and Leon, A. (1987). An early onset retinal dystrophy with dominant inheritance in the Abyssinian cat. *Investigations in Ophthalmology and Visual Science*, **28**, 131–139.

Danforth, C.H. (1947a). Heredity of polydactyly in the cat. *Journal of Heredity*, **38**, 107–112.

Danforth, C.H. (1947b). Morphology of the feet in polydactyl cats. *American Journal of Anatomy*, **80**, 143–171.

Deforest, M.E. and Basur, P.K. (1979). Malformation and the Manx syndrome in cats. *Canadian Veterinarian*, **7(20)**, 304–314.

Desnick, R.J., Mcgovern, M.M., Schuch, E.H. and Haskins, M.E. (1982). Animal analogues of human inherited metabolic diseases. In: *Animal Models of Inherited Metabolic Diseases*, Desnick, R.J., Pattison, D.F., and Scarpelli, D.G. (eds). Alan R. Liss Inc.

DiBartola, S.P., Hill, R.L., Fechheimer, N.S. and Powers, J.D. (1986). Pedigree analysis of Abyssinian cats with familial amyloidosis. *American Journal of Veterinary Research*, **47**, 2666–2668.

Dodds, W.J. (1981). Haemophilia B. *ILAR News*, **24(4)**, R8.

Dorn, C.R., Taylor, D.O.N. and Schneider, R. (1997). Sunlight exposure and risk of developing cutaneous and oral squamous cell carcinomas in white cats. *Journal of the National Cancer Institute*, **46**, 1073–1078.

Elverand, H.H. and Mair, I.W.S. (1980). Hereditary deafness in the cat. *Acta Otolaryngologica*, **90**, 360–369.

Falconer, D.S. (1998). *Introduction to Quantative Genetics*. Longman.

Flecknell, P.A. and Gruffydd-Jones, T.J. (1979). Congenital luxation of the patella in the cat. *Feline Practice*, **9**, 18–20.

Gasper, P.W., Thrall, M.A. and Wenger, D.A. (1984). Correction of feline mucopolysaccharidosis VI by bone marrow transplantation. *Nature*, **312**, 467–469.

Georges, M., Hilbert, P., Lequarre, A.S., Leclerc, V., Hanset, R. and Vassart, G. (1988). Use of DNA bar codes to resolve a canine paternity dispute. *Journal of the American Veterinary Medical Association*, **193**, 1095–1098.

Gillespie, T.H. (1954). Cats – wild and domestic. *Scotsman*, November 27, 1954.

Glenn, B.L., Glenn, H.G. and Omtvedt, I.T. (1968). Congenital porphyria in the domestic cat. *American Journal of Veterinary Research*, **29**, 1653–1657.

Guillery, R.W. (1974). Visual pathways in albinos. *Scientific American*, **230**, 44–54.

Guillery, R.W., Hicker, T.L. and Spear, P.D. (1980). Do blue eyed white cats have normal or abnormal retinofugal pathways? *Investigations in Ophthalmology and Visual Science*, **21**, 27–33.

Hamilton, E. (1986). *The Wild Cat of Europe*. Porter.

Haskins, M.E., Jezyk, P.F., Desnick, R.J., Mcdonough, S.K. and Patterson, D.F. (1979). Alpha-L-iduronidase deficiency in a cat. *Pediatric Research*, **13**, 1294–1297.

Haskins, M.E., Jezyk, P.F., Desnick, R.J., Mcgovern, M.M., Vine, D.T. and Patterson, D.F. (1982). In *Animal Models of Inherited Metabolic Diseases*, Desnick, R.J. (ed.), Alan R. Liss Inc.

Haskins, M.E., Jezyk, P.F. and Patterson, D.F. (1979). Mucopolysaccharide storage disease in three families of cats. *Pediatric Research*, **13**, 1203–1210.

Hendy-Ibbs, P.M. (1984). Hairless cats in Great Britain. *Journal of Heredity*, **75**, 506–507.

Hendy-Ibbs, P.M. (1985). Familialfeline epibulbar dermoids. *Veterinary Record*, **116**, 13–14.

Henricson, B. and Bornstein, S. (1965). Hereditary umbilical hernia in cats. *Svensk. Vet. Tid.*, **17**, 95–97.

Howell, J.M. and Siegel, P. (1966). Morphological effects of the Manx factor in cats. *Journal of Heredity*, **57**, 100–104.

Hutt, F.B. (1964). *Animal Genetics*. Ronald Press.

Iljin, N. and Iljin, V.N. (1930). Temperature effects on the color of the Siamese cat. *Journal of Heredity*, **21**, 309–318.

Jackson, J.M. and Jackson, J. (1967). The hybrid jungle cat. *Newsl. Long Island Ocelot Club*, **11**, 45.

Jackson, O.F. (1975). Congenital bone lesions in cats with folded ears. *Bulletin of the Feline Advisory Bureau*, **14(4)**, 2–4.

James, C.C., Lassman, L.P. and Tomlinson, B.E. (1969). Congenital anomalies of the lower spine and spinal cord in Manx cats. *Journal of Pathology*, **97**, 269–276.

Jeffreys, A.J. and Morton, D.B. (1987). DNA fingerprints of dogs and cats. *Animal Genetics*, **18**, 1–15.

Johnson, K.H. (1970). Globoid leukodystrophy in the cat. *Journal of the American Veterinary Medical Association*, **157**, 2057–2064.

Johnston, S.D., Bouen, L.C., Madl, J.E., Weber, A.F. and Smith, F.O. (1983). X chromosome monosomy (37,XO) in a Burmese cat with gonadal dysgenesis. *American Veterinary Medical Association*, **182**, 986–989.

Jones, B.R., Johnstone, A.C., Hancock, W.S. and Wallace, A. (1986). Inherited hyperchylomicronemia in the cat. *Feline Practice*, **16**, 7–12.

Jones, G.R., Johnstone, A.C., Cahill, J.I. and Hancock, W.S. (1986). Peripheral neuropathy in cats with inherited primary hyperchylomicronaemia. *Veterinary Record*, **119**, 268–272.

Kier, A.B., Bresnahan, J.F., White, F.J. and Wagner, J.E. (1980). The inheritance pattern of factor XII (Hageman) deficiency in domestic cats. *Canadian Journal of Comparative Medicine*, **44**, 309–314.

Kramer, J.W., Davis, W.C. and Prieur, D.J. (1977). The Chediak-Higashi syndrome of cats. *Laboratory Investigations*, **36**, 554–562.

Kuhn, A. and Kroning, F. (1928). Ueber der vererbung der weisezchung bei der hauskatze. *Zuchtungskunde*, **3**, 448–454.

Lange, A.I., Berg, P.B.V. and Baker, M. (1977). A suspected lysosomal storage disease in Abyssinian cats. *Journal of the South African Veterinary Association*, **48**, 201–209.

Latimer, K.S., Rakich, P.M. and Thompson, D.F. (1985). Pelger-Huet anomaly in cats. *Veterinary Pathology*, **22**, 370–374.

Leipold, H.W., Huston, K., Blauch, B. and Guffy, M.M. (1974). Congenital defects of the caudal vertebral column and spinal cord in Manx cats. *Journal of the American Veterinary Medical Association*, **164**, 520–623.

Letard, E. (1938). Hairless Siamese cats. *Journal of Heredity*, **29**, 173–175.

Leventhal, A.G. (1982). Morphology and distribution of retinal ganglion cells projecting to different layers of the dorsal lateral geniculate nucleus in normal and Siamese cats. *Journal of Neuroscience*, **8**, 1024–1042.

Leventhal, A.G., Vitek, D.J. and Creel, D.J. (1985). Abnormal visual pathways in normally pigmented cats that are heterozygous for albinism. *Science*, **229**, 1395–1397.

Little, C.C. (1957). Four ears, a recessive mutation in the cat. *Journal of Heredity*, **48**, 57.

Littlewood, D.J. (1986). Haemophilia A (factor VIII deficiency) in the cat. *Journal of Small Animal Practice*, **27**, 541–546.

Livingston, M. (1965). A possible hereditary influence in feline urolithiasis. *Veterinary Medicine Small Animal Clinic*, **60**, 705.

Lomax, T.D. and Robinson, R. (1988). Tabby alleles of the domestic cat. *Journal of Heredity* **79**, 21–23.

Lush, J.L. (1945). *Animal Breeding Plans*. Iowa State College Press.

Mair, I.W.S. and Elverland, H.H. (1977). Hereditary deafness in the cat. *Archives in Oto-Rhino-Laryngology*, **217**, 199–217.

Mason, K. (1988). A hereditary disease in Burmese cats manifested as an episodic weakness with head nodding and neck ventroflexion. *Journal of the American Animal Hospital Association*, **24**, 147–151.

Mather, K. (1977). *Introduction to Biometrical Genetics*. Chapman and Hall.

Mcgovern, M.M., Mandell, N., Haskins, S. and Desnick, R.J. (1985). Animal model studies on allelism. *Genetics*, **110**, 733–749.

Mcgovern, M.M., Vine, D.T., Haskins, M.E. and Desnick, R.J. (1981). An improved method for heterozygous identification in feline and human mucopolysaccharidosis VI. *Enzyme*, **26**, 206–210.

Mckerrell, R.E., Blakemore, W.F., Heath, M.F., Plumb, J., Bennett, M.J., Pollitt, R.J. and Danpure, C.J. (1989). Primary hyperoxaluria in the cat. *Veterinary Record*, **125**, 31–34.

Meyers-Wallen, V.N., Wilson, J.D., Griffin, J.E., Fisher, S., Moorhead, P.H., Goldschmidt, M.H., Haskins, M.E. and Patterson, D.F. (1989). Testicular feminization in a cat. *Journal of the American Veterinary Medical Association*, **195**, 631–634.

Moran, C., Gillies, C.B. and Nicholas, F.W. (1984). Fertile male tortoise-shell cats. *Journal of Heredity*, **75**, 397–402.

Morrison-Scott, T.C.S. (1952). The mummified cats of ancient Egypt. *Proceedings of the Zoological Society of London*, **121**, 861–867.

Moutschen, J. (1950). Quelques particularites hereditaires du chat siamois. *Nature Belges*, **31**, 200–203.

Murray, J.A., Blakemore, W.J. and Barnett, K.C. (1977). Ocular lesions in cats with GM1 gangliosidosis with visceral involvement. *Journal of Small Animal Practice*, **18**, 1–10.

Narfstrom, K. (1983). Hereditary progressive retinal atrophy in the Abyssinian cat. *Journal of Heredity*, **74**, 273–276.

Narfstrom, K. (1985). Progressive retinal atrophy in the Abyssinian cat. *Investigations in Ophthalmology and Visual Science*, **26**, 193–200.

Noden, D.M. and Evans, H. (1986). Inherited homeotic midfacial malfor-mations in Burmese cats. *J Craniof. Genet. Devel. Biol.* (Supplement), **2**, 249–266.

Norby, D.E. and Thuline, H.C. (1965). Gene action in the X chromosome of the cat. *Cytogenetics*, **4**, 240–244.

Norby, D.E. and Thuline, H.C. (1970). Inherited tremor in the domestic cat. *Nature*, **227**, 1262–1263.

Patterson, D.F. and Minor, R.F. (1977). Hereditary, fragility and hyper-extensibility of the skin of cats. *Laboratory Investigations*, **37**, 129.

Pearson, H., Gaskell, C.J., Gibbs, C. and Waterman, A. (1974). Pyloric and oesophageal dysfunction in the cat. *Journal of Small Animal Practice*, **15**, 487–501.

Pocock, R.I. (1907). Crosses between *Felis silvestris* and *Felis acreata ugandae*. *Proceedings of the Zoological Society of London*, **1907**, 749–750.

Prieur, D.J. and Collier, L.L. (1981a). Inheritance of the Chediak-Higashi syndrome in cats. *Journal of Heredity*, **72**, 175–177.

Prieur, D.J. and Collier, L.L. (1981b). Morphologic basis of inherited coat colour dilutions of cats. *Journal of Heredity*, **72**, 178–82.

Prieur, D.J. and Collier, L.L. (1984). Maltese dilution of domestic cats. *Journal of Heredity*, **75**, 41–44.

Prieur, D.J., Collier, L.L., Bryan, G.M. and Meyers, K.M. (1979). The diagnosis of feline Chediak-Higashi syndrome. *Feline Practice*, **9**, 26–32.

Pujol, R., Rebillard, M. and Rebillard, G. (1977). Primary neural disor-ders in the deaf white cat cochlea. *Acta Otolaryngologica*, **83**, 59–64.

Rebillard, M., Pujol, R. and Rebillard, G. (1981a). Variability of hered-itary deafness in the white cat. Histology. *Hearing Research*, **5**, 189–200.

Rebillard, M., Rebillard, G. and Pujol, R. (1981b). Variability of hereditary deafness in the white cat. Physiology. *Hearing Research*, **5**, 179–187.

Robinson, R. (1959). Genetics of the domestic cat. *Bibliography of Genetics*, **18**, 273–362.

Robinson, R. (1973). The Canadian hairless or Sphinx cat. *Journal of Heredity*, **64**, 47–49.

Robinson, R. (1976). Genetic aspects of umbilical hernia incidence in cats and dogs. *Veterinary Record*, **100**, 9–10.

Robinson, R. (1981). A third hypotrichosis in the domestic cat. *Genetica*, **55**, 39–40.

Robinson, R. (1985). Fertile male tortoiseshell cats. *Journal of Heredity*, **76**, 137–138.

Robinson, R. (1989). The American Curl cat. *Journal of Heredity*, **80**, 474–475.

Rubin, L.F. (1986). Hereditary cataract in Himalayan cats. *Feline Practice*, **26**, 14–15.

Rubin, L.F. and Lipton, D.E. (1937). Retinal degeneration in kittens. *Journal of American Veterinary Medical Association*, **162**, 467–469.

Schwangart, F. and Grau, H. (1931). Ueber entformung, besonders die vererbbaren Schwangmissbildungen bei des Hauskatze. *Z. Tierz. Zuchtsbiol.*, **21**, 203–249.

Searle, A.G. (1953). Hereditary 'split-hand' in the domestic cat. *Ann. Eugenics*, **17**, 279–282.

Searle, A.G. (1968). *Comparative Genetics of Coat Colour in Mammals*. Logos Press.

Silson, M. and Robinson, R. (1969). Hereditary hydrocephalus in the cat. *Veterinary Record*, **84**, 477.

Sponenberg, D.P. and Graf-Webster, E. (1986). Hereditary meningoencephalocele in Burmese cats. *Journal of Heredity*, **77**, 60.

Thibos, L.N., Levick, W.R. and Morstyn, E. (1980). Ocular pigmentation in white and Siamese cats. *Investigations in Ophthalmology and Visual Science*, **19**, 475–482.

Thompson, J.C., Cobb, V.C., Keeler, C.V. and Dmytryk, M. (1943). Genetics of the Burmese cat. *Journal of Heredity*, **34**, 119–123.

Tjebbes, K. (1924). Crosses with Siamese cats. *Journal of Genetics*, **14**, 355–366.

Todd, N.B. (1951). A pink eyed dilution in the cat. *Journal of Heredity*, **52**, 202.

Turner, P. and Robinson, R. (1973). Melanin inhibitor: a dominant gene in the cat. *Journal of Heredity*, **71**, 427–428.

Turner, P., Robinson, R. and Dyte, C.E. (1981). Blue eyed albino: a new albino allele in the domestic cat. *Genetica*, **56**, 71–73.

Ullman, E. and Hargreaves, A. (1958). New coat colours in domestic cats. *Proceedings of the Zoological Society of London*, **130**, 606–609.

Vandevelde, M., Frankhauser, R., Wiesmann, U. and Erschkowitz, N. (1982). Hereditary neurovisceral mannosidosis associated with alpha-mannosidase deficiency in a family of Persian cats. *Acta Neuropathologica*, **58**, 64–65.

Vawer, G.D. (1981). Corneal mummification in colourpoint cats. *Veterinary Record*, **109**, 413.

Weigel, L. (1961). Das Fellmuster der wildebenden Katzenarten und der Hauskatze in wergleichender und stammesgeschtlicher Hinsicht. *Saugetierk. Mitt.*, **9** (Supplement), 120.

Wenger, D.A., Sattler, M., Kudoh, T., Snyder, S.P. and Kingston, R.S. (1980). Niemann-Pick disease: a genetic model in Siamese cats. *Science*, **208**, 1471–1473.

West-Hyde, L. and Buyukmihci, N. (1982). Photoreceptor degeneration in a family of cats. *Journal of the American Veterinary Medical Association*, **181**, 243–245.

Whiting, P.W. (1919). Inheritance of white spotting and other coat characters in cats. *American Nature*, **53**, 433–482.

Wilkinson, G.T. and Kristensen, T.S. (1989). A hair abnormality in Abyssinian cats. *Journal of Small Animal Practice*, **30**, 27–28.

William-Jones, H.E. (1944). Arrested development of the long bones of the fore limbs in a female cat. *Veterinary Record*, **56**, 449.

Woodard, J.C., Collins, G.H. and Hessler, J.R. (1974). Feline hereditary-neuroaxonal dystrophy. *American Journal of Pathology*, **74**, 551–566.

Zeuner, F.E. (1963). *A History of Domestic Animals*. Hutchinson.

Zook, B.C., Sostaric, B.R., Draper, D.J. and Graf-Webster, E. (1983). Encephalocele and other congenital craniofacial anomalies in Burmese cats. *Veterinary Medicine Small Animal Practice*, **75**, 675–701.

Index